Introduction to Clinical Methods in Communication Disorders

Introduction to Clinical Methods in Communication Disorders

edited by

Rhea Paul, Ph.D.
Southern Connecticut State University
and Yale Child Study Center, New Haven

with invited contributors

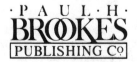

Baltimore • London • Toronto • Sydney

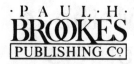

Paul H. Brookes Publishing Co.
Post Office Box 10624
Baltimore, Maryland 21285-0624

www.brookespublishing.com

Typeset by Pro-Image Corp., York, Pennsylvania.
Manufactured in the United States of America by
Sheridan Books, Fredericksburg, Virginia.

All of the case studies in this book are completely fictional. Any similarity to actual
individuals or circumstances is coincidental, and no implications should be inferred.

Several of the definitions in the glossary are from Dirckx, J. (Ed.). (1997). *Stedman's
Concise Medical Dictionary* (3rd ed.). Baltimore: Lippincott Williams & Wilkins;
reprinted by permission.

Library of Congress Cataloging-in-Publication Data

Introduction to clinical methods in communication disorders/[edited] by Rhea Paul,
   with invited contributors
      p. ;   cm.
   Includes bibliographical references and index.
   ISBN 1-55766-526-5
   1. Speech therapy.   2. Audiology.   I. Paul, Rhea.
   [DNLM: 1. Communication Disorders—therapy.   2. Clinical Medicine—methods.   3.
   Speech-Language Pathology—methods. WL 340.2 I618 2002]
   RC423 .I545 2002
   616.85'506—dc21

                                                                    2001037592

British Library Cataloguing in Publication data are available from the British Library.

Contents

About the Editor

Rhea Paul, Ph.D., received her bachelor's degree from Brandeis University in Waltham, Massachusetts, in 1971, her master's degree from Harvard Graduate School of Education in 1975, and her doctorate in communication disorders from the University of Wisconsin–Madison in 1981. Dr. Paul has published more than 60 journal articles and has authored six books. Her research on language development in toddlers with delayed language acquisition was funded by the National Institutes of Health. She has also held grants from the Meyer Memorial Trust, the American Speech-Language-Hearing Association (ASHA) Foundation, the Medical Research Foundation, and the National Association for Autism Research. Dr. Paul has been a fellow of ASHA since 1991 and received the 1996 Editor's Award from the *American Journal of Speech-Language Pathology*. In September 1997, she accepted a joint appointment in the Communication Disorders Department at Southern Connecticut State University and the Child Study Center at Yale University. She spent the summer of 1998 as a visiting professor at the University of Sydney in Australia. Dr. Paul received a Yale Mellon Fellowship for 1998–1999 and the Southern Connecticut State University Faculty Scholar Award for 1999. She was recently awarded an Erskine Fellowship to spend a semester as a visiting scholar at Canterbury University in Christchurch, New Zealand. The second edition of her textbook, *Language Disorders from Infancy Through Adolescence: Assessment and Intervention,* was published in 2001 by Mosby in St. Louis, Missouri. Dr. Paul has been teaching child language development and disorders courses for 20 years.

Contributors

G. Robert Buckendorf, Ph.D.
Speech-Language Pathologist
Oregon Health Sciences University
Box 574
Portland, Oregon 97207

Paul W. Cascella, Ph.D.
Associate Professor
Southern Connecticut State University
501 Crescent Street
New Haven, Connecticut 06515

James J. Dempsey, Ph.D.
Associate Professor/Coordinator of
	Audiology
Southern Connecticut State University
501 Crescent Street
New Haven, Connecticut 06515

Brian Goldstein, Ph.D.
Associate Professor
Temple University
13th and Cecil B. Moore Avenues
Philadelphia, Pennsylvania 19122

Candace J. Gordon, M.A.
Clinic Supervisor
Portland State University
Post Office Box 751
Portland, Oregon 97207

Yvette D. Hyter, Ph.D.
Assistant Professor
Western Michigan University
1201 Oliver Street
Kalamazoo, Michigan 49008

Aquiles Iglesias, Ph.D.
Professor
Temple University
13th and Cecil B. Moore Avenues
Philadelphia, Pennsylvania 19122

Marianne Kennedy, Ph.D.
Associate Professor
Southern Connecticut State University
501 Crescent Street
New Haven, Connecticut 06515

Ann K. Lieberth, Ph.D.
Assistant Professor
Texas Woman's University
Post Office Box 425737
Denton, Texas 76204

Douglas Martin, Ph.D.
Associate Professor
Portland State University
Post Office Box 751
Portland, Oregon 97207

Kevin M. McNamara, M.A.
Clinical Director
Southern Connecticut State University
501 Crescent Street
New Haven, Connecticut 06515

Nickola Wolf Nelson, Ph.D.
Professor
Western Michigan University
1201 Oliver Street
Kalamazoo, Michigan 49008

Mary H. Purdy, Ph.D.
Assistant Professor
Southern Connecticut State University
501 Crescent Street
New Haven, Connecticut 06515

Ellen S. Reuler, M.A.
Clinic Director and Senior Instructor
Portland State University
Post Office Box 751
Portland, Oregon 97207

Denise LaPrade Rini, M.A.
Adjunct Faculty
Southern Connecticut State University
501 Crescent Street
New Haven, Connecticut 06515

Froma P. Roth, Ph.D.
Associate Professor
University of Maryland
Lefrak Hall
Room 0100
College Park, Maryland 20742

John A. Tetnowski, Ph.D.
Assistant Professor
University of Louisiana at Lafayette
Post Office Box 43170
Lafayette, Louisiana 70504

Acknowledgments

The completion of this book owes much to its outstanding contributors who met deadlines and incorporated editorial suggestions with efficiency and good grace that are as rare as they are appreciated. To my colleagues at the Yale Child Study Center—Donald Cohen, Fred Volkmar, and Ami Klin—I express my thanks for their forbearance, as I devoted time to this project while putting others on the back burner. I also thank Stephanie Miles for all of her support, assistance, and friendship.

To the loving memory of my husband, Charles Isenberg,
whose commitment to teaching endures as my constant inspiration

Introduction

Rhea Paul

I was once supervising a first-term student clinician by the name of Jane. Jane was working on articulation with Mike, a pixie-faced 3½-year-old with almost completely unintelligible speech. Mike had a lot to say, but Jane could not understand much of it. He was trying to tell her something about the toy dinosaur he'd brought from home, and, try as she might, she just was not getting it. After attempting three or four times to get the same message across, poor little Mike burst into tears of frustration. Jane was, naturally, taken aback. Sitting behind the mirror, I saw her trying to "talk" the little boy into feeling better. Finally, I was unable to contain my own distress at seeing him so miserable, and I went into the room and took him on my lap, holding and rocking him until he finished his jag. He was soon able to resume his work. In our conference following this incident, Jane said to me, "I was so glad when you came in and held him. I didn't think I was allowed to do that; it didn't seem like the kind of thing a clinician is supposed to do."

That is what this book is all about—the kinds of things that clinicians are supposed to do. And this incident highlights something essential about clinical practice: Even the clinician with the highest level of technical training and the most scientific outlook has to remember that our clients are first and foremost *people*—people with complicated, sometimes conflicting feelings and needs; people who sometimes do not use their clinical time efficiently; and people whose motivation to improve their communication skills is sometimes overwhelmed by their emotions or the broader circumstances of their lives. This means that a good clinician must be part scientist and also part humanist.

But, you may be thinking, how can I learn to be a scientist, a humanist, and an expert on normal and disordered communication before I see my first client NEXT SEMESTER? Well, fortunately for all of us, there is one more thing that every clinician needs to be, and that is a human being. Neither your supervisor, your client, nor anyone else will expect you to be a fully evolved clinician your first term. With your first client, and probably with some of your later ones, too, you will make mistakes. Like any other human being, you will have to make amends for these mistakes, try to learn from them, and do better the next time. Still, the purpose of this book is to help you begin to make the transition from a student of communication disorders to a speech, language, and/or hearing clinician.

Being a clinician entails some qualities that probably cannot be taught by your professors. These are the qualities that we identify with the humanist and to some extent they arise out of your own beliefs, needs, desires, and personality. It is these qualities that probably brought you to consider a career in communication disorders. These qualities include:

- A desire to help others

- Strengths in social interactions

- Enjoyment of close contact with people

- Strong communication skills

- The ability to take pleasure in "just talking"

- An interest in the various processes by which communication takes place

- A level of comfort with people with disabilities

These qualities are not present in everyone, but as a starting point for becoming a clinician, they are essential. As you must know by now, though, these qualities play a limited role in making you a good clinician. But more is needed. Part of the "more" is the in-depth knowledge about the normal processes and development of communication and the characteristics, causes, and correlates of the various kinds of communication disorders that you will be learning about in your academic classes throughout your preparation. Yet another part is the knowledge that you will be introduced to in this book. Here you will learn about the kinds of behaviors and activities in which a clinician engages and about the contexts in which these behaviors and activities take place. The goal is that when you are through, you will have a better sense of what it is a clinician does; where he or she does it; and what general principles of ethics, public policy, cultural sensitivity, and respect for clients and families guide your behaviors and activities.

SCOPE OF PRACTICE

What do speech-language pathologists (SLPs) and audiologists do? Where do they do it? With and for whom? These are the questions that define our scope of practice. SLPs and audiologists work with clients of all ages, from birth through old age. Audiologists screen newborns for hearing loss; SLPs work with premature infants to develop feeding, swallowing, and early parent–child communication skills. Audiologists and SLPs work with infants and toddlers with a variety of developmental disabilities, including hearing impairments, mental retardation, pervasive developmental disorders, congenital anomalies such as cleft palate, congenital disorders such as cerebral palsy or fetal alcohol syndrome, feeding and swallowing problems, and children with cochlear implants who are a relatively new group of clients. Clinicians working with this age range are often engaged in *secondary prevention,* assessment, and intervention aimed at limiting the impact of disorders on communication and development. SLPs and audiologists also work with preschool children who have these kinds of problems. Additional disabilities that tend to surface between the ages of 3 and 5 include problems in the development of speech and/or language associated with various conditions including articulation disorders and specific language delays. We also, unfortunately, see children in this age range whose communication has been affected by abuse or neglect or whose development has been affected by parental substance abuse.

SLPs and audiologists often work with school-age populations. In this age range, we see children similar to those already described, as well as children who stutter, abuse their voices, or endanger their hearing through noise exposure. A large part of an SLP's practice in schools deals with students who have language-based learning disorders that affect their ability to master the curriculum. These students require support to enhance their language so that they can use it more effectively to succeed in school. SLPs also sometimes provide management for students with socioemotional disorders that affect communication, such as Asperger syndrome or selective mutism.

Many SLPs and audiologists work with adult clients as well. Adults with various developmental disabilities continue to require the services of communication specialists. Some young and middle-age adults have communication disabilities as a result of illnesses or traumatic brain injury. Older adults are especially vulnerable to acquiring communication disorders. Many audiologists work with older adults experiencing age-related hearing loss. SLPs serve older clients who lose speech and language skills due to neurological diseases such as strokes.

The recommended practice for clients along the spectrum of development includes close collaboration with their families and with other professionals who are involved in their care. When someone receives services from several professionals, it serves the client best if these professionals are aware of each other's goals and methods and can coordinate services for the client. Many professionals "cross-train" each other to help deliver services in a more integrated manner so that the client receives consistent feedback and reinforcement and has more opportunities for generalization. Clinical practice in communication disorders often involves collaboration with teachers and special educators; physical and occupational therapists; psychologists and social workers; recreational and vocational counselors; nurses and physicians; as well as with the staff of schools, residential centers, group homes, rehabilitation facilities, hospitals, and nursing facilities in which clients are placed.

SCOPE OF TEXT

In this book, we attempt to introduce you to the processes, settings, and issues involved in clinical practice in communication disorders. In Chapter 2, we talk about the Code of Ethics disseminated by the American Speech-Language-Hearing Association (ASHA) that guides our practice. This code is central to the practice of our profession because it lays out our obligations to our clients, our payers, and our colleagues and provides guidelines to help us make the sometimes difficult clinical decisions with which our practice may confront us. In

Chapter 3, you learn about basic principles of assessment. We discuss the properties that make standardized tests fair and accurate. We talk about the times when
it is appropriate to use tests and when other methods of assessment come to the
fore. Chapter 4 provides information on the physical examination of the speech
mechanism and the methods of assessing its functional status. We are the only
professionals who do this examination, so it is especially important to be confident and capable in this aspect of our work. Chapter 5 addresses the issue of the
assessment of samples of communicative behavior. These include samples of
speech and language, nonverbal communication, and the use of augmentative
and alternative communication such as Sign and picture boards. The ability to
sample communicative behavior adequately and analyze it in order to determine
appropriate goals and methods for intervention is one of the most important
functions of the SLP.

Chapter 6 moves our discussion from assessment to the domain of intervention. Here we talk about the range of intervention procedures used to help people with communication disorders improve their functioning. We discuss a
continuum of approaches and show how they apply across a variety of communication disorders. In Chapter 7, we address our own communication skills—
those we use in interacting with clients, families, and other professionals. We
learn about the various kinds of documentation that our profession requires and
the importance of acquiring skills not only in assessment and intervention but
also in collaborating with families and colleagues to ensure our clients' progress.
We are reminded, too, of our role not so much as professional counselors but as
humanists—caring individuals who listen to the concerns of clients and families,
even when they extend beyond speech, hearing, and language issues. Chapter 8
provides information on the laws, rules, and regulations that govern our practice.
We find out about clients' rights, our own responsibilities, and the emerging public policies that affect our practice. In Chapter 9, the varied environments in
which communication disorders professionals practice is our topic. We learn
about the kinds of practice options each provides, the kinds of documentation
each requires, and the various roles communication professionals can play in
each one. This may give you the first sense of the setting in which you might like
to anchor your own practice. Chapter 10 addresses the thorny issues involved
when helping clients who come from cultural and linguistic backgrounds different from your own. This issue has become increasingly important as the demographic trends in our society reflect greater diversity. As you can imagine,
facilitating communication is complicated when the client and clinician speak different languages or have different cultural rules for communicating. Chapter 11
reviews some of the many ways new technologies are affecting our practice.
Because many of these new technologies are *information* systems, it is not surprising that they will have a great impact on how we deliver services. Finally, in
Chapter 12, we discuss the important role that families play in the clinical
process. We consider ways of including families at every stage of our decision
making in order to maximize the impact of our treatments beyond the clinical
setting and into the real, integrated life of the clients that we serve.

Our hope is that after completing your studies with this book, you will have
a greater sense of what a clinician does and does not do and a greater confidence
that you will be able to make the correct choices with your first client and with

every one thereafter. Although mastering both the science and the art of clinical practice will take much longer than the time that you spend in school, your clinical education will provide you with the tools that you need to continue learning and improving your service to clients. We hope that you will consider this book a useful part of that education. Yet another part, though, will be the support that you receive after you graduate from the national organization that represents our professions in the United States of America. We would like to take the opportunity at this juncture to introduce you to this as well.

THE AMERICAN SPEECH-LANGUAGE-HEARING ASSOCIATION AND THE CLINICIAN

ASHA is a professional and scientific association that credentials nearly 100,000 communication disorders professionals around the world. Its mission is to "promote the interests of and provide the highest quality services for professionals in communication disorders and to advocate for people with communication disabilities" (ASHA web site, http://professional.asha.org). ASHA disseminates standards of ethical conduct, publishes original research in its journals, and provides continuing education programs to its members. It advocates for our clients by monitoring and participating in the development and implementation of health care reform proposals and programs at the federal and state levels.

ASHA provides the standards for earning the clinical credential in our field, the Certificate of Clinical Competence (CCC), which can be earned in either speech-language pathology, audiology, or both. Current standards for ASHA certification in speech-language pathology and audiology are outlined in the appendixes at the end of this chapter, but you should be aware that these standards change from time to time and, in fact, revisions are being considered by the ASHA Council on Academic Accreditation (CAA) as of this writing. In addition, many states require SLPs and audiologists to be *licensed* with the state board of health, with the teacher certification agency, or both. In many cases, licensing and teacher certification requirements overlap with ASHA certification, but it is important to check on the licensing and certification requirements for the state in which you plan to practice and for the practice settings (schools, hospitals, home health agencies, etc.) in which you intend to participate.

In addition to providing national certification for its members, there are a variety of other benefits that membership in a national professional organization provides. These include:[1]

- *Political advocacy:* ASHA tracks issues of concern to our clients and colleagues in legislatures, courts, and regulatory agencies at state and federal levels.

- *Opportunities to shape the profession:* Members who take an active role in their professional organization can affect their profession's future and make changes that benefit clients and colleagues.

---

[1]©American Speech-Language-Hearing Association; adapted with permission.

- *Professional contacts:* Attending state and national conferences and reading newsletters and journals helps keep members "plugged in" once they leave the university environment.

- *Professional visibility:* Members who are active have a high profile among peers and are known outside their own practice setting.

- *Multicultural initiatives:* ASHA provides support for members who need to deal with multicultural issues in their practice, from lists of tests and resources to educating citizens from minority groups about the importance of communicative health.

- *Research:* ASHA supports an extensive research database available to help members write grants, business plans, and reports or update their knowledge in particular clinical areas. ASHA's foundation supports members' research by offering competitive grant opportunities for students, new researchers, and more senior investigators.

- *Professional publications:* Membership includes subscription to one of the journals ASHA publishes, which include the *Journal of Speech, Language, and Hearing Research; Language, Speech, and Hearing Services in Schools; American Journal of Audiology* (http://professional.asha.org/aja); and *American Journal of Speech-Language Pathology.* In addition, ASHA publishes a newsletter, the *ASHA Leader,* for all members.

- *Technical assistance:* Members can receive information about funding agencies, developing proposals, and other professional issues.

- *Referral service:* ASHA maintains a referral list of clinical programs and private practitioners who have asked to be listed. It is grouped by state and available to individuals who request referrals.

- *Employment service:* Members seeking new positions may use ASHA's job placement services both on-line and at professional meetings.

- *Professional development opportunities:* ASHA provides members with many options for continuing education, including meetings, audio and video conferences, and printed materials. It can also serve as a repository for members' Continuing Education Units, which are required for maintaining licensure/certification in many states.

- *Specialty recognition:* ASHA maintains a group of 16 Special Interest Divisions (SIDs) that focus on particular aspects of practice, such as language learning and education, aural rehabilitation and its instrumentation, and augmentative and alternative communication, to name a few. Membership in an SID provides access to colleagues who practice in similar settings or with similar populations and the opportunity to share experiences and information with them through SID listservs and newsletters; some have developed standards for recognition of the specialty with an endorsement, beyond the terminal degree.

- *National office:* ASHA maintains a full-time staff that provides publications, advice, and various services by e-mail (actioncenter@asha.org), by telephone (800-498-2071), or by fax (877-541-5035). ASHA also maintains a web site (http://professional.asha.org) with a great deal of current information on a variety of topics relevant to communication disorders professionals.

Clearly, membership in a professional organization confers numerous benefits. Perhaps the most important, though, is the commitment it represents to your clients. Clinicians who align themselves formally with their colleagues do so not only for the direct benefits that this membership offers them, but also because they want to be affiliated in an active way with their profession and its development. These clinicians know that we get more from our profession, both for ourselves and for our clients, when we are part of a larger whole.

MOVING FORWARD/LOOKING BACK

We have begun to talk here about what it means to be a clinician. What it means for you personally will unfold as you consolidate your knowledge and test it in your practicum experiences. It is our hope that you will acquire some of that knowledge from the chapters in this book. But as you acquire this new knowledge, do not let yourself forget the things you have always known. When you begin to feel overwhelmed by all of the new things that you must learn, by all of the facts that you must amass, by the equipment that you must master, and by the papers and reports and lesson plans, remember to look back. Look back to the reasons why you entered into this process, and remember what motivated you to go through such a long and rigorous training program in the first place. You do not need to leave your humane instincts behind. If you find yourself faced with a situation like the one Jane encountered, trust your intuition. As you move forward in your clinical education, your newly gained knowledge will inform your actions; but it will never replace the humane motive of bringing the birthright of communication to every individual. This is the impulse that first set you on your present path and it should continue to guide your steps throughout your career.

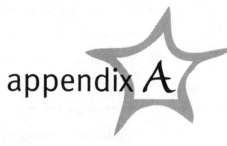

appendix A

An Outline of Standards for the Certificate of Clinical Competence in Audiology

Effective January 1, 2007

STANDARD I: THE DEGREE

- Candidates must have a minimum of 75 semester credit hours of postbaccalaureate education culminating in a recognized graduate degree. As of January 2012, applicants must have a doctoral degree.

STANDARD II: THE INSTITUTION

- The graduate degree must be completed in a program accredited by the Council on Academic Accreditation (CAA) in audiology and speech-language pathology of ASHA.

STANDARD III: PROGRAM OF STUDY

- Candidates must complete a minimum of 75 semester credit hours that include academic coursework and a minimum of 12 months' full-time equivalent supervised clinical practicum. Supervision must be provided by an individual that holds the appropriate CCC.

The information in this appendix can be found at http://professional.asha.org. ©American Speech-Language-Hearing Association; adapted with permission.

STANDARD IV: KNOWLEDGE AND SKILLS

- Candidates must have a foundation of prerequisite knowledge and skills
  - Oral and written communication
  - Knowledge and coursework in
    - Life sciences
    - Physical sciences
    - Behavioral sciences
    - Mathematics
- Candidates must have acquired knowledge in foundations of practice
  - Professional codes of ethics and credentialing
- Patient characteristics (e.g., age, demographics, cultural and linguistic diversity, medical history and status, cognitive status, physical and sensory abilities) and how they relate to clinical services
- Educational, vocational, and social and psychological effects of hearing impairment and their impact on the development of a treatment program
- Anatomy and physiology, pathophysiology and embryology, and development of the auditory and vestibular systems
- Normal development of speech, language, and hearing
- Phonologic, morphologic, syntactic, and pragmatic aspects of human communication associated with hearing impairment
- Normal processes of speech and language production and perception over the life span
- Normal aspects of auditory physiology and behavior over the life span
- Principles, methods, and applications of psychoacoustics
- Effects of chemical agents on the auditory and vestibular systems; instrumentation and bioelectrical hazards
- Infectious/contagious diseases and universal precautions
- Physical characteristics and measurement of acoustic stimuli
- Physical characteristics and measurement of electric and other nonacoustic stimuli
- Principles and practices of research, including experimental design, statistical methods, and application to clinical populations
- Medical/surgical procedures for treatment of disorders affecting auditory and vestibular systems

- Health care and educational delivery systems

- Ramifications of cultural diversity on professional practice

- Supervisory processes and procedures

- Laws, regulations, policies, and management practices relevant to the profession of audiology

- Manual communication, use of interpreters, and assistive technology

Prevention and Identification

- Interact effectively with patients, families, other appropriate individuals, and professionals

- Prevent the onset and minimize the development of communication disorders

- Identify individuals at risk for hearing impairment

- Screen individuals for hearing impairment and disability using clinically appropriate and culturally sensitive screening measures

- Screen individuals for speech and language impairments and other factors affecting communication function using clinically appropriate and culturally sensitive screening measures

- Administer conservation programs designed to reduce the effects of noise exposure and of agents that are toxic to the auditory and vestibular systems

Evaluation

- Interact effectively with patients, families, other appropriate individuals, and professionals

- Evaluate information from appropriate sources to facilitate assessment planning

- Obtain a case history

- Perform an otoscopic examination

- Determine the need for cerumen removal

- Administer clinically appropriate and culturally sensitive assessment measures

- Perform audiologic assessment using physiologic, psychophysical, and self-assessment measures

- Perform electrodiagnostic test procedures

- Perform balance system assessment and determine the need for balance rehabilitation

- Perform aural rehabilitation assessment

- Document evaluation procedures and results
- Interpret results of the evaluation to establish type and severity of disorder
- Generate recommendations and referrals resulting from the evaluation process
- Provide counseling to facilitate understanding of the auditory or balance disorder
- Maintain records in a manner consistent with legal and professional standards
- Communicate results and recommendations orally and in writing to the patient and other appropriate individual(s)
- Use instrumentation according to manufacturer's specifications and recommendations
- Determine whether instrumentation is in calibration according to accepted standards

Treatment

- Interact effectively with patients, families, other appropriate individuals, and professionals
- Develop and implement treatment plan using appropriate data
- Discuss prognosis and treatment options with appropriate individuals
- Counsel patients, families, and other appropriate individuals
- Develop culturally sensitive and age-appropriate management strategies
- Collaborate with other service providers in case coordination
- Perform hearing aid, assistive listening device, and sensory aid assessment
- Recommend, dispense, and service prosthetic and assistive devices
- Provide hearing aid, assistive listening device, and sensory aid orientation

Conduct Aural Rehabilitation

- Monitor and summarize treatment progress and outcomes
- Assess efficacy of interventions for auditory and balance disorders
- Establish treatment admission and discharge criteria
- Serve as an advocate for patients, families, and other appropriate individuals
- Document treatment procedures and results
- Maintain records in a manner consistent with legal and professional standards

- Communicate results, recommendations, and progress to appropriate individual(s)

- Use instrumentation according to manufacturer's specifications and recommendations

- Determine whether instrumentation is in calibration according to accepted standards

STANDARD V: OUTCOMES ASSESSMENT

- The candidate must successfully complete formative (ongoing) and summative (final) assessment of the knowledge and skills in Standard IV.

STANDARD VI: MAINTAINING CERTIFICATION

- As of January 1, 2007, audiologists must accumulate three continuing education credits (30 contact hours) from approved providers every 3 years.

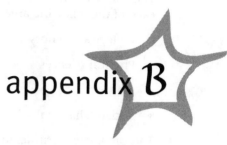

appendix B

An Outline of Standards for the Certificate of Clinical Competence in Speech-Language Pathology

Effective January 1, 2005

STANDARD I: THE DEGREE

- Candidates must have a master's or doctoral degree.

- Graduate work must be in the area of certification and completed in a Council on Academic Accreditation (CAA) accredited program.

- A minimum of 75 semester credit hours must be completed in speech-language pathology.

- A minimum of 36 hours must be earned at the graduate level.

STANDARD II: THE INSTITUTION

- The graduate degree must be at an accredited institution of higher education.

- The graduate degree must be completed in a program accredited by the CAA in audiology and by ASHA in speech-language pathology.

The information in this appendix can be found at http://professional.asha.org. ©American Speech-Language-Hearing Association; adapted with permission.

STANDARD III: KNOWLEDGE OUTCOMES

- The candidate must present skills in oral and written communication sufficient for clinical practice.

- The candidate must demonstrate knowledge and show transcript credit in each of the following areas:

  - Biological sciences

  - Physical sciences

  - Mathematics

  - Social/behavioral sciences

- The candidate must demonstrate knowledge of human communication and swallowing processes.

- The candidate must demonstrate knowledge of the nature of speech, language, hearing, swallowing, and communication disorders, specifically in:

  - Articulation

  - Fluency

  - Voice and resonance

  - Receptive and expressive language in speaking, listening, reading, and writing modalities

  - Hearing

  - Swallowing

  - Cognitive aspects of communication (e.g., attention, memory, sequencing, problem solving, executive function)

  - Social aspects of communication (e.g., mulitcultural aspects, challenging behaviors, lack of communication opportunities)

  - Nonoral communicative modalities

  - The candidate must demonstrate knowledge of prevention, assessment, and intervention for communication and swallowing disorders.

  - The candidate must demonstrate knowledge of standards of ethical conduct.

  - The candidate must demonstrate knowledge of processes used in research and the integration of research principles in clinical practice.

  - The candidate must demonstrate knowledge of contemporary professional issues.

- The candidate must demonstrate knowledge of certification, specialty recognition, licensure, and other professional credentials.

STANDARD IV: SKILL OUTCOMES

- The candidate must complete at least 400 clock hours of supervised clinical practicum; 25 of these must be spent in clinical observation and 375 in client contact.

- At least 325 hours must be completed at the graduate level.

- Practicum must be supervised by an appropriately certified individual, at a level appropriate to the student's development, but not less than 25% of the student's client contact time.

- Practicum must include experience with clients across the life span and from culturally different backgrounds, with various types and severities of communication disorders.

- Supervised clinical experiences must include:
  - Evaluation
  - Prevention and screening
  - Case history and report writing
  - Selection and administration of tests, behavioral observation, and other nonstandardized procedures
  - Adaptation of evaluation procedures to meet client needs
  - Interpretation and synthesis of information for diagnosis and recommendations
  - Completion of administration and reporting functions
  - Client referral
  - Intervention
  - Development of intervention plans with measurable, appropriate goals by collaborating with families
  - Implementation of intervention plans
  - Selection of appropriate materials and instrumentation
  - Measurement of performance and progress
  - Completion of administration and reporting functions
  - Identification and referral of clients

- Interaction
- Communication about effectively recognizing needs, values, and cultural background of clients and others
- Collaboration with other professionals
- Provision of counseling regarding communication and swallowing disorders
- Adherence to the Code of Ethics

STANDARD V: ASSESSMENT

- The candidate must successfully complete formative (ongoing) and summative (final) assessment of the knowledge and skills in Standards II and IV.

STANDARD VI: CLINICAL FELLOWSHIP YEAR

- The candidate must complete a year (36 weeks) of full-time supervised professional employment in clinical service delivery or clinical research.

STANDARD VII: MAINTAINING CERTIFICATION

- As of January 1, 2005, SLPs must accumulate three continuing education credits (30 contact hours) from approved providers every 3 years.

Ethical and Professional Practices

Paul W. Cascella

CASE EXAMPLE 1

Michelle is a speech-language pathologist (SLP) at a local rehabilitation center in a busy urban New England community. Because of ongoing expansion in the rehabilitation agency over the past 5 years, the speech-language pathology department has employed speech therapy assistants to help manage the clinical caseload. As a supervisor, Michelle has found that these assistants are dedicated and are able to implement treatment plans and procedures that she has taught them. Of late, Michelle has found that her own job has spread her thin across agency committees, task forces, and the new satellite birth-to-three program across town. As a result, she finds that she often is less able to directly supervise the speech therapy assistants and she relies on telephone and e-mail consultation to review client data sheets and case notes. After talking with Nicole, one of her most talented speech therapy assistants, Michelle has allowed her to modify a treatment plan for three adults with aphasia even though Michelle has not directly seen these patients in the past 4 weeks.

CASE EXAMPLE 2

Tom is an audiologist who works at a local teaching hospital that contracts with four skilled nursing home facilities. In this contract, nursing home residents participate in audiological evaluations and follow-up, usually the first and third Tuesdays of every month. On any of these days, Tom may see up to 20 people from any or all of the four nursing homes. On one particularly busy day, Tom has a list of patients who are scheduled for appointments but loses track of which patients kept their appointments, which patients canceled, and who was added at the last minute. At the end of the day,

Tom sits down to write his case notes about the patients. Unfortunately, because the day was so busy, Tom cannot be sure of which patients were seen and which ones had canceled. When he goes to complete his billing, he accidentally bills for services for two patients who were not actually seen that day.

As a beginning clinician in speech-language pathology or audiology, you may confront clinical situations like the ones described for Michelle and Tom. These two case examples provide an opportunity for you to think about issues that involve professional ethics. Later in this chapter, guidelines and a summary are provided for analysis.

INTRODUCTION

Each of us has our own personal standards and perceptions of ethical behavior. When thinking about the term **ethics,** it is common to consider the moral and/or civil codes of conduct for a particular person, situation, community, religious group, organization, or society. These codes evolve from a philosophy of human interaction that values behaviors that are personally or collectively regarded as good, honest, proper, and respectable. Each of us has a set of **personal ethics** that have been formed from our upbringing, acculturation, life experiences, and education. As children, our parents were likely to stress that certain behaviors were right or wrong. Some of us were taught to follow the Golden Rule (i.e., "Do unto others. . ."), to treat older adults with respect, to tell the truth, to play fairly in sports competitions, and to never cheat on an examination. As adults, we consciously choose our own individual ethics and values, which guide us to interact with our families and our friends in what we personally consider the *right* way to behave—our sense of duty and obligation.

Personal ethics are important because they enable individuals to make choices about their own behavior. Personal ethics differ from person to person, and not everyone with similar ethical tenets applies them in the same way. Therefore, many professions abide by a set of **professional ethics** that establish right and

---

REASONS FOR A PROFESSIONAL CODE OF ETHICS

1. Consumer protection and client welfare are safeguarded.

2. The professional reputation of the discipline is maintained.

3. Professional behavior is regulated.

4. Objective guidance is provided for ethical dilemmas and deliberation.

5. Practitioners can rely on an external code to complement their own values.

6. Clients have an objective standard against which to evaluate their clinician's behavior.

wrong actions in the workplace. Professional ethics publicly state the common core values and collective obligations shared by people in a particular discipline. Although each of us brings our personal ethics to clinical practice, the American Speech-Language-Hearing Association (ASHA) and the American Academy of Audiology (AAA) have codified a set of standards for ethical behavior. Each organization has its own **Code of Ethics** that includes tangible expectations that define acceptable conduct and conscientious judgment. As members of the communication disorders discipline, each of us is expected to accept these tenets and apply them to clinical settings. By having professional ethical standards, practitioners can look to a common set of core values when confronted with ethical dilemmas in the workplace.

This chapter introduces the ethical standards that are the foundation of clinical practice in speech-language pathology and audiology. Ethical principles are presented and case situations are described that may raise ethical dilemmas. As you read the examples of ethical dilemmas, take a moment to pause and consider your personal response. The AAA and ASHA Codes of Ethics are reprinted in their entirety in Appendixes A and B at the end of this chapter.

SYNOPSES OF THE ASHA AND AAA CODES OF ETHICS

ASHA Code of Ethics

The ASHA (1994b) Code of Ethics applies to people who are already credentialed (i.e., the CCC-SLP [Certificate of Clinical Competence—Speech-Language Pathology]; CCC-A [Certificate of Clinical Competence—Audiology]), candidates in the process of earning those credentials (i.e., students, CFY [Clinical Fellowship Year] participants), and members of the organization. The ASHA Code of Ethics consists of three parts: the Preamble, Principles of Ethics, and Rules of Ethics. The Preamble introduces the philosophy of ethical service delivery and the overall content, principles, and structure of the code. Principles of Ethics are divided into four parts, each of which provides a broad statement about ethical conduct. Principles of Ethics I and II relate to the delivery of services to clients. Principle of Ethics III outlines standards related to interaction with the public, and Principle of Ethics IV outlines standards and responsibilities to the profession. Within each Principle of Ethics there are Rules of Ethics, which are statements that articulate acceptable and restricted actions pertaining to each principle. In matters in which ethical violations may occur, ASHA has separate documents (ASHA, 1998a, 1998b) concerned with due process and the consequences of unethical behavior. (From ©1994 American Speech-Language-Hearing Association; reprinted by permission.)

AAA Code of Ethics

The AAA (1991) Code of Ethics applies to current and potential members of the organization. The AAA Code of Ethics consists of three parts: the Preamble,

Statement of Principles and Rules, and Procedures for the Management of Alleged Violations. The Preamble outlines the overall philosophy of the code and identifies its content. Statement of Principles and Rules highlights specific actions deemed ethically acceptable to audiology practice. Procedures for the Management of Alleged Violations outlines the due process format when violations are suspected, as well as the penalties that can be assigned (i.e., reprimand, cease and desist order, suspension of membership, revocation of membership). This section also outlines record keeping and public disclosure.

ETHICAL PRINCIPLES IN PROFESSIONAL PRACTICE

To begin our discussion of ethics, we start by considering some of the common core principles shared by AAA and ASHA.

The Principle of Safeguarding Client Welfare

At the core of ethical practice is a guarantee that clinicians will act to ensure the dignity, protection, and autonomy of client rights. Let us look at some concrete examples of how clinicians can guarantee client welfare.

Beneficence and Nonmaleficence **Beneficence** means that professionals promote the interests and welfare of others, whereas **nonmaleficence** means that professionals deliberately avoid inflicting potential or actual harm (e.g., emotional harm, physical harm) on clients. These principles compel professionals to monitor their own behavior as well as that of caregivers who interact with clients. For example, we are expected to report situations in which we perceive that clients may be victims of physical, emotional, and/or sexual abuse, as well as neglect by their caregivers.

Nondiscrimination How would you feel if a transgendered client came to see you for services so that his or her voice would sound more like that of the sex to which he or she is being surgically altered? Or, how would you feel about working with a child whose parent asks if "you have found Jesus in your life?" Or, how would you feel if you were assigned to work with a class of preschoolers, one of whom is being raised by her grandparents because her mother is incarcerated? These may be difficult questions for you to answer based on your own personal ethical values; still, every client's right to quality services is guaranteed because clinicians must practice **nondiscrimination.** This means that clinicians do not exclude clients from their professional practice for reasons other than the person's potential to benefit from their services. Ethical practice is compromised when a clinician discriminates by making a clinical decision based on a client's race, gender, ethnicity, religion, age, national origin, sexual orientation, or disability status.

Referral   Another example of securing a client's welfare is the use of **referrals.** This occurs when an SLP or audiologist feels that a client presents a communication disorder or situation beyond the clinician's level of expertise. Professional referrals safeguard a client's right to appropriate clinical services. Take our example of the **transgendered** client: A referral would be appropriate if a clinician has no experience in gender-appropriate voice treatment approaches and, thus, would be unable to provide him or her with competent voice services. In contrast, when clinicians receive a referral, they are expected to exercise independent judgment about the content, frequency, and duration of services that may be recommended. In other words, outside influences should not interfere with evaluation and treatment decisions. For example, an audiologist may receive a physician referral to fit a client with a hearing aid because the physician noted that the client had some difficulty hearing case history questions during a physical examination. Before proceeding with a hearing aid, the audiologist should first complete an independent hearing evaluation to assess client need and/or potential to benefit from such equipment. For either type of referral (i.e., *by* the clinician or *to* the clinician), clinicians are prohibited from receiving a commission.

Informed Consent   **Informed consent** means that clients are told about their speech-language or hearing condition and are informed about the relative strengths, weaknesses, and risks (i.e., side effects) associated with a recommended plan of action or inaction. For people who are unable to understand legal consent, informed consent must be obtained from family members or legal guardians. With informed consent, the clinician enables the client to exercise autonomy during the course of treatment. This principle also guarantees that clients can voluntarily withdraw from a treatment protocol at any point during its course. For example, think about how you would react to a middle school child who decides that he no longer wants stuttering therapy even though his speech continues to include blocks, prolongations, and repetitions. How might you attempt to guarantee his welfare if he voluntarily withdraws from treatment?

Confidentiality   In daily practice, we often hear clinical and personal information about clients (i.e., health status, medical history, educational background, cognitive status, financial status, family structure). The principle of **confidentiality** means that professionals take this privileged information and share it only with people directly responsible for client management and care, and only for purposes related to the client's welfare. As professionals, we are bound neither to use privileged information for gossip within a work setting, nor to repeat any confidential information outside of the clinical environment. This requires some self-control on the clinician's part, as it is too easy to start talking about clients in the lunchroom when others, who should not be privy to the information, may be within earshot. Client confidentiality may become an ethical dilemma when the client's right to confidentiality is overridden by precedents in law or other compelling circumstances. This might arise, for example, if you are working with an adult with aphasia who expresses in therapy that he wants to kill himself. It might come up, too, if a mother confides to a child's clinician that the stepfather has repeatedly hit the child. Should statements such as these compel you to breach your client's right to confidentiality?

Prognosis and Cures   Implicit in ethical practice is that professionals must not imply or guarantee cures. Instead, clinicians are expected to make a reasonable **prognosis,** or a statement that describes the likelihood that a benefit will be gained from treatment. If a person is not likely to benefit from initial or ongoing treatment, intervention should not be recommended or continued. In practice, this means that we do not recommend treatment for every person who has a speech-language or hearing disorder. Instead, we exercise professional judgment about the likelihood that treatment will yield benefits for a client. For example, how would you handle a situation in which family members insist on speech therapy services for a person with advanced dementia residing in a nursing home?

Infection Control   Clinicians are expected to safeguard their clients and themselves from infectious diseases by maintaining **infection control** and prevention procedures (see Table 2.1). Hygienic precautions usually include hand washing and the use of barriers (e.g., gloves, masks). In addition, clinicians are expected to disinfect equipment and know the proper procedures for the disposal of bodily fluids (e.g., saliva, blood). All clinicians are expected to practice universal precautions, whether their work setting has a medical orientation. In other words, universal precautions apply to preschools and schools, child care settings, home health, university clinics, birth-to-three programs, group homes, and pri-

Table 2.1.   Infection control and prevention procedures

Hand washing	You must vigorously lather and rub your hands, your wrists, and your forearms with warm water and liquid antibacterial soap before each clinical session.
Disposable gloves	You must wear disposable gloves when you have contact with clients' bodily fluids or substances (e.g., saliva, blood, cerumen, vomit).
Contaminated items	Consumable items (e.g., gloves, tongue depressors) that contacted clients' bodily fluids or substances must be disposed of into a plastic bag with a tie. Nonconsumable items (e.g., eartips, specula) must be decontaminated.
Decontamination/disinfecting	Disinfectant must be strongly rubbed onto all nonconsumable items, clinical materials, and clinical furniture. A solution of one tenth bleach and nine tenths water is recommended.
Illness	Clinical sessions should be rescheduled when either the clinician or the client has an infectious illness or condition.
Vaccinations	Clinicians should seriously consider vaccination for hepatitis B, rubella, and the mumps. Clinicians are also encouraged to have a yearly tuberculosis test.

vate practice. For example, it would be typical for you to handle bodily fluids if you are working with an infant-toddler early intervention group.

The Principle of Competence

A second core principle critical to SLPs and audiologists is **competent practice.** This occurs when a clinician provides effective diagnostic procedures, accurate prognosis, and appropriate therapy strategies for the particular disorder, as well as ongoing analysis of client outcomes. Ethical practice requires clinicians to keep equipment in working order and to maintain accurate and accessible records for clients.

Ethical practice obligates that each of us clearly understand our own strengths and limitations and that we practice only in those areas in which we regard ourselves as competent. Except for clinical screenings, clinicians are only able to practice in their particular profession (e.g., speech-language pathology, audiology) unless credentials are held in more than one profession. Although our education and clinical preparation lead to a credential (i.e., CCC, state licensure, teaching certification), many of us become specialists for a particular population, disorder, and/or service delivery model. **Specialization** occurs with in-depth experience, advanced knowledge, and training beyond the initial credential. Whether a specialist or a generalist, each of us is expected to maintain our overall clinical competency through **continuing education.** Continuing education enables clinicians to update their skills by keeping abreast of the latest trends and advances in their discipline. This can be achieved by reading textbooks and journal articles,

---

CONTEMPORARY ISSUES THAT INFLUENCE ETHICAL COMPETENCE

Competition: Clinicians must balance ethics with competition for employment and the market share (i.e., competitive bidding, marketing, advertising).

Resources: When resources are lacking in public education (e.g., small budget, shortage of personnel), clinicians must continue to act competently.

Health care: Clinicians must balance ongoing changes in medical reimbursement and the cost of health care with the needs presented by clients.

Scope of practice: Clinicians must stay current on and judicious of the latest technologies within clinical practice.

Paraprofessionals: Clinicians must be able to carefully judge the utilization of speech assistants and aides in service delivery.

attending workshops, shadowing professional colleagues, and participating in research activities.

Ethical clinicians judge their own fitness for providing services and withdraw from practice if their own conduct is influenced by substance abuse or related health conditions. Similarly, it is expected that clinicians will monitor the ethical compliance of other SLPs and audiologists. Finally, ethical compliance relies on clinicians who keep up-to-date on contemporary issues that influence clinical practice. The chart on page 25 provides examples of issues that have uniquely challenged us to maintain our ethics and competency.

The Principle of Acting without a Conflict of Interest

A **conflict of interest** occurs when an SLP or audiologist accepts personal or financial gifts from clients or manufacturers that compromise professional judgment because there are strings attached. When a conflict of interest arises, clinicians can lose their sense of objectivity and their decision making becomes clouded. Examples of potential conflicts of interest include self-dealing (i.e., utilizing commercial enterprises in which you have a financial stake) and self-referral (i.e., referring patients between two work settings, both of which employ the same clinician). A conflict of interest might also occur when a clinician draws cases for private practice from his or her primary place of employment. This can occur especially when school-based clinicians provide privately based services to children during summer recess. In and of itself, this is not a conflict of interest as long as the school administration is aware of these services, and clients are fully informed about service options and costs.

The Principle of Acting without Misrepresentation

CASE EXAMPLE 3

Adele is an SLP at a local community hospital whose staff is developing a marketing plan to attract more business. Because there are many community-based speech-language-hearing providers, an advertising strategy that "catches the eye" is being sought. After a morning meeting, it has been decided that more consumers will be drawn to this hospital if Adele's auditory processing remediation program is advertised as one of the best in the state. Adele does not feel right about this decision, even though she is confident that the program is effective. Adele knows that she has not done efficacy research or published her results for professional review.[1]

Later that day, Adele participates in a meeting with hospital administration where it is noted that patient billable hours have decreased with the implementation of a new insurance reimbursement system. At the meeting, Adele is informed that without this reimbursement, the speech pathology staff is likely to lose personnel. Adele also

---

[1]From American Speech-Language-Hearing Association. (1993a). *Ethics: Resources for professional preparation and practice.* Rockville, MD: Author; reprinted by permission.

learns that particular diagnoses are guaranteed reimbursement, as are people for whom the prognosis for improvement is rated as "good." Although never directly stated, Adele feels as though she is encouraged to reconsider the diagnostic criteria for particular diagnoses, as well as the factors that relate to prognosis.

How would you respond if you were Adele? Because of her morning meeting, she is concerned that the hospital advertising strategy may be a form of misrepresentation. **Misrepresentation** is a type of dishonesty that occurs when truth is distorted or falsified. In this case, misrepresentation occurs because there is an exaggerated description of Adele's auditory processing program. Even though Adele has observed the benefits of the program, she knows that its efficacy has not been scientifically tested. Another example of misrepresentation can occur if clinicians exaggerate their own personal levels of training, experience, and expertise, or that of people who provide clinical services (e.g., CFY participants, graduate students, speech assistants, aides). Clients should be specifically informed about the educational level of the person providing services.

Because of her afternoon meeting, Adele continues to be concerned about misrepresentation. She is being asked to ignore competent clinical diagnostic procedures (i.e., criteria, prognosis) to secure insurance reimbursement. In effect, Adele would be misrepresenting the client's status by making a diagnosis and a prognosis solely to maintain the financial solvency of her employer.

Finally, another form of misrepresentation occurs when a clinician unfairly influences client decisions by "stacking the deck" a particular way. Ethically, clients are guaranteed access to all of the information necessary for making decisions about their care and rehabilitation. We are not supposed to unfairly mislead a client by omitting information that would be helpful in client decision making. For example, for consumers with a hearing loss, audiologists should provide information about the variety of hearing aids (e.g., brand, type, cost, size) that might be beneficial to a particular client.

Ethical Practice within Professional Supervision

SLPs and audiologists often supervise as part of their job description. We may supervise people who are already credentialed (i.e., people with the CCC or state license), CFY participants, student-clinicians, and speech assistants/aides. Clinical supervisors should model ethical standards, and they are expected to monitor the ethical compliance of the people that they supervise. When an unethical behavior is suspected or obvious, the supervisor must take concrete actions to prevent violation of ethical standards, whether the person supervised is credentialed or an ASHA or AAA member.

For CFY participants, it is expected that the supervisor will make a genuine effort to meet the terms (i.e., expectations, follow-up) outlined in the CFY contract. For student-clinicians, ASHA guidelines require that supervisors hold the appropriate CCC credential, provide appropriate diagnostic and clinical supervision, and provide ongoing written and oral feedback to the student. In 1995 and 2000, ASHA published guidelines about the duties of a speech-language pathology assistant, the amount and type of supervision that he or she needs, and the professional experience of the supervisor.

Ethical Behavior within Professional Relationships

Clinicians are expected to maintain **professional relationships** with other communication specialists, as well as with personnel from other professions. There are many ways to demonstrate collegial behavior. First, we can work to understand the nature of related disciplines and the particular skills that a colleague tests and treats. Second, professional behavior includes a give-and-take open communication style so that all team members have the opportunity to discuss pertinent issues in a client's treatment plan. Third, education and rehabilitation professionals are expected to work in a climate of mutual respect and cooperation by avoiding personal conflict. This is especially true given recent efforts in transdisciplinary and team teaching models.

THE IMPLEMENTATION OF ETHICS FOR CLINICIANS

With a foundation in ethical principles, it is important that practicing and future clinicians understand how to judge their own compliance with ethical practice standards. Beginning and seasoned clinicians benefit from having a framework in which ethical situations can be discussed and debated. One such approach has been developed by Seymour (1994) as the **Ethics Calibration Quick Test** (ECQT; see Figure 2.1). Using the ECQT, we are able to analyze the ethical propriety of a situation by considering the ethical conflict, the values that are involved, the evidence, the possible plans of action, and the decision-making process. After you review the ECQT, return to Case Examples 1 and 2 at the beginning of the chapter and make a judgment about Michelle and Tom's ethical compliance. In the first case, you should be concerned about the degree of supervision Michelle provides to the speech assistants and whether she should allow a speech assistant, even a talented one, to modify a treatment program. In the second situation, Tom has billed for services not rendered and unintentionally committed fraud. In addition, because Tom cannot be certain about which clients received which services, his ability to keep accurate records should be questioned.

In addition to our own evaluation of ethical scenarios, both AAA and ASHA have centralized committees that address ethical situations. The AAA committee is called the **Ethical Practice Board** and the ASHA committee is called the **Board of Ethics.** One role of these committees is to develop position statements that further define particular ethical rules already cited in each code. A second role of these committees is to handle the adjudication process when violations are alleged. Through a due process format, complaints can be heard, evidence can be admitted, sanctions or penalties can be applied, and appeals can be processed. A third role of these committees is to educate ASHA and AAA members about ethics. One example of this is the "Ethics Roundtable" previously published in the ASHA magazine and presently available through the ASHA web site (http://professional.asha.org). Here, case situations are described in which a particular ethical dilemma is highlighted. Responses to the situation are debated by clinicians

Ethics Calibration Quick Test (ECQT)

1. What is the problem/conflict/dilemma?

    Is it a professional violation, a legal violation, or both?

2. What values are in conflict?

    Under these circumstances, what do I value the most?

    Will my feelings interfere with my judgment?

3. What evidence is provided by the parties involved?

    Whose evidence is most convincing?

    Is there a consistency in the facts?

    Have I heard all of the facts?

    What is acceptable practice in this situation?

    Who is most believable?

    Have I considered other viewpoints?

4. What courses of action can I take or recommend?

    Do I need outside consultation?

    Have I considered the social, cultural, and political impact of the consequences?

    Have I considered the short-term and long-term impact of the consequences?

5. In whose best interest is the decision?

    Will the decision be fair to all parties concerned?

    If yes, why? If not, why?

6. How will the decision make me feel about myself today and tomorrow?

Figure 2.1.   Using the ECQT, clinicians are able to analyze the ethical propriety of a situation by considering the ethical conflict, the values that are involved, the evidence, the possible plans of action, and the decision-making process. (From *Professional Issues in Speech-Language Pathology and Audiology, 1st edition*, by Lubinski. ©1994. Reprinted with permission of Delmar, a division of Thomson Learning. Fax: 800-730-2215.)

> ### Ethics Roundtable Example
>
> Ms. Robertson, a 78-year-old woman, is hospitalized after a hip fracture. A speech-language consultation is requested because her physician is concerned about her cognitive abilities. The evaluation is conducted by Scott, a student clinician. He observes mild cognitive impairments but also notes that Ms. Robertson coughs immediately after taking sips of water and that she has a wet voice quality for several minutes after drinking. From the medical record, Scott notes that she had pneumonia on admission to the hospital and has been treated for pneumonia at least three times in the past 9 months.
>
> Scott discusses his observations with his supervisor and recommends a swallowing evaluation. His supervisor suggests Ms. Robertson coughs because she is recovering from pneumonia. Furthermore, the supervisor says that they were consulted for a cognitive assessment and thus Scott's observations about her swallowing are inappropriate to include in his report. Scott is concerned about the patient but unsure of his role as a student and questions how to interpret his own observations.[2]

and/or ethicists who are familiar with the particular circumstance portrayed (i.e., the disorder, the service delivery model). Examples of some situations that have been discussed include interpretation of a living will after a stroke, sales quotas, refusal by patients to tube feedings, the limitations of health care plans, ethical issues in randomized clinical trials, and disagreement about patient care between a supervisor and student (reprinted in the box above). As a final task, try using the ECQT to analyze this example.

CONCLUSION

By introducing you to ethical practice, this chapter probably causes you to think about your own personal ethics and the degree to which they are consistent with professional ethics set by ASHA and AAA. Ethical guidelines will enable you to protect the rights and welfare of your clients and to construct your own personal ethics in regard to your profession. The AAA and ASHA Codes of Ethics provide you with an objective set of standards against which to compare your day-to-day professional actions. By adhering to standards and ethical principles, we are collectively able to promote our clients' welfare, as well as safeguard our own professional reputations and those of the professions of speech-language pathology and audiology.

---

[2]From Blake, A. (1999). When student and supervisor disagree about patient care. *ASHA, 41*(6), 65. ©1999 American Speech-Language-Hearing Association; reprinted by permission.

REFERENCES

American Academy of Audiology. (1991). *Code of ethics*. Houston: Author.

American Speech-Language-Hearing Association. (1993a). *Ethics: Resources for professional preparation and practice*. Rockville, MD: Author.

American Speech-Language-Hearing Association. (1993b). Statements of practices and procedures. *ASHA, 35,* 19–20.

American Speech-Language-Hearing Association. (1994a). Code of ethics. *ASHA, 36* (Suppl. 13), 1–2.

American Speech-Language-Hearing Association. (1994b). Code of ethics. *ASHA, 40* (Suppl. 18), 43–45.

American Speech-Language-Hearing Association. (1995). Position statement for the training, credentialing, use and supervision of support personnel in speech-language pathology. *ASHA, 37* (Suppl. 14), 21.

American Speech-Language-Hearing Association. (1998a). Statement of practices and procedures of the Board of Ethics. *ASHA, 40* (Suppl. 18), 46–49.

American Speech-Language-Hearing Association. (1998b). Practices and procedures for appeals of the Board of Ethics decisions. *ASHA, 40* (Suppl. 18), 50.

American Speech-Language-Hearing Association. (2000). Background information and criteria for the registration of speech-language pathology assistants. Available online at http://www.professional.asha.org.

Blake, A. (1999). When student and supervisor disagree about patient care. *ASHA, 41*(6), 65.

Buie, J. (1997). Medicare fraud probe pressure felt by members. *ASHA Leader, 2*(18), 1–8.

Freeman, N.K. (1997, September). Mama and daddy taught me right from wrong—isn't that enough? *Young Children, 52,* 64–67.

Heron, T., Martz, S.A., & Margolis, H. (1996, November). Ethical and legal issues in consultation. *Remedial and Special Education, 17,* 377–385.

Pannbacker, M., Middleton, G.F., & Vekovius, G.T. (1996). *Ethical practices in speech-language pathology and audiology: Case studies*. San Diego: Singular Publishing Group.

Resnick, D.M. (1993). *Professional ethics for audiologists and speech-language pathologists*. San Diego: Singular Publishing Group.

Rowland, R.C. (1988). Malpractice in audiology and speech-language pathology. *ASHA, 30*(1), 45–48.

Seymour, C.M. (1994). Ethical considerations. In R. Lubinski & C. Frattali (Eds.), *Professional issues in speech-language pathology and audiology: A textbook* (pp. 61–74). San Diego: Singular Publishing Group.

Silverman, F.H. (1999). *Professional issues in speech-language pathology and audiology*. Needham Heights, MA: Allyn & Bacon.

1. Why is it important to have ethical standards in professional practice?

2. Give three examples of how an SLP or an audiologist can safeguard a client's welfare.

3. Identify two ways in which a clinician can maintain his or her competence.

4. Describe three external factors that influence clinical competence.

5. Define and give an example of each of the following terms: misrepresentation, conflict of interest, nondiscrimination, infection control, informed consent, and referral.

6. What is the role of the clinical supervisor in ethical practice?

7. Why is it necessary for ASHA and AAA to have committees that review ethical standards and actions?

8. Describe the ECQT.

9. What revisions would you make to the ASHA Code of Ethics?

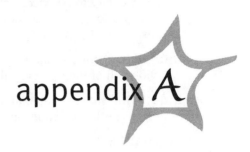

appendix A

The AAA Code of Ethics

PREAMBLE

The Code of Ethics of the American Academy of Audiology specifies professional standards that allow for the proper discharge of audiologists' responsibilities to those served, and that protect the integrity of the profession. The Code of Ethics consists of two parts. The first part, the Statement of Principles and Rules, presents precepts that members of the Academy agree to uphold. The second part, the Procedures, provides the process that enables enforcement of the Principles and Rules.

PART I : STATEMENT OF PRINCIPLES AND RULES

PRINCIPLE 1: Members shall provide professional services with honesty and compassion, and shall respect the dignity, worth, and rights of those served.

Rule 1a: Individuals shall not limit the delivery of professional services on any basis that is unjustifiable or irrelevant to the need for the potential benefit from such services.

PRINCIPLE 2: Members shall maintain high standards of professional competence in rendering services, providing only those professional services for which they are qualified by education and experience.

Rule 2a: Individuals shall use available resources, including referrals to other specialists, and shall not accept benefits or items of personal value for receiving or making referrals.

Rule 2b: Individuals shall exercise all reasonable precautions to avoid injury to persons in the delivery of professional services.

From the American Academy of Audiology. (1998). *Code of ethics.* McLean, VA: Author; reprinted by permission.

Rule 2c: Individuals shall not provide services except in a professional relationship, and shall not discriminate in the provision of services to individuals on the basis of sex, race, religion, national origin, sexual orientation, or general health.

Rule 2d: Individuals shall provide appropriate supervision and assume full responsibility for services delegated to supportive personnel. Individuals shall not delegate any service requiring professional competence to unqualified persons.

Rule 2e: Individuals shall not permit personnel to engage in any practice that is a violation of the Code of Ethics.

Rule 2f: Individuals shall maintain professional competence, including participation in continuing education.

PRINCIPLE 3: Members shall maintain the confidentiality of the information and records of those receiving services.

Rule 3a: Individuals shall not reveal to unauthorized persons any professional or personal information obtained from the person served professionally, unless required by law.

PRINCIPLE 4: Members shall provide only services and products that are in the best interest of those served.

Rule 4a: Individuals shall not exploit persons in the delivery of professional services.

Rule 4b: Individuals shall not charge for services not rendered.

Rule 4c: Individuals shall not participate in activities that constitute a conflict of professional interest.

Rule 4d: Individuals shall not accept compensation for supervision or sponsorship beyond reimbursement of expenses.

PRINCIPLE 5: Members shall provide accurate information about the nature and management of communicative disorders and about the services and products offered.

Rule 5a: Individuals shall provide persons served with the information a reasonable person would want to know about the nature and possible effects of services rendered, or products provided.

Rule 5b: Individuals may make a statement of prognosis, but shall not guarantee results, mislead, or misinform persons served.

Rule 5c: Individuals shall not carry out teaching or research activities in a manner which constitutes an invasion of privacy, or that fails to inform persons fully about the nature and possible effects of these activities, affording all persons informed free choice of participation.

Rule 5d: Individuals shall maintain documentation of professional services rendered.

PRINCIPLE 6: Members shall comply with the ethical standards of the Academy with regard to public statements.

Rule 6a: Individuals shall not misrepresent their educational degrees, training, credentials, or competence. Only degrees earned from regionally accredited institutions in which training was obtained in audiology, or a directly related discipline, may be used in public statements concerning professional services.

Rule 6b: Individuals' public statements about professional services and products shall not contain representations or claims which are false, misleading, or deceptive.

PRINCIPLE 7: Members shall honor their responsibilities to the public and to professional colleagues.

Rule 7a: Individuals shall not use professional or commercial affiliations in any way which would mislead or limit services to persons served professionally.

Rule 7b: Individuals shall inform colleagues and the public in a manner consistent with the highest professional standards about products and services they have developed.

PRINCIPLE 8: Members shall uphold the dignity of the profession and freely accept the Academy's self-imposed standards.

Rule 8a: Individuals shall not violate these Principles and Rules, nor attempt to circumvent them.

Rule 8b: Individuals shall not engage in dishonesty or illegal conduct that adversely reflects on the profession.

Rule 8c: Individuals shall inform the Ethical Practice Board when there are reasons to believe that a member of the Academy may have violated the Code of Ethics.

Rule 8d: Individuals shall cooperate with the Ethical Practice Board in any matter related to the Code of Ethics.

Signature: _____ Date: _____

PART II: PROCEDURES FOR THE MANAGEMENT OF ALLEGED VIOLATIONS

Introduction

Members of the American Academy of Audiology are obligated to uphold the Code of Ethics of the Academy in their personal conduct and in the performance of their professional duties. To this end it is the responsibility of each Academy member to inform the Ethical Practice Board of possible Ethics Code violations. The processing of alleged violations of the Code of Ethics will follow the procedures specified below in an expeditious manner to ensure that violations of ethical conduct by members of the Academy are halted in the shortest time possible.

Procedures

1. Suspended violations of the Code of Ethics should respond in letter formt— giving documentation sufficient to support the alleged violation. Letters must be signed and addressed to:

> Chair, Ethical Practice Board
> American Academy of Audiology
> 8201 Greensboro Drive, Suite 300
> McLean, VA 22102

2. Following receipt of the alleged violation the Board will request from the complainant a signed Waiver of Confidentiality indicating that the complainant will allow the Ethical Practice Board to disclose his or her name should this become necessary during investigation of the allegation. The Board may, under special circumstances, act in the absence of a signed Waiver of Confidentiality.

3. On receipt of the Waiver of Confidentiality signed by the complainant, or on the decision of the Board to assume the role of active complainant, the member(s) implicated will be notified by the Chair that an alleged violation of the Code of Ethics has been reported. Circumstances of the alleged violation will be described and the member(s) will be asked to respond fully to the allegation.

4. The Chair may communicate with other individuals, agencies, and/or programs, for additional information as may be required for Board review. The accumulation of information will be accomplished as expeditiously as possible to minimize the time between initial notification of possible Code violation and final determination by the Ethical Practice Board.

5. All information pertaining to the allegation will be reviewed by members of the Ethical Practice Board and a finding reached regarding infractions of the Code. In cases of Code violation, the section(s) of the Code violated will be cited, and a sanction specified when the Ethical Practice Board decision is disseminated.

   Members found to be in violation of the Code may appeal the decision of the Ethical Practice Board. The route of Appeal is by letter format through the Ethical Practice Board to the Executive Committee of the Academy. Requests for Appeal must:

   a. be received by the Chair, Ethical Practice Board, within 30 days of the Ethical Practice Board notification of violation.

   b. state the basis for the appeal, and the reason(s) that the Ethical Practice Board decision should be changed.

    c. not offer new documentation.

The decision of the Executive Committee regarding Appeals will be considered final.

SANCTIONS

1. *Reprimand.* The minimum level of punishment for a violation consists of a reprimand. Notification of the violation and the sanction is restricted to the member and the complainant.

2. *Cease and Desist Order.* Violator(s) may be required to sign a Cease and Desist Order which specifies the non-compliant behavior and the terms of the Order. Notification of the violation and the sanction is made to the member and the complainant, and may on two-thirds vote of the Ethical Practice Board be reported in an official publication.

3. *Suspension of Membership.* Suspension of membership may range from a minimum of six (6) months to a maximum of twelve (12) months. During the period of suspension the violator may not participate in official Academy functions. Notification of the violation and the sanction is made to the member and the complainant and is reported in official publications of the Academy. Notification of the violation and the sanction may be extended to others as determined by the Ethical Practice Board. No refund of dues or assessments shall accrue to the member.

4. *Revocation of Membership.* Revocation of membership will be considered as the maximum punishment for a violation of the Code. Individuals whose membership is revoked are not entitled to a refund of dues or fees. One year following the date of membership revocation the individual may reapply for, but is not guaranteed, membership through normal channels and must meet the membership qualifications in effect at the time of application. Notification of the violation and the sanction is made to the member and the complainant and is reported in official publications of the Academy for at least three (3) separate issues during the period of revocation. Special notification, as determined by the Ethical Practice Board, may be required in certain situations.

RECORDS

1. A Central Record Depository shall be maintained by the Ethical Practice Board which will be kept confidential and maintained with restricted access.

2. Complete records shall be maintained for a period of five years and then destroyed.

3. Confidentiality shall be maintained in all Ethical Practice Board discussion, correspondence, communication, deliberation, and records pertaining to members reviewed by the Ethical Practice Board.

4.   No Ethical Practice Board member shall give access to records, act or speak independently, or on behalf of the Board, without the express permission of the Board members then active, to impose the sanction of the Board, or to interpret the findings of the Board in any manner which may place members of the Board, collectively or singly, at financial, professional, or personal risk.

5.   A Book of Precedents shall be maintained by the Ethical Practice Board which shall form the basis for future findings of the Board.

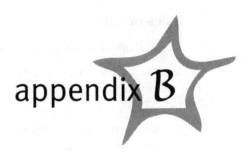

appendix B

The ASHA Code of Ethics

PREAMBLE

The preservation of the highest standards of integrity and ethical principles is vital to the responsible discharge of obligations in the professions of speech-language pathology and audiology. This Code of Ethics sets forth the fundamental principles and rules considered essential to this purpose.

Every individual who is (a) a member of the American Speech-Language-Hearing Association, whether certified or not, (b) a nonmember holding the Certificate of Clinical Competence from the Association, (c) an applicant for membership or certification, or (d) a Clinical Fellow seeking to fulfill standards for certification shall abide by this Code of Ethics.

Any action that violates the spirit and purpose of this Code shall be considered unethical. Failure to specify any particular responsibility or practice in this Code of Ethics shall not be construed as denial of the existence of such responsibilities or practices.

The fundamentals of ethical conduct are described by Principles of Ethics and by Rules of Ethics as they relate to responsibility to persons served, to the public, and to the professions of speech-language pathology and audiology.

Principles of Ethics, aspirational and inspirational in nature, form the underlying moral basis for the Code of Ethics. Individuals shall observe these principles as affirmative obligations under all conditions of professional activity.

Rules of Ethics are specific statements of minimally acceptable professional conduct or of prohibitions and are applicable to all individuals.

From American Speech-Language-Hearing Association. (1994a). Code of ethics. *ASHA, 36*(Suppl. 13), 1–2. Last revised January 1, 1994; reprinted by permission.

not the most up to date version

PRINCIPLE OF ETHICS I

Individuals shall honor their responsibility to hold paramount the welfare of persons they serve professionally.

Rules of Ethics

A. Individuals shall provide all services competently.

B. Individuals shall use every resource, including referral when appropriate, to ensure that high-quality service is provided.

C. Individuals shall not discriminate in the delivery of professional services on the basis of race or ethnicity, gender, age, religion, national origin, sexual orientation, or disability.

D. Individuals shall fully inform the persons they serve of the nature and possible effects of services rendered and products dispensed.

E. Individuals shall evaluate the effectiveness of services rendered and of products dispensed and shall provide services or dispense products only when benefit can reasonably be expected.

F. Individuals shall not guarantee the results of any treatment or procedure, directly or by implication; however, they may make a reasonable statement of prognosis.

G. Individuals shall not evaluate or treat speech, language, or hearing disorders solely by correspondence.

H. Individuals shall maintain adequate records of professional services rendered and products dispensed and shall allow access to these records when appropriately authorized.

I. Individuals shall not reveal, without authorization, any professional or personal information about the person served professionally, unless required by law to do so, or unless doing so is necessary to protect the welfare of the person or of the community.

J. Individuals shall not charge for services not rendered, nor shall they misrepresent[1], in any fashion, services rendered or products dispensed.

K. Individuals shall use persons in research or as subjects of teaching demonstrations only with their informed consent.

L. Individuals whose professional services are adversely affected by substance abuse or other health-related conditions shall seek professional assistance and, where appropriate, withdraw from the affected areas of practice.

---

[1]For purposes of this Code of Ethics, misrepresentation includes any untrue statements or statements that are likely to mislead. Misrepresentation also includes the failure to state any information that is material and that ought, in fairness, to be considered.

PRINCIPLE OF ETHICS II

Individuals shall honor their responsibility to achieve and maintain the highest level of professional competence.

Rules of Ethics

A. Individuals shall engage in the provision of clinical services only when they hold the appropriate Certificate of Clinical Competence or when they are in the certification process and are supervised by an individual who holds the appropriate Certificate of Clinical Competence.

B. Individuals shall engage in only those aspects of the professions that are within the scope of their competence, considering their level of education, training, and experience.

C. Individuals shall continue their professional development throughout their careers.

D. Individuals shall delegate the provision of clinical services only to persons who are certified or to persons in the education or certification process who are appropriately supervised. The provision of support services may be delegated to persons who are neither certified nor in the certification process only when a certificate holder provides appropriate supervision.

E. Individuals shall prohibit any of their professional staff from providing services that exceed the staff member's competence, considering the staff member's level of education, training, and experience.

F. Individuals shall ensure that all equipment used in the provision of services is in proper working order and is properly calibrated.

PRINCIPLE OF ETHICS III

Individuals shall honor their responsibility to the public by promoting public understanding of the professions, by supporting the development of services designed to fulfill the unmet needs of the public, and by providing accurate information in all communications involving any aspect of the professions.

Rules of Ethics

A. Individuals shall not misrepresent their credentials, competence, education, training, or experience.

B. Individuals shall not participate in professional activities that constitute a conflict of interest.

C. Individuals shall not misrepresent diagnostic information, services rendered, or products dispensed or engage in any scheme or artifice to defraud in connection with obtaining payment or reimbursement for such services or products.

D. Individuals' statements to the public shall provide accurate information about the nature and management of communication disorders, about the professions, and about professional services.

E. Individuals' statements to the public—advertising, announcing, and marketing their professional services, reporting research results, and promoting product—shall adhere to prevailing professional standards and shall not contain misrepresentations.

PRINCIPLE OF ETHICS IV

Individuals shall honor their responsibilities to the professions and their relationships with colleagues, students, and members of allied professions. Individuals shall uphold the dignity and autonomy of the professions, maintain harmonious interprofessional and intraprofessional relationships, and accept the professions' self-imposed standards.

Rules of Ethics

A. Individuals shall prohibit anyone under their supervision from engaging in any practice that violates the Code of Ethics.

B. Individuals shall not engage in dishonesty, fraud, deceit, misrepresentation, or any form of conduct that adversely reflects on the professions or on the individuals fitness to serve persons professionally.

C. Individuals shall assign credit only to those who have contributed to a publication, presentation, or product. Credit shall be assigned in proportion to the contribution and only with the contributor's consent.

D. Individuals' statements to colleagues about professional services, research results, and products shall adhere to prevailing professional standards and shall contain no misrepresentations.

E. Individuals shall not provide professional services without exercising independent professional judgment, regardless of referral source or prescription.

F. Individuals shall not discriminate in their relationships with colleagues, students, and members of allied professions on the basis of race or ethnicity, gender, age, religion, national origin, sexual orientation, or disability.

G. Individuals who have reason to believe that the Code of Ethics has been violated shall inform the Ethical Practice Board.

H. Individuals shall cooperate fully with the Ethical Practice Board in its investigation and adjudication of matters related to this Code of Ethics.

Principles
of Assessment

Marianne Kennedy

CASE EXAMPLE 1

Darrell is 4 years, 6 months old, but his speech is more like that of a much younger child. His parents report that he is very difficult to understand and they feel that he is becoming frustrated. They want him to improve his speech before he begins kindergarten next year.

CASE EXAMPLE 2

Jonah is 7 years old and has a severe bilateral sensorineural hearing loss. He uses behind-the-ear hearing aids at home and an auditory trainer at school. His school district has referred him for re-evaluation of his hearing, speech, and language and to determine whether his amplification equipment continues to be appropriate for him.

CASE EXAMPLE 3

Anna is a seventh-grade student with significant learning disabilities. She received speech and language therapy when she was younger but was dismissed from services in third grade. Although she receives special education assistance with reading and math, her current teacher believes that she needs more help and wonders whether language therapy would be beneficial at this time.

CASE EXAMPLE 4

Marlene is a 50-year-old woman who has had significant difficulty with communication since her stroke 8 months ago. She received speech and language therapy only for a short time, and her family would like to pursue more therapy now. They believe that she could continue to make improvements in her ability to communicate.

CASE EXAMPLE 5

Richard, 62 years old, recently underwent a total laryngectomy. He would like to learn to use esophageal speech.

CASE EXAMPLE 6

Thomas is a 27-year-old man with a history of severe stuttering. He feels that his speech disorder is interfering with his ability to advance in his career.

The six individuals described previously all appear to have a communication disorder, but they have little else in common. You have been asked to evaluate and make recommendations for these individuals. How will you provide an appropriate assessment for each of these potential clients given the large differences in their problems and the varied assessment protocols that will be necessary to complete the task competently? These examples are provided not to overwhelm the beginning clinician, but to illustrate the breadth of the field of communication disorders. As different as the clients described previously may seem, they are but a sample of the variety of ages, functional levels, and types of disorders to which you will be exposed during training and later in practice. How is it possible to competently assess such a range of problems?

Despite the fact that the needs of these clients are indeed diverse, as are the assessment instruments you will use, there are some general principles that apply. This chapter introduces you to these general principles that guide the process of assessing any communication disorder and provides examples of assessment tools for a variety of communication disorders.

When you hear the word *assessment,* you may think of testing, but the two are not really the same. Testing is only one part of assessment. **Assessment** is the process of collecting and interpreting relevant data for clinical decision making. The process includes a series of problem-solving activities to assist in making decisions that will result in effective management and intervention for clients with communication disorders. In this chapter, the terms **diagnostic, evaluation,** and **assessment** are used interchangeably to denote the problem-solving and descriptive process.

Various approaches to assessment in communication disorders have been described in the literature. One approach, derived from the medical model, makes a distinction between **appraisal** and **diagnosis** (e.g., Darley & Spriestersbach, 1978; Peterson & Marquardt, 1994). Appraisal is seen as the collection of both quantitative and qualitative data about the client. Diagnosis involves interpretation of these data in order to decide whether a problem exists and then differentiating the problem from other similar problems (i.e., **differential diagnosis**). In a medical model, emphasis is also put on identification of possible causes (i.e., **etiology**) and maintaining factors. Another approach is what Miller (1978) and Paul (1995) described as a **descriptive-developmental model** of assessment. In this orientation, the two phases are less distinct. Emphasis is placed on description of the client's present communication behaviors rather than on causal factors or categorization of the disorder. Tomblin (2000) also described a **systems model** of assessment. This model stresses the importance of the family and the cultural context in which the client must function. In this model, there is much emphasis on including the "significant others" in the assessment process to get information about the dynamics of the communication problem. There is a great deal of overlap among the various approaches, and there is no one correct model. For example, use of the descriptive-developmental model certainly does not preclude family involvement or consideration of the client's cultural background. It is more of a question of relative emphasis. The specific model (or combination of models) to be used will depend on the philosophical orientation of the clinician, the setting, and the type of communication problem demonstrated by the client. For example, clinicians who work in medical settings may be more likely than other clinicians to perform assessments that fit the appraisal and diagnosis model. Clinicians who work primarily in educational settings may find the descriptive-developmental approach more useful.

No matter which setting you work in, you will be involved with professionals from other disciplines. Teaming and collaboration among professionals is recognized as the best practice for meeting the needs of clients with a variety of disabilities. Various models of teaming are used in the assessment process, including **multidisciplinary, interdisciplinary,** and **transdisciplinary.** Regardless of the model used, remember that the client and the family are partners in the assessment process; that is, they are critical team members.

Before we can proceed further, several concepts derived from the medical model that are important to the diagnostic process must be discussed. The World Health Organization (WHO; 1980) differentiated among the terms **impairment, disability,** and **handicap.** (In 2001, the WHO proposed modification of these terms, and they may be changed.) Impairment refers to a disruption or abnormality in the physiologic structure or function. The impairment is usually labeled or named by the disease state. Disability is a loss in function or the inability to perform certain activities as a result of the impairment, such as **aphasia** following a stroke. A handicap is the effect or negative consequence that the impairment or disability may have on the individual. The handicap may be a result of environmental or social barriers and expectations. Although it may seem that we should be able to infer disability and handicap from a known impairment, this is not always the case, and it can be illustrated in Richard, the man who underwent a total laryngectomy. Consider two different scenarios: first, that Richard is a computer programmer by profession, and second, that Richard is a trial attorney by profession. Although Richard's disability (the inability to produce speech following the laryngectomy), which is secondary to the impairment (laryngeal cancer treated with surgery), is the same in both cases, the degree of handicap relative to his career may be quite different. In the first scenario, Richard may very well be able to continue his career with minor adaptations and compensations. Resuming his career in the second scenario might be more difficult and would most likely require major adaptations and compensation. Knowledge of the impairment is important in describing prognosis and determining an optimal intervention strategy. For example, in Richard's case, we know that barring other medical problems his status should be stable, and we make prognostic statements and intervention recommendations based on that knowledge. In other cases, with individuals who have neurologic impairments known to be degenerative, it is equally important to be familiar with the associated symptoms in order to make appropriate prognostic statements and intervention recommendations. Thus, these issues of impairment, disability, and handicap must be considered in a comprehensive assessment.

PURPOSES OF ASSESSMENT

Assessments are completed for various purposes. Understanding the purpose or goal of the assessment is important because it will affect the types of instruments and protocols chosen. The most common reasons for assessment described in this chapter are based on the works of Miller (1978, 1983) and Paul (1995).

Screening

Screening involves the collection of data to decide whether there is a strong likelihood that an individual does or does not have a problem that will require more in-depth assessment. Screening has its roots in medical practices used to identify those who are at risk for a particular disease or disorder (Salvia & Ysseldyke, 1995). Rather than yielding scores, screening results are generally described as "pass" or "fail" based on a predetermined **cut-off score.** A "fail" will typically result in a referral for more intensive follow-up assessment. You may be familiar with one common use of screening. Most school districts screen children before they enter kindergarten in a number of areas including speech, language, readiness skills, hearing, and vision. Children who fail one or more of these screenings are referred for further evaluation. Examples of frequently used screening procedures in communication disorders are provided in Table 3.1. As Paul (1995) pointed out, it is not always necessary to use a test published as a screening instrument. Any standardized test that samples the relevant areas efficiently and meets certain psychometric criteria can be used.

Screening is also an important component of comprehensive communication assessments. In addition to addressing the presenting concerns, it is important to screen other aspects of speech, language, and communication as well as selected collateral areas. You will see how screening procedures are included into the assessment of Darrell, the 4-year-old whose speech sounds immature. Most likely, you will decide to assess articulation and language skills in depth using several different instruments, both formal and informal. You will also need to screen other areas, however, such as fluency, voice, hearing, and the oral mechanism in order to determine the possibility that a problem in these areas is also

Table 3.1. Examples of screening instruments used in speech, language, and communication assessment

Test	Area	Ages	Comments
Bedside Evaluation Screening Test, Second Edition (West, Sands, & Ross-Swain, 1998)	Aphasia: Speaking, comprehension, reading	Adult	Yields severity ratings Normed on 200 individuals with aphasia
Boone Voice Program for Children (Boone, 1993)	Voice	School-age children	Program includes a voice screening protocol that uses clinician rating scale and s/z ratio
Brief Test of Head Injury (Helm-Estabrooks & Hotz, 1991)	Cognitive, linguistic, communicative abilities	14-0 to adult	Yields standard score, percentile, and severity rating Assesses postcoma abilities following brain injury
Clinical Evaluation of Language Fundamentals–3 Screening Test (Semel, Wiig, & Secord, 1996)	Language: Receptive and expressive morphology, syntax, semantics	6-0 to 21-0 years	Yields criterion-referenced score
Early Language Milestones Scale, Second Edition (ELM-2; Coplan, 1993)	Language: Receptive and expressive semantics, syntax; phonology	Birth to 3-0 years	Pass/fail or point scoring method available Latter yields standard, percentile, or age scores
Fluharty Preschool Speech and Language Screening Test (Fluharty, 1978)	Language: Vocabulary, articulation, syntax	2-0 to 6-0 years	Cut-off score for each subtest is provided based on age
Kindergarten Language Screening Scale, Second Edition (KLS-2; Gauthier & Madison, 1998)	Language: Receptive and expressive semantics, syntax	3-6 to 6-11 years	Yields percentile rank and stanine Cut-off score based on stanine is recommended
Oral Speech Mechanism Screening Exam, Third Edition (OSMSE-3; St. Louis & Ruscello, 2000)	Oral motor mechanism	Preschool to 70-0 years	Yields +/− scores Provides checklist for noting appropriate structure and function
Quick Screen of Phonology (Bankson & Bernthal, 1990)	Articulation, phonological processes	3-0 to 7-11 years	Yields ranks and standard scores Cut-off scores for different ages available
Screening Test for Developmental Apraxia of Speech (Blakeley, 1980)	Apraxia	4-0 to 12-0 years	Yields criterion-referenced score Has eight subtests
Screening Test of Adolescent Language (Prather, Beecher, Stafford, & Wallace, 1980)	Language: Vocabulary, auditory memory span, language processing, proverb explanation	Grades 6 to 12	Yields pass/fail cut-off score

47

contributing to the concerns that Darrell's parents have described. In addition, you may need to get information about related areas such as play and cognitive skills. These areas will be discussed in more detail later in the chapter. If the examiner suspects any problems in these areas, a more in-depth evaluation should follow.

Determining a Diagnosis or Differential Diagnosis

In some cases, it may be important or useful to label the communication problem or to distinguish the disorder from another disorder with similar symptoms (Emerick & Hatten, 1974). Consider Marlene, the woman who had a stroke 8 months ago. In order to recommend an appropriate course of treatment, we need to understand the basis for her communication problems. Does Marlene's communication problem stem from aphasia, **dysarthria, apraxia,** or some form of **dementia?** In many cases, a diagnostic label may be a prerequisite to obtaining funding for services.

Before assigning a diagnostic label, though, it is always important to ascertain whether the communication issues presented are the result of a *difference* rather than a *disorder.* In other words, is it possible that the client's communication differs from the norm because the individual's environment and experiences have been different from the norm? For example, if Darrell's family speaks a language other than English at home, then we must consider the possibility that his current language status is related to the different linguistic experiences he has had rather than a language disorder (see Chapter 10). If we find that the presenting concern is a disorder, then it will be important to carefully describe his current level of performance in the various language and communication areas.

Determining Eligibility for Services

Intervention services, which are supported by public or third-party funding, may have specific guidelines and eligibility requirements that must be met before those sources of funding can be accessed. For example, the Individuals with Disabilities Education Act (IDEA) of 1990 (PL 101-476) requires local school districts to provide free special education and related services to those children whose problems have a negative impact on their ability to profit from general education. In many school districts, this means that in order to qualify for services, a child must perform below a predetermined level (usually 1.5 to 2 standard deviations below the mean for his or her age) on an assessment. This point is illustrated by Anna's case. As you will recall, she already receives special education services for her learning disability. Following the referral from her teacher, Anna will have to undergo assessment. In order to qualify for additional services from the school's speech-language pathologist (SLP), the assessment results will have to demonstrate that her performance is significantly below average. These conclusions must be based on several different types of assessment data, never solely on the basis of one test.

Establishing a Baseline

Once we have ascertained that a client has a problem and is eligible for services, it is important to describe the individual's current functioning in all areas of communication. This description, which, as you will see later, can include both qualitative and quantitative data, will serve as a **baseline** or reference point for measuring progress during treatment. It is important to describe what the client is able to do as well as what the client cannot do. So, the baseline information should be a profile of the client's strengths and weaknesses. Furthermore, because the client's behavior in a clinical setting may not represent typical behavior, baseline information should be gathered in various settings and contexts. To illustrate, consider the cases of Richard and Thomas. Both clients clearly have a communication problem and both already have a diagnosis. For these clients, the purpose of the current assessment is to document and describe their present level of communication functioning. This description not only will serve as a baseline for comparison with subsequent performance, but it also will lay the basis for the next phase of assessment.

Developing Intervention Targets

Once the client's present status has been described, the next step is to identify potential targets or goals for intervention. Many factors are considered to determine goals and intervention priorities, including developmental appropriateness, targets that would have the greatest impact on the individual's communication, and client and family priorities. As part of this process, the assessment may include **stimulability** testing to determine which communication behaviors can be easily modified or elicited through the use of various levels of cueing or prompting. Similarly, the examiner may use some trial teaching or facilitating techniques to gauge the client's responsiveness. This is often referred to as **dynamic assessment** (e.g., Lidz, 1987). When developing goals and intervention methods, it is also important to consider how the client's areas of strength can be used to facilitate or compensate for areas of weakness.

Tracking and Documenting Progress

Finally, assessment procedures are used throughout intervention in order to measure progress toward the stated goals and to assess the effectiveness of the intervention itself. Ongoing assessment is necessary so that adjustments can be made as needed in the intervention targets and techniques. It is also important when you are making decisions about when to dismiss a client from therapy. Just as it was important to sample communication behaviors in a variety of settings when determining baseline functioning, it is also important to document progress in a variety of real-life situations. Tracking and documenting progress will be used as part of the clinical process with all of the clients described previously during the course of their therapy.

Periodic re-evaluation, a somewhat more formal process than the ongoing assessment described previously, is another way to document changes over time.

Table 3.2. Types of assessment instruments and their primary use in assessment

	Norm-referenced	Criterion-referenced	Behavioral observation	Instrumental
Screening	✓	✓		✓
Determine existence of a problem, diagnosis, differential diagnosis	✓			✓
Determine eligibility for services	✓			✓
Establish baseline		✓	✓	✓
Determine intervention goals		✓	✓	✓
Document or track progress		✓	✓	✓

This is one reason that Jonah, the boy who has a severe hearing loss, gets a referral for testing. Tracking his hearing levels is an essential part of ensuring that he gets the most benefit from his hearing aids and auditory trainer.

METHODS OF ASSESSMENT

Assessment instruments generally fall into one of three main groups: norm-referenced or standardized tests, criterion-referenced tests, and observational tools. Each group has advantages and disadvantages that must be considered in light of the questions being asked of the assessment. Table 3.2 summarizes the major types of instruments and their primary uses in assessment.

Norm-Referenced Tests

Norm-referenced tests are standardized instruments that can be used to compare an individual's performance to the performance of others with similar demographic characteristics such as age and gender. This type of test is useful for determining the existence of a problem and establishing eligibility for services. Norm-referenced instruments have certain statistical properties that allow meaningful comparisons among individuals and allow us to determine if an individual's performance is significantly different from typical performance on a given trait or skill. Examples of frequently used norm-referenced tests in the field of communication disorders are provided in Table 3.3. In order to use tests appropriately, clinicians must be informed consumers. This includes investigating the relevant properties of tests and using only those that meet acceptable psychometric criteria. Although detailed explanations of psychometric and statistical theories underlying norm-referenced tests are beyond the scope of this chapter, a brief summary of key characteristics follows (McCauley & Swisher, 1984; Paul, 1995; Salvia & Ysseldyke, 1995).

Reliability **Reliability** refers to the consistency or dependability with which a test measures what it is supposed to be measuring. When we administer a test, we should be able to make some assumptions about the results that we get. First, we want to be sure that an individual's performance is not unduly influenced by some examiner characteristics. In other words, a different examiner should be able to get the same results, either by administering the test directly or

Table 3-3. Examples of norm-referenced tests used in speech, language, and communication assessments

Test	Area	Ages	Comments
Arizona Battery for Communication Disorders of Dementia (ABCD; Bayles & Tomoeda, 1991)	Language (dementia): Auditory comprehension, verbal episodic and semantic memory, oral expression, visual spatial skills	Adult	Yields criterion scores which can be converted to 5-point scaled score. Standardized on patients with Alzheimer's disease and Parkinson's disease as well as younger and older individuals without disabilities. Has 14 subtests.
Boston Diagnostic Aphasia Examination, Second Edition (BDAE; Goodglass & Kaplan, 1983)	Language (aphasia): Auditory and written language comprehension, oral expression, writing	Adult	Yields percentile ranks and severity ratings. A profile can be developed from subtest rating scores.
Clinical Evaluation of Language Fundamentals-3 (CELF-3; Semel, Wiig, & Secord, 1995)	Language: Receptive and expressive semantics, syntax, morphology; auditory memory	6-0 to 21-0 years	Yields standard, percentile, and age-equivalent scores (CELF-3 Clinical Assistant). Spanish edition available. Has 10 subtests.
Communication Abilities in Daily Living, Second Edition (CADL-2; Holland, Frattali, & Fromm, 1999)	Language (aphasia/brain damage): Semantics, pragmatics, reading, writing	Adult	Yields percentile scores and stanines. Normed on 175 adults with neurogenic communication disorders.
Expressive One Word Picture Vocabulary Test, 2000 Edition (EOWPVT; Gardner, 2000)	Language: Expressive vocabulary	2-0 to 18-11 years	Yields standard, percentile, and age-equivalent scores.
Expressive Vocabulary Test (Williams, 1997)	Language: Expressive vocabulary, synonyms	2-6 to 90-0 years	Yields standard, percentile, and age-equivalent scores. Computer scoring program available.
Goldman-Fristoe Test of Articulation, Second Edition (Goldman & Fristoe, 2000)	Articulation	2-0 to 21-0 years	Yields standard scores. Separate gender norms are available.
Khan-Lewis Phonological Analysis (Khan & Lewis, 1986)	Phonological processes	2-0 to 5-11 years	Yields composite, percentile, and age-equivalent scores. Speech simplification rating.
MacArthur Communicative Development Inventories (Fenson et al., 1993)	Language: Receptive and expressive vocabulary; gestures, syntax, morphology	0-8 to 2-6 years	Yields percentile ranks. Parent report format. Two versions: "Words and Gestures" for ages 8–16 months and "Words and Sentences" for 16–30 months.
Oral and Written Language Scales (OWLS; Carrow-Woolfolk, 1996)	Language: Receptive and expressive semantics, syntax, morphology; written language	3-0 to 21-11 years	Yields standard, percentile, age, and grade equivalent scores. Computer scoring program is available.
Peabody Picture Vocabulary Test-III (Dunn & Dunn, 1997)	Language: Receptive vocabulary	2-6 to 90-0 years	Yields standard, percentile, and age-equivalent scores. Equivalent forms A and B. Computer scoring program is available. Spanish version (TVIP) is available.

Table 3.3. *(continued)*

Test	Area	Ages	Comments
Preschool Language Scales-3 (PLS-3; Zimmerman, Steiner, & Pond, 1992)	Language: Receptive and expressive semantics, syntax, morphology; articulation	Birth to 6-11 years	Yields standard, percentile, and age-equivalent scores. Spanish version available.
Reynell Developmental Language Scales, U.S. Edition (Reynell & Gruber, 1990)	Language: Receptive and expressive semantic, syntax	1-0 to 6-11 years	Yields standard, percentile, and developmental level. Adaptation for children with severe oral impairment. Uses pictures and objects.
Stuttering Severity Instrument for Children & Adults, Third Edition (SSI-3; Riley, 1994)	Fluency	2-10 to adult	Yields criterion scores, percentile ranks, and severity rating. Computer scoring program available.
Test of Adolescent and Adult Language-3 (TOAL-3; Hammill, Brown, Larsen, & Wiederholt, 1994)	Language: Receptive and expressive semantics, syntax; reading; writing; auditory comprehension	12-0 to 24-11 years	Yields standard, percentile, and age-equivalent scores. Software scoring program is available.
Test of Auditory Comprehension of Language, Third Edition (TACL-3; Carrow-Woolfolk, 1999)	Language: Auditory comprehension of semantics, syntax, morphology	3-0 to 9-11 years	Yields standard, percentile, and age-equivalent scores.
Test of Language Development P-3 (TOLD-P:3; Newcomer & Hammill, 1997)	Language: Receptive and expressive semantics, syntax, morphology; phonology; articulation	4-0 to 8-11 years	Yields standard, percentile, and age-equivalent scores. Has nine subtests.
Test of Language Development—Intermediate (TOLD-I:3; Hammill & Newcomer, 1997)	Language: Receptive and expressive syntax and semantics	8-0 to 12-11 years	Yields standard, percentile, and age scores. Computer scoring program available.
Test of Pragmatic Language (TOPL; Phelps-Terasaki & Phelps-Gunn, 1992)	Language: Pragmatics	5-0 to 13-11 years	Yields standard and percentile scores. Can also be used for adult remedial, English as a Second Language, and aphasic population.
Western Aphasia Battery (WAB; Kertesz, 1982)	Language (aphasia): Auditory comprehension, verbal fluency, naming, information content	Adolescent to adult	Yields aphasia quotient to indicate severity.
Woodcock Language Proficiency Battery, Revised (Woodcock, 1991)	Language: Auditory comprehension, oral expression, reading, writing	2-0 to 95-0 years	Yields standard, percentile, age, and grade equivalent scores. Separate norms for college students provided. Computer scoring program available.

by rescoring a test given by another examiner. This is called **interrater reliability.** Second, if the test is given to an individual on two separate occasions, theoretically, the results should be identical. This property speaks to the stability of the test and is referred to as **test–retest reliability.** Finally, we want to assume that similar test items would yield similar results and that there is agreement among items within different parts of the test. This third type of reliability is demonstrated in several ways. Some tests have two forms that measure the same skills. This is called **equivalent** or **alternate form reliability.** A commonly used example in speech-language pathology is the Peabody Picture Vocabulary Test-III (PPVT) that has Forms A and B (Dunn & Dunn, 1997). This type of reliability can also be demonstrated by correlating one half of the test with the other half; this is referred to as **internal consistency.** The test can be split by comparing the first half of the items to the second half (**split-half reliability**), by comparing the even items to the odd numbered items (**odd-even reliability**), or by using a statistical procedure that compares all possible divisions of a test into two parts (**Cronbach's coefficient alpha**). Reliability data are reported in correlation coefficients and range from .00 (no reliability) to 1.00 (perfect reliability). These coefficients should be clearly presented in the test manual. Salvia and Ysseldyke (1995) recommended .90 correlation coefficient as a minimum standard for a test to be considered reliable.

Validity   The extent to which a test measures what it claims to measure is known as **validity.** We must be able to make accurate inferences from test results; thus, the tests we use must have a high degree of validity. Validity subsumes other characteristics such as reliability, adequacy of norms, and lack of bias. In addition, several types of validity should be reported in the test manual. First, a test has **content validity** when test items actually represent an adequate sample of the domain being measured. This kind of validity is usually judged by experts in the field and is based on the following factors: appropriateness of the items included, completeness of the sample, and the manner in which the items assess the content. Another type of validity is **criterion-related validity,** the extent to which performance on a test is correlated with performance on another instrument (i.e., criterion measure) believed to measure the same skill or behavior. Criterion-related validity should be presented as a correlation coefficient in the test manual and can be measured in two ways. **Concurrent validity** refers to the relationship between an individual's performance on the test and a criterion measure when they are administered at the same time, whereas **predictive validity** refers to how well the individual's current performance on the test predicts future performance on a criterion measure. The third major type of validity is **construct validity.** This refers to how a test measures the theoretical trait or construct that it is supposed to measure. This is particularly important for characteristics, such as comprehension, that cannot be directly observed or measured. For example, the PPVT was once used as a measure of IQ. Because the test is designed to measure receptive vocabulary (which is only one aspect of verbal intelligence), it is not surprising that it is not a good measure of overall intelligence. Evidence for construct validity comes from examination of the theory underlying the construct and the ability of the theory to predict performance. If a test does not have strong construct validity, it may not be measuring the underlying characteristic in question. Again, it is the examiner's responsibility to be clear about which skills or behaviors are being measured and to choose tests with high levels of validity for measuring the desired areas.

Standardization   Because it is impossible to test everyone in a given population, test developers rely on a subset of the population from whom the characteristics of the population can be estimated. An individual's performance is then compared with this **norming sample.** The characteristics of the norming or standardization sample are very important because all of the norm-referenced scores are based on the performance of this group. Adequate norms depend on several factors. First, the norming sample must be representative; that is, it must include a wide range of people with characteristics similar to those who will take the test. These characteristics include age, gender, race, ethnicity, socioeconomic background, and geographic distribution in the same proportion as in the general population. McCauley and Swisher (1984) emphasized the importance of noting whether people with disabilities or nonnormal language and communication abilities have been included in the standardization sample. Although the exclusion of such people seems to make intuitive sense, it presents problems. For one thing, if all the people in the standardization sample are considered normal, then even the lowest score in the sample represents a *normal* performance. This makes it very difficult to interpret scores, especially those at or below the lowest score of the norming sample. A second factor affecting the adequacy of norms is the number of people included in the sample. There must be adequate cases at each age level tested. Test experts recommend a minimum of 100 people at each age tested (Salvia & Ysseldyke, 1995). The final factor to be considered is the relevance of the norms to the purpose of the test. In most cases, we will be using national norms based on the general population in a particular age range. In some cases, local norms will be more appropriate. For example, some school districts with high percentages of children with limited English proficiency have developed local norms for language assessment. Yet, in other cases, we may wish to use norms based on particular groups. Examples include the Hiskey-Nebraska Test of Learning Aptitude (Hiskey, 1966) that is standardized on people who are deaf and the Communication Abilities in Daily Living test battery (Holland, Frattali, & Fromm, 1999) that is standardized on adults with neurogenic disorders.

Descriptive Statistics   In order to correctly interpret test scores, it is important to understand a few basic concepts of descriptive statistics, which is a way to describe or summarize quantitative data. If a test is given to a sufficiently large number of people, the resulting scores should form a **normal distribution.** This is usually depicted as a symmetrical or "bell-shaped" curve as shown in Figure 3.1. The advantage of this distribution is that the number of cases falling between any two points is known; therefore, scores can be interpreted relative to the distribution. We usually assume that the norming sample for a standardized test had a normal distribution. In a normal distribution, most scores will be clustered close to the **mean,** that is, the arithmetic average of the scores. The mean is known as a **measure of central tendency.** As you move away from the mean, there are fewer scores in either direction. You can see this in the bell curve—as you move

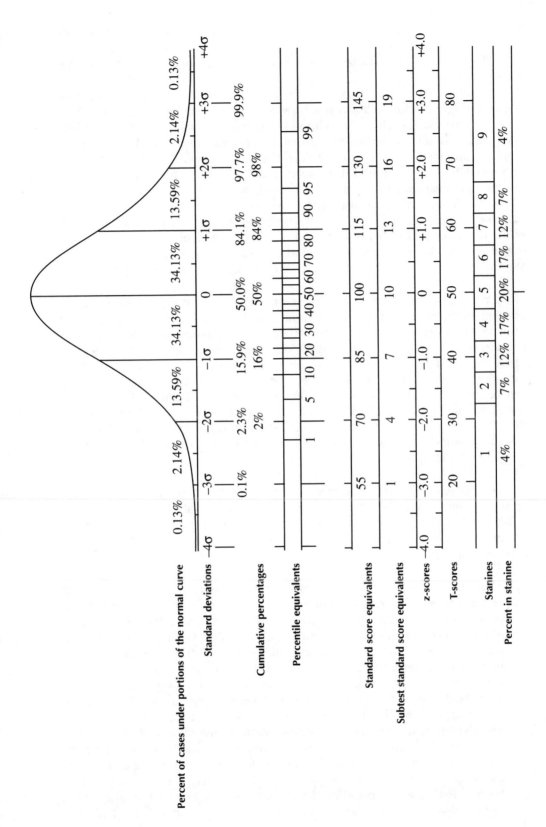

Figure 3.1. Relationship of the normal curve to various types of standard scores.

away from the middle, the area between the curve and the horizontal axis becomes smaller.

Although the mean tells us about the average performance of the group, we need more information to know just how close to the average the individuals in the group scored. Therefore, in addition to knowing the measure of central tendency, we must also know the measure of dispersion or variability. How were the scores of the norming group spread out? The most frequently reported measure of dispersion is the **standard deviation.** Mathematically, this measure is based on another measure of dispersion (variance), but in essence, it represents the average difference of scores from the mean score. In a normal distribution, we expect that approximately 68% of the scores will fall within 1 standard deviation of the mean on either side. Half the scores (34%) will be higher and half will be lower. About 96% of scores will be within 2 standard deviations of the mean. When using a test, it is critical to be aware of the means and standard deviations.

Error   All measurement contains error. Any score that we obtain is only an estimate of the person's true score. Test manuals for norm-referenced tests should provide the examiner with the **standard error of measurement (SEM),** which takes into account the variability that is inherent in human behavior. The SEM is really the standard deviation of error around a person's true score. Because we never really know a person's true score, we use the SEM to determine a **confidence interval** around the person's obtained test score. Figure 3.2 shows how the SEM aids in interpreting test results as it presents results for Darrell on the PPVT. You can see the confidence interval around his observed standard score of 83. This means that we can say with 68% confidence that Darrell's true score falls between 79 and 87.

Test Norms and Scores   The raw score obtained on a test has little usefulness in and of itself; it must be interpreted in reference to the test's norms. Test manuals provide tables that allow the examiner to convert raw scores into derived scores. There are two types of derived scores: developmental scores and scores of relative standing.

1.   The most common kinds of **developmental scores** are **age equivalents** and **grade equivalents.** Age equivalents are expressed in years and months, usually with a hyphen between the two (e.g., 3-8 means 3 years, 8 months old). Age equivalent means that a person's raw score is the average performance for that age group. Grade equivalents mean that a person's raw score is the average performance for a given grade; they are expressed in grades and tenths of grades, with a decimal point between the two (e.g., 6.2 means sixth grade, second month). Although developmental scores seem easy to understand, they should only be used with great caution. Salvia and Ysseldyke (1995) listed several problems with the use of these derived scores. First, they are easily misinterpreted. Darrell has earned an age-equivalent score of 3-0 (see Figure 3.2). This means that he has answered correctly as many items as the average 3-year-old child. He may not necessarily have "performed" as a 3-year-old child would. Let us suppose that another child, James, also received an age-equivalent score of 3-0 on the PPVT-III. But

Peabody Picture Vocabulary Test–Third Edition
by Lloyd M. Dunn & Leota M. Dunn

PPVT-III

Performance Record

FORM III A

Name Darrell Thompson   Sex: ☐F ☒M

Home Address 18 Main St   Phone (210) 451-3701

City Southwick   State CT   ZIP 06610

School Jackson   (or agency)   Grade Preschool   (or education)

Language of the Home ☒Standard English ☐Other _____
(specify: foreign language, or type of English dialect spoken)

Teacher Ms Phely   (or counselor)   Examiner MK

Date & Age Data

	Year	Month	Day
Date of testing	01	9	29
Date of birth	97	4	3
Chronological age*	4	6	

*Disregard extra days.

Reason for testing Parents concerned about speech development — hard to understand

Other information on test taker Being treated (with antibiotics) for ear infection

RECORD OF SCORES

Raw Score
(from oval on page 2) **38**

Deviation-type Norms

Standard Score
(Norms Table 1) **83**

Percentile Rank
(Norms Table 2) **13**

Normal Curve Equivalent
(Norms Table 2) **26**

Stanine
(Norms Table 2) **3**

Developmental-type Norms

Age Equivalent
(Norms Table 3) **3-0**

Graphic Display of Deviation-type Norm Scores

Mark the obtained standard score on the appropriate line below. Draw a straight vertical line through it and across the other scales. (See manual for more information.)

Optional confidence intervals also may be plotted. To do so, draw two lines vertically across all the scales, one on either side of the obtained standard score line. For the 68 percent band width, use ± 4 standard score units. (See manual for other options.)

	0.13%	2.15%	13.59%	34.13%	34.13%	13.59%	2.15%	0.13%
	-4σ	-3σ	-2σ	-1σ $\bar{X}$	$+1\sigma$	$+2\sigma$	$+3\sigma$	$+4\sigma$
Standard Score Equivalents	40	50	60	70	80	90	100	110	120	130	140	150	160
Percentile Ranks				1	5	10	20 30 40 50 60 70 80	90 95	99
Normal Curve Equivalents			1	10	20	30	40	50	60	70	80	90	99
Stanines			1	2	3	4	5	6	7	8	9
Score Range Descriptions		Extremely Low Score	Moderately Low Score	Low / High Average Score	Moderately High Score	Extremely High Score

Copyright 1997, Lloyd M. Dunn, Leota M. Dunn and Douglas M. Dunn. It is illegal to reproduce this form for testing. However, permission is granted to reproduce a completed front page to convey an examinee's scores to other qualified personnel. Unless this form is printed in violet and black, it is not an original and is an illegal photocopy.

For additional forms, call or write AGS, 4201 Woodland Road, Circle Pines, MN 55014-1796; toll-free 1-800-328-2560. In Canada, 1-800-263-3558. Ask for item #12004 (25 per package).

Figure 3.2.   Darrell's PPVT-III results. (From Dunn, L.M., & Dunn, L.M. [1997]. *Peabody Picture Vocabulary Test-III* [p. 1]. Circle Pines, MN: American Guidance Service; permission to reprint this sample page granted by publisher.)

James is 7 years old. Most likely, Darrell and James have not performed identically! Furthermore, in the construction of the norms, average age and grade scores may be estimated for groups of individuals that were never actually tested. The "average" 3-year-old is really a statistical abstraction. Real average 3-year-old children represent a range of performance, as you will recall from our previous discussion about normal distributions. In fact, the way that equivalent scores are constructed ensures that 50% of any age or grade group will perform below age or grade level. Because developmental scores are not based on equal interval measures (e.g., a 1 year delay in a 3-year-old is quite different from a 1 year delay in a 10-year-old), they cannot be added or subtracted. That means if we retest Darrell next year on the PPVT and he receives an age-equivalent score of 3-8, we *cannot* conclude that he has made 8 month's progress. Unfortunately, you will probably see this type of misinterpretation during your career.

2. **Scores of relative standing,** however, do allow us to make comparisons among individuals of different ages as well as among scores on various tests taken by the same person. There are several types of scores of relative standing and they can be seen in Figure 3.1.

   a. **Percentile ranks** indicate the percentage of people in the norming sample who scored *at or below* a given raw score. We see in Figure 3.2 that Darrell's PPVT raw score converts to the 13th percentile. This means that of 100 children his age who were in the norming sample, 13 of them earned the same or lower raw score than Darrell. Percentile scores are easy to understand and explain to families, but a caution is in order. In looking back at Figure 3.1, note that percentile scores are not equal interval scores. For example, the distance between the 5th and 10th percentiles is larger than the difference between the 45th and 50th percentiles. Therefore, as with developmental scores, you cannot add or subtract them.

   b. **Standard score** is the name for a derived score that has been standardized or transformed so that the mean and standard deviation have predetermined (i.e., standard) values. Standard scores are based on equal interval units so that they can be combined mathematically. Several different standard score distributions are commonly used. The most basic is the **z-score,** which tells us how many standard deviation units a person's score falls from the mean for the particular population. Z-distributions have a mean of 0 and a standard deviation of 1. In Figure 3.1, you can see that a z-score of −1 means that an individual's score fell 1 standard deviation below the mean, whereas a z-score of +2 means that an individual's score was 2 standard deviations above the mean. **T-scores** are much like z-scores, except that the mean is 50 and the standard deviation is 10. So the z-score of −1 above would convert to a T-score of 40, meaning that the individual scored 1 standard deviation below the mean. Many tests use **scaled scores** (sometimes called *deviation IQ scores* because they were first used as standard scores for IQ tests) with a mean of 100 and a standard deviation of 15. This means that scores between 85 and 115 are considered to be in the average range, that is, within 1 standard deviation of the mean. Returning to Darrell's PPVT results, you can see that his standard score of 83 places him slightly more than 1 standard deviation below the mean. Tests with subtests frequently use scaled scores with a mean of 10 and a standard deviation of 3 for subtests. The advantage of T-scores and scaled scores is that you do not have to deal with negative numbers or decimals. Although standard scores may be more difficult to understand and explain to people without some statistical knowledge, they are the best method for deciding whether a client demonstrates a significant deviation from the norm.

Test Administration Procedures   Finally, standardized tests should have clear and sufficiently detailed descriptions of administration procedures so that the clinician can administer the test in the same manner as during test standardization. It is essential that the test be administered exactly as described in the administration manual. Any deviation from the standardized administration can affect the results and must be reported. In such cases, interpretation of the scores must be done with great caution.

Criterion-Referenced Procedures

Rather than measure an individual's performance in comparison to others, **criterion-referenced** procedures allow us to measure skills in terms of absolute levels of mastery. These measures do not tell us whether an individual differs significantly from the norm. However, they are extremely useful in helping to establish baseline functioning, developing intervention targets, and in documenting progress. Criterion-referenced procedures include commercially available instruments as well as clinician-constructed procedures. Examples of the former include **developmental scales,** which sample behaviors from specific developmental periods. These scales frequently rely on observational or interview techniques to gather data. Although many of these instruments do yield equivalency score information (usually age scores), they do not meet the strict psychometric criteria for norm-referenced tests. Many commercially available criterion-referenced instruments are standardized in the sense that they have standard procedures for administration and scoring but as mentioned previously do not provide scores of relative standing. Examples of criterion-referenced procedures frequently used in communication assessments are provided in Table 3.4.

A great advantage of other criterion-referenced procedures is that administration procedures can be modified to suit the needs of the individual client. Tasks can sample **decontextualized** behaviors (i.e., without the support of the context, as in norm-referenced tests) as well as communication behaviors in naturalistic situations. Knowledge about a client's performance in both of these contexts is important in order to get a complete picture. Many sources are available to help clinicians with developing appropriate tasks. For example, Miller and Paul (1995) discussed the development of criterion-referenced procedures to assess language comprehension in young children. Figure 3.3 is an example of a task for assessing comprehension of prepositions. A variety of procedures are also available for the assessment of speech and language formulation and production. Analyzing samples of a client's speech, language, and communication is an excellent way of gathering information about the individual's current skills in real-life situations (see Chapter 5).

Criterion-referenced assessments are scored differently than norm-referenced tests. Remember that these procedures do not yield scores of relative standing but are compared with an absolute standard. Types of scores that you will use include pass/fail, +/−, percentage correct, performance rate, and simple rating scales. For example, the following information shows procedures and scoring for frequently used procedures in voice assessment.

Table 3.4. Examples of criterion-referenced tests used in speech, language, and communication assessments

Test	Area	Ages	Comments
Apraxia Battery for Adults, Second Edition (Dabul, 2000)	Apraxia	Adult	Yields criterion-referenced score and level of impairment profile. Has six subtests.
Assessment of Phonological Processes, Revised (Hodson, 1986)	Phonology	3-0 to 12-0 years	Yields criterion-referenced scores: total number of occurrences, percentage of occurrence. Screening version available.
Deep Test of Articulation (McDonald, 1964)	Articulation	4-0 to Adult	Yields percentage correct score. Used to get information about the phonetic context of misarticulated sounds.
Frenchay Dysarthria Assessment (Enderby, 1983)	Dysarthria	12-0 to Adult	Yields criterion-referenced severity rating and profile of strengths and weaknesses. Data on persons with dysarthrias as well as typical individuals are provided. Has 11 sections.
Minnesota Test for Differential Diagnosis of Aphasia (Schuell, 1973)	Aphasia	Adult	Yields percentage correct and clinical ratings in each area. Results can be used to assist in making a differential diagnosis of different types of aphasia.
Multilevel Informal Language Inventory (Goldsworthy, 1982)	Language: Syntax, semantics, and morphology	4-0 to 12-0 years	Yields a profile that can be used to select intervention targets.
Preschool Language Assessment Instrument (Blank, Rose, & Berlin, 1978)	Language: Comprehension and production of discourse	3-0 to 6-0 years	Yields scores on a three-point scale. Tests information at four levels of abstraction.
Rossetti Infant-Toddler Language Scale (Rossetti, 1990)	Language and related areas: Interaction-attachment, pragmatics, gesture, play, language comprehension, language expression	Birth to 3-0 years	Yields basal and ceiling levels for each developmental area and global development. A compilation of caregiver reporting, interview, and child observation.
Sequenced Inventory of Communication Development—Revised (SICD-R; Hedrick, Prather, & Tobin, 1984)	Language: Receptive and expressive vocabulary, syntax, semantics	0-4 to 4-0 years	Yields age-equivalent scores. Combines parent report and observations of child.
Voice Assessment Protocol for Children and Adults (VAP; Pindzola, 1987)	Voice	Children and adults	Yields ratings and descriptions of voice parameters.
Wiig Criterion Referenced Inventory of Language (Wiig, 1990)	Language: Semantics, pragmatics, syntax, morpholog	4-0 to 13-0	Yields raw score and percentage correct. Record forms are available for each area and allow for tracking progress over time.

Comprehension of Locatives: Search Task

◇

DEVELOPMENTAL LEVEL	30–48 months
LINGUISTIC LEVEL	Lexical
LINGUISTIC STIMULI	Prepositions *in, on, under, behind, in front of,* and *beside*
RESPONSE TYPE	Natural—behavioral compliance
MATERIALS	• Toy mailbox or egg carton for reference object • Six small boxes and six raisins, peanuts, or small candies • A piece of cardboard for use as a screen
PROCEDURE	1. Place the six small boxes in the six locative positions (indicated by the prepositions above) relative to the toy mailbox. 2. Introduce the toy mailbox and the screen to the child. 3. Give the child the following instructions: "Here is a raisin (or peanut or candy). I'm going to hide it and I'll tell you where to find it." 4. Put up the screen between the child and the test items. 5. Hide one raisin (or peanut or candy) under the small box *in* the mailbox. 6. Remove the screen. 7. Tell the child, "The candy is in the mailbox." 8. Record the child's response on a score sheet like the one on page 126. Normative data from Hodun (1975) appear there. 9. Put the screen up again and repeat the procedure using the next stimulus locative. The stimulus locatives must be presented in the following order: *in, on, under, behind, in front of, beside.* Because the first three locatives are the easiest, they are presented first to ensure some success. Alter the stimulus sentence as appropriate for each locative preposition.
PASSING RESPONSE	The child finds the prize (raisin, peanut, or candy) under the appropriate box. Response is repeated on several trials with different target objects.
RESPONSE STRATEGY	• "Probable location" (i.e., child searches for objects where they are usually found)
DEVELOPMENTAL NOTE	Although *in, on,* and *under* are understood by 50%–85% of children at 30 months of age, *in front of* and *beside* are not comprehended by most children until 42 months (Hodun, 1975). Hodun (1975) reports that this search task is easier for children than the placement task (see Procedure 3.5).

Figure 3.3.   Example of a criterion-referenced task. (From Miller, J.F., & Paul, R. [1995]. *The clinical assessment of language comprehension* [p. 47]. Baltimore: Paul H. Brookes Publishing Co.; reprinted by permission.)

CALCULATING THE S/Z RATIO

The s/z ratio is a frequently used task in voice assessment. The ratio shows whether there is a difference in the client's ability to sustain voiced and voiceless expiration. The task is used to help assess respiratory and phonatory efficiency.

Procedure

Ask the client to take a deep breath and say /s/ (or /z/) for as long as possible. You can present a model first. Have the client repeat each phoneme three times. Vary the order of /s/ and /z/. Time each performance with a stopwatch.

Scoring

Use the longest production for each phoneme to compute a ratio as follows:

$$\frac{\text{Longest /s/}}{\text{Longest /z/}} = \text{s/z ratio}$$

Interpretation

- A ratio of 1.0 with normal duration (approximately 10 seconds for children and 20–25 seconds for adults) indicates normal respiration ability and no vocal fold pathology.

- A ratio of 1.0 with shortened duration of /s/ and /z/ suggests possible inefficiency of respiration.

- A ratio of 1.2 or greater suggests possible vocal fold pathology.

Sources: Boone & McFarlene, 2000; Deem & Miller, 2000.

Clinician-constructed instruments are sometimes referred to as *informal assessments*. Witt, Elliott, Gresham, and Kramer (1988) pointed out that informal assessment is actually anything but informal. The "informal" refers to the content rather than the process of the assessment. These techniques, which represent a structured and systematic approach, allow us to examine specific communication behaviors or skills in detail and in a way that is individualized to the client's particular needs. Many clinicians call these *probes*.

Behavioral Observation

The testing methods that we have discussed so far were designed to compare an individual's performance against some standard, whether that standard is the performance of others with similar demographic characteristics or some predetermined criterion. Observational techniques, however, provide a means for describing behavior in a systematic fashion without reference to any predetermined standard. They are useful for measuring the presence or absence of a behavior; the frequency, rate, magnitude, or duration of its occurrence; and the situations in which it is likely to occur. Observations can be made in real time (as they occur) or can be videotaped or audiotaped for later analysis. There are qualitative and quantitative approaches to systematic observation; both have specific, albeit quite different, methodologies associated with them in order to gather meaningful information.

Qualitative systematic observation is primarily descriptive, although it should not be confused with anecdotal records. The latter often precedes quantitative assessment, with the observer watching the individual to get a general impression and recording a description of the behaviors and the contexts in which they occurred (Salvia & Ysseldyke, 1995). Qualitative methodology involves prolonged observation by highly trained observers with prescribed ways of interpreting results and ensuring reliability and validity (Marshall & Rossman, 1995). **Ethnography,** one type of qualitative methodology, is particularly effective for obtaining information about children and families from different cultural groups (e.g., Crago & Cole, 1991; Hammer, 1998). Another method, **conversation analysis,** has been found to be useful in describing the conversational competence of individuals with aphasia (e.g., Damico, Oelschlaeger, & Simmons-Mackie, 1999).

For the most part, in communication assessments, you will be using quantitative approaches to systematic observation. In order to be useful and meaningful, a few guidelines should be kept in mind. First, you must identify the purpose of the observation and be clear about the behaviors that you wish to observe. Define the behaviors and select the contexts in which you will observe. Next, it is important to have a recording system that is appropriate to the behavior you wish to measure. Your recording system can be as simple as a tally sheet with a checkmark every time the behavior of interest is observed. Other recording methods include rankings (e.g., frequently, seldom, never), ratings (e.g., scale of 1–5), and duration (e.g., how many seconds the behavior lasted). An example of a scale for rating speech intelligibility is provided in Table 3.5.

Sometimes it is important to assess affective behaviors, such as attitudes. In many cases, there may be a direct link between a communication disorder and a person's feelings and attitudes. For example, in the case of stuttering, feelings and attitudes are considered to be part of the disorder (Guitar, 1998). In other cases, they may have a direct impact on a person's ability to communicate, as in the effect of stress on a person's voice (e.g., Case, 1996). Thus, information about affective behaviors is helpful in understanding the level of handicap that individuals experience as a result of their disability. Checklists or surveys completed by the client or a family member can be good sources of information about these areas. A number of surveys are commonly used in communication assessments. An example that is frequently used in fluency assessments is shown in Figure 3.4. Overall, behavioral observations can be an invaluable source of information in establishing baselines, determining targets for intervention, and gauging progress.

Use of Instrumentation in Communication Assessment

Although instrumentation has always been essential in hearing assessment and certain types of speech assessment, such as voice, recent advances in technology have resulted in its increased availability and usefulness in the assessment process. Technological tools for assessment include instrumentation for actual

Table 3.5. Intelligibility rating scale for motor speech disorders

Rating	Dimension	Intelligibility
10	Environment[a] Content[b] Efficiency[c]	Normal in all environments without restrictions on content without need for repairs
9	Environment Content Efficiency	Sometimes[d] reduced under adverse conditions when content is unrestricted but adequate with repairs
8	Environment Content Efficiency	Sometimes reduced under ideal conditions when content is unrestricted but adequate with repairs
7	Environment Content Efficiency	Sometimes reduced under adverse conditions even when content is restricted but adequate with repairs
6	Environment Content Efficiency	Sometimes reduced under ideal conditions when content is unrestricted even when repairs are attempted
5	Environment Content Efficiency	Usually[e] reduced under adverse conditions when content is unrestricted even when repairs are attempted
4	Environment Content Efficiency	Usually reduced under ideal conditions even when content is restricted but adequate with repairs
3	Environment Content Efficiency	Usually reduced under adverse conditions even when content is restricted even when repairs are attempted
2	Environment Content Efficiency	Usually reduced under ideal conditions even when content is restricted even when repairs are attempted
1	Speech is not a viable means of communication in any environment, regardless of restrictions in content or attempts at repair	

From Duffy, J.R. (1995). *Motor speech disorders: Substrates, differential diagnosis, and management* (p. 90). St. Louis: Mosby; reprinted by permission.

[a]Environment may be "ideal" (e.g., face to face, without visual or auditory deficits in the listener, without competition from noise or visual distractions) or "adverse" (e.g., at a distance, with visual or auditory deficits or distractions).

[b]Content may be "unrestricted" (include all pragmatically appropriate content, new topics, lengthy narratives, etc.) or "restricted" (e.g., limited to brief responses to questions or statements by the listener that allow for some degree of prediction or response content).

[c]Efficiency may be "normal" (rarely in need of repetition or clarification because of poor motor speech production) or "repairs" may be necessary (repetition, restatement, responses to clarifying questions, modified production such as oral spelling, word-by-word confirmation of listener's repetition, spelling, etc.).

[d]Intelligibility is reduced in 25% or less of the individual's utterances.

[e]Intelligibilty is reduced in 50% or more of the individual's utterances, but not for all utterances.

Note: Not all possible combinations of deviant dimensions can be captured by a 10-point scale, and there is an obvious "gray area" between the meaning of *sometimes* and *usually*. The point on the scale that most closely approximates the clinician's judgment should be used. Many patients will fit into more than one point on the scale. It may be prudent to assign a range rather than a single point in such cases (e.g., 5–6).

Modified Erickson Scale of Communication Attitudes (S-24)

Name: _____ Date: _____ Score: _____

Directions: Mark the "true" column with a check (✓) for each statement that is true or mostly true for you and mark the "false" column with a check (✓) for each statement that is false or not usually true for you.

	True	False
1. I usually feel that I am making a favorable impression when I talk.	____	____
2. I find it easy to talk with almost anyone.	____	____
3. I find it very easy to look at my audience while speaking to a group.	____	____
4. A person who is my teacher or my boss is hard to talk to.	____	____
5. Even the idea of giving a talk in public makes me afraid.	____	____
6. Some words are harder than others for me to say.	____	____
7. I forget all about myself shortly after I begin a speech.	____	____
8. I am a good mixer.	____	____
9. People sometimes seem uncomfortable when I am talking to them.	____	____
10. I dislike introducing one person to another.	____	____
11. I often ask questions in group discussions.	____	____
12. I find it easy to keep control of my voice when speaking.	____	____
13. I do not mind speaking before a group.	____	____
14. I do not talk well enough to do the kind of work I'd really like to do.	____	____
15. My speaking voice is rather pleasant and easy to listen to.	____	____
16. I am sometimes embarrassed by the way I talk.	____	____
17. I face most speaking situations with complete confidence.	____	____
18. There are few people I can talk to easily.	____	____
19. I talk better than I write.	____	____
20. I often feel nervous while talking.	____	____
21. I find it hard to make small talk when I meet new people.	____	____
22. I feel pretty confident about my speaking ability.	____	____
23. I wish that I could say things as clearly as others do.	____	____
24. Even though I knew the right answer, I have often failed to give it because I was afraid to speak out.	____	____

Figure 3.4.   Example of a self-report checklist used in stuttering assessment. Score 1 point for each answer that matches the following: 1. False, 2. False, 3. False, 4. True, 5. True, 6. True, 7. False, 8. False, 9. True, 10. True, 11. False, 12. False, 13. False, 14. True, 15. False, 16. True, 17. False, 18. True, 19. False, 20. True, 21. True, 22. False, 23. True, 24. True. For stutterers the mean is 19.22 and the range is 9–24; for nonstutterers the mean is 9.14 and the range is 1–21. (From Andrews, G., & Cutler, J. [1974]. Stuttering therapy: The relation between changes in symptom level and attitudes. *Journal of Speech and Hearing Disorders, 39,* 318–319. ©American Speech-Language-Hearing Association; reprinted by permission.)

testing as well as computer software for scoring and analyzing data. Examples of the former include equipment used for behavioral and **electrophysiologic** measures of hearing such as the audiometer and **immittance** meter. It also includes instruments for speech assessment, such as the Computerized Speech Lab (Kay Elemetrics, Bridgewater Lane, Lincoln Park, NJ 07035; telephone: 800-289-5297) for acoustic analysis of speech. Examples of technology helpful in data scoring and analysis include software programs for scoring tests (e.g., Clinical Evaluation of Language Fundamentals-3 [CELF-3 Clinical Assistant; Semel, Wiig, & Secord, 1998]) and language sample analysis (e.g., Systematic Analysis of Language Transcripts [SALT; Miller & Chapman, 1983–2000]; see Chapter 11).

AREAS OF ASSESSMENT

In this section, we discuss the areas that you will be covering in an assessment. As illustrated in the beginning of the chapter, assessments may include the evaluation of many different communication disorders. Although the emphasis will be on the area of concern, other speech, language, communication, and related areas must also be considered during the assessment. This is necessary to get as complete a picture as possible of the individual's communication profile and to make a differential diagnosis when necessary. Many types of speech and language disorders have a high probability of occurring together. For example, articulation disorders are frequently seen in children with language disorders (Bernthal & Bankson, 1998), and children with fluency disorders have a higher than typical rate of associated articulation disorders (Yairi, Ambrose, Paden, & Throneburg, 1996). Motor speech disorders affect not only articulation but all speech systems, resulting in voice and resonance abnormalities (Kent, 1994). Other speech and language disorders have been shown to have high rates of **comorbidity** with other developmental problems. For example, individuals with Down syndrome are at high risk not only for language disorders but also motor speech problems and hearing loss (Miller, Leddy, & Leavitt, 1999). Specific areas to be assessed follow, and Tables 3.3 and 3.4 show examples of commonly used instruments for assessment of the various areas.

Language

Domains A useful paradigm for language assessment is to consider an individual's performance in the areas of **content, form,** and **use** (Bloom & Lahey, 1978; Lahey, 1988). Effective communicators demonstrate competence in all three areas, and there is interaction among the three areas. Language content, or **semantics,** includes the areas of vocabulary, concepts, and linkages of ideas. Form includes rules of **syntax, morphology, phonology,** and **prosody.** Language use, or **pragmatics,** includes interactional aspects such as being able to express a variety of communicative intentions (e.g., requests, protests, comments), using conversational rules (e.g., turn-taking, asking for clarification when necessary, initiating conversation, maintaining a topic), and taking the listener's perspective.

Modalities   Each of these domains consists of a receptive and an expressive component. Individuals must both comprehend and be able to produce the elements of content, form, and use in their native language. For older children and adults, language assessment should also include consideration of literacy skills. The following are some specific issues in each major modality of language.

1. *Comprehension.* Because we cannot directly observe comprehension and must rely on various behaviors from which we make inferences about an individual's comprehension, assessment in this area can be challenging, especially in young children and those people whose production skills are impaired. Much has been written in the literature about what constitutes proof of comprehension (e.g., Bates, Bretherton, & Snyder, 1988; Hirsh-Pasek & Golinkoff, 1996). We typically assess comprehension in terms of some motor production, such as pointing to a picture or object or acting out a command or sentence. Consider a young child who does not carry out a command that we give him during an assessment. Is it because he does not understand the words? Is it because he is not compliant? Is it because he does not have the necessary motor skills? It can be difficult to sort out! In such a situation, additional assessment methods such as parent report, dynamic assessment techniques, and observation may be helpful in formulating a hypothesis about the possible reasons for the child's performance.

   One important distinction to make in assessing comprehension is the difference between *contextualized* (in the presence of routines and nonlinguistic cues) and *decontextualized* (as in formal testing) tasks. Many authors, including Chapman (1978) and Paul (1990), have noted the differences in performance between the two. Gathering information about both, in other words, using both standardized and nonstandardized procedures, can be helpful in getting a more complete picture of the client's skills. Specific areas to be assessed include receptive vocabulary and concepts, knowledge of syntactic and morphological forms, and comprehension of discourse-level language and social aspects of language use.

2. *Formulation and production.* Although measuring expressive language may appear to be more straightforward than comprehension, it presents its own set of challenges. As Paul (1995) and others have pointed out, the nature of the task may influence the amount and complexity of language that is produced. For example, several studies have noted differences in performance between imitated and spontaneous productions in children (Prutting, Gallagher, & Mulac, 1975; Siegel, Winitz, & Conkey, 1963). Because language is a transactional process, the communication partners influence each others' productions. The types of questions and directions given by the examiner will have an impact on the client's response. Consider the following brief examples:

   Examiner: What color is your car?
   Client: Red.
   Examiner: Tell me about your car.
   Client: It's a red convertible.

It would be a mistake to conclude that the second example represents a more complex response. Both clients were fulfilling their obligations as communication partners by responding contingently. Open-ended questions and requests for information are preferable when trying to elicit multiword utterances.

Assessment of language production and formulation skills includes size and usage of vocabulary, semantic relations in word combinations, usage of grammatical and morphological structures, phonology, pragmatic skills, and prosody. Typical tasks to assess these areas include labeling pictures or objects, describing action in pictures, defining words, filling in the blanks, constructing sentences with a stimulus word, and imitating sentences. Although these types of tasks are useful in testing expressive language skills in a decontextualized manner, more information is needed to describe the person's expressive abilities in actual conversations. For this purpose, language sampling is the most valid and useful method of assessment (see Chapter 5).

Motor Speech

Speech intelligibility is an important factor in communication effectiveness. When intelligibility is affected, the relative contributions of linguistic (i.e., phonologic) and motor (i.e., articulation) skills to the problem must be considered. A variety of perceptual, acoustic, and physiologic instruments are available for assessing motor speech status (Duffy, 1995). Typical perceptual tasks involve naming pictures or objects and reading sentences (for clients who are literate). Again, analysis of spontaneous speech will provide the most valuable information regarding overall intelligibility (see Table 3.5 for an example of an intelligibility rating scale). Examining the oral mechanism and assessing the client' s performance in nonspeech tasks are both critical in the investigation of the structure and function of the articulators. Specialized tests are also available to help identify symptoms of *dysarthria* (weakness or incoordination of the speech musculature) or *apraxia* (motor speech impairment in the absence of weakness or incoordination of muscles). See Chapter 4 for an in-depth discussion of the speech-mechanism assessment.

Voice

Voice assessment also includes analysis of various perceptual, acoustic, and physiologic factors. The assessment should include evaluation of the individual's pitch, loudness, vocal quality, resonance, speaking rate, phonation, and respiration. These areas can be assessed noninstrumentally through perceptual measures, such as criterion-referenced tasks (see boxed information on page 62) and rating scales, and with a variety of instrumentation, such as the Computerized Speech Lab. **Videostroboscopy,** a way of viewing the anatomy and physiology of the larynx and surrounding structures, has become an invaluable tool in the diagnosis of voice disorders. The American Speech-Language-Hearing Association (ASHA; 1998) has affirmed the use of this technique to be within the scope of practice for SLPs, but specialized training is required. Teamwork between the SLP and the otolaryngologist is essential in the assessment process. Whereas the physician makes the medical diagnosis, the SLP makes the diagnosis of a voice disorder. The voice assessment may either precede or follow the medical evaluation, but under no circumstance can therapy be initiated before a complete laryngeal examination by the otolaryngologist is completed (Boone & McFarlene, 2000).

Fluency

Assessment of fluency disorders includes the careful observation and measurement of the client's speech behaviors as well as the assessment of various aspects of the client' s feelings and attitudes about communication and stuttering (Guitar, 1998; Zebrowski, 2000). Speech samples should be obtained in several different situations. This usually includes at least a reading and a conversational sample. Analysis of the samples will include calculating the percentage of syllables stuttered and speech rate, timing the duration of any blocks, and describing the relative percentages of different types of disfluencies (**repetitions, prolongations, blocks**). Physical concomitants such as eye blinks and head nods should be described and rated as to their severity. A variety of surveys and questionnaires are available to assess attitudes and feelings (see Figure 3.4). In the evaluation of a client referred for disfluencies, it is always important to make a differential diagnosis between normal disfluency and stuttering, particularly in young children (Guitar, 1998).

Hearing

The impact of hearing impairment on communication functioning is well documented. Audiologists are the professionals responsible for the evaluation of hearing and hearing impairment. The scope of practice of audiology includes the use of a variety of behavioral, electroacoustic, and electrophysiologic methods to assess hearing, balance, and neural system function (ASHA, 1996).

Early diagnosis of hearing loss is crucial to speech and language development. Testing the hearing of young children, however, can be quite challenging. Based on the child's age and developmental level, behavioral testing techniques would consist of behavioral observation, **visual reinforcement audiometry,** or **play audiometry** techniques. Electrophysiological testing procedures, which measure involuntary responses and therefore do not rely on the child's cooperation, are used to confirm or rule out a hearing loss and to estimate the type and degree of a hearing loss. These procedures include **auditory brain stem evoked response audiometry** and the measurement of **otoacoustic emissions (OAEs).** With older children and adults who are able to cooperate in the assessment, audiological evaluation usually consists of **pure tone audiometry, speech audiometry,** and immittance testing.

Because of the critical importance of hearing, all communication assessments should include at least a hearing screening. The scope of practice of speech-language pathology includes pure-tone hearing screening and screening **tympanometry** (ASHA, 1996). ASHA has developed guidelines for the screening of

Hearing Screening (Adults)

Name: _____ Date: _____

Date of birth: _____ Age: _____ Gender: ___ Male ___ Female

Screening unit/examiner: _____ Calibration date: _____

Case history (circle the appropriate answers)

Do you think you have a hearing loss?	Yes	No
Have hearing aid(s) ever been recommended for you?	Yes	No
Is your hearing better in one ear?	Yes	No
If yes, which is the better ear? Right Left		
Have you ever had a sudden or rapid progression of hearing loss?	Yes	No
If yes, which ear? Right Left		
Do you have ringing or noises in your ears?	Yes	No
If yes, which ear? Right Left Both		
Do you consider dizziness to be a problem for you?	Yes	No
Have you had recent drainage from your ear(s)?	Yes	No
If yes, which ear? Right Left		
Do you have pain or discomfort in your ear(s)?	Yes	No
If yes, which ear? Right Left		
Have you received medical consultation for any of the above conditions?	Yes	No

PASS   **REFER**

Visual/otoscopic inspection

PASS   **REFER**   Right   Left

_____ Referral for cerumen management   _____ Referral for medical evaluation

---

Pure-tone screen (25 decibel [dB] hearing level [HL]) (R = Response, NR = No Response)

Frequency	1000	2000	4000 Hz
Right Ear			
Left Ear			

PASS   **REFER**

Hearing-disability index

Score: HHIE-S _____ SAC _____ Other _____ Score _____

PASS   **REFER**

Discharge ____ Medical examination   ____ Counsel

____ Cerumen management   ____ Audiologic evaluation

Comments: _____

Patient signature: _____ Date: _____

Figure 3.5.   Protocol for adult hearing screening. (From American Speech-Language-Hearing Association Audiologic Assessment Panel 1996. [1997]. *Guidelines for audiologic screening* [pp. iv–74vv]. Rockville, MD: Author. © American Speech-Language-Hearing Association; reprinted by permission.)

individuals of all ages (ASHA, 1997). Different techniques and criteria are used for pediatric and adult populations. The following information summarizes criteria for the audiologic screening of children ages 5–18, and Figure 3.5 summarizes recommended screening practices for adults. Any client who is unable to participate or who fails the hearing screening must be referred for a full audiological evaluation.

PROCEDURES FOR SCREENING THE HEARING OF SCHOOL-AGE CHILDREN

Clinical indications

1. Screen school-age children on initial entry to school, annually in kindergarten through third grade, and in seventh and eleventh grades.

2. Screen school-age children as needed, requested, or mandated. In addition, children should be screened upon entrance to special education, in the case of grade repetition, new entry to the school system without evidence of having passed a previous hearing screening, or absence during a previously scheduled screening.

3. The following risk factors suggest the need for a hearing screening in other years:

   a. Parent/care provider, health care provider, teacher, or other school personnel have concerns regarding hearing, speech, language, or learning abilities

   b. Family history of late or delayed onset hereditary hearing loss

   c. Recurrent or persistent otitis media with effusion for at least 3 months

   d. Craniofacial anomalies, including those with morphological abnormalities of the pinna and ear canal

   e. Stigmata or other findings associated with a syndrome known to include sensorineural and/or conductive hearing loss

   f. Head trauma with loss of consciousness

   g. Reported exposure to potentially damaging noise levels or ototoxic drugs

4. School-age children who receive regular audiologic management need not participate in a screening program.

Clinical process

1. These guidelines recommend obtaining informed consent, or, in the case of children, informed parental/legal guardian permission; however, extant state statutes or regulations, or institutional policies, supersede this recommendation.

2. Conduct screening in a manner congruent with appropriate infection control and universal precautions.

3. Conditioned play audiometry (CPA) or conventional audiometry are the procedures of choice.

4. Conduct screening under earphones using 1000, 2000, and 4000 hertz (Hz) tones at 20 dB HL.

5. All hearing screening programs should include an educational component designed to provide parents with information, in lay language, on the process of hearing screening, the likelihood of their child having a hearing impairment, and follow-up procedures.

Pass/refer criteria

1. Pass if responses are judged to be clinically reliable at criterion dB level at each frequency in each ear.

2. If a child does not respond at criterion dB level at any frequency in either ear, reinstruct, reposition earphones, and rescreen within the same screening session in which the child fails.

3. Pass children who pass the rescreening.

4. Refer children who fail the rescreening or fail to condition to the screening task.[1]

Two other areas of assessment fall within the domain of the SLP: **augmentative and alternative communication** (AAC) assessment and swallowing (**dysphagia**) evaluation. To competently assess a client in these areas, additional specialized expertise and instrumentation are required.

Collateral Areas

In getting a complete picture of the client's communication status, it is frequently necessary to gather information about other areas of development or functioning that impact communication. In many settings, you will be working as part of a team, so team members from other professions will also be evaluating the client simultaneously or will be available for consultation to obtain the relevant data. Some or all of this information may be already available from records or, if you are not working in a team setting, it may be necessary to refer the client to another professional in order to get the required information. Collateral areas include the following:

---

[1]From American Speech-Language-Hearing Association Audiologic Assessment Panel 1996. (1997). *Guidelines for audiologic screening.* Rockville, MD: Author. ©American Speech-Language-Hearing Association; reprinted by permission.

1. *Cognitive status:* Because cognitive status can have an impact on aspects of language, it is helpful to have at least a general sense of the individual's nonverbal cognitive status. Ideally, you will have this information from psychological assessment, but in many instances, this information will not be available. SLPs are not qualified to do IQ testing; however, there are informal screening measures that can help establish whether the client is functioning at or near age level in the nonverbal cognitive area. For children, Paul (1995) suggested play assessments, Piagetian tasks, and drawing as screenings. For adults with suspected cognitive impairments, a combination of informal tasks and a general screening instrument, such as the Mini Mental State exam (Folstein, Folstein, & McHugh, 1975), may be used. In either case, if you have concerns about the client's performance, a referral for cognitive testing should be made.

2. *Literacy:* When testing adults and older children, reading and writing skills should always be considered as part of a comprehensive assessment. In test batteries designed for adults with neurogenic-based language disorders, such as the Western Aphasia Battery (Kertesz, 1982) and the Boston Diagnostic Aphasia Examination (Goodglass & Kaplan, 1983), reading comprehension and written expression subtests are essential components of the test. In testing older children and adults, a variety of tests, such as the Oral and Written Language Scales (Carrow-Woolfolk, 1996) and the Woodcock Language Proficiency Battery (Woodcock, 1991), are available to assess reading and writing skills.

3. *Social/emotional/behavioral:* Because communication is an interactive process, it is important to know something about our clients' social environment in order to understand their needs (Paul, 1995). Paul cautioned that communication patterns in families may be an adaptation to the needs of the individual with a disability rather than a cause of the communication problem. Information about the client's social functioning can be obtained through the interview process, review of records, self-report surveys, and observation of the client. Instruments, such as the Vineland Adaptive Behavior Scales (Sparrow, Balla, & Cicchetti, 1984), can be administered by a trained SLP and can yield important information about the client's status in this domain. Gathering information in this area will also help you in determining the degree of handicap experienced by the client. Referrals to or consultation with mental health professionals such as social workers, psychologists, or psychiatrists may be necessary.

4. *Motor functioning:* Information about the client's gross and fine motor skills may be very relevant to the communication assessment, particularly in making realistic recommendations. For clients with significant motor problems, knowing about the client's motor status is crucial as proper positioning and use of adaptive equipment are important in getting valid and reliable data during the assessment. Physical and occupational therapists may be part of your team, in which case, they may already be involved in the case or readily accessible to you for consultation. If not, a referral may be in order.

PLANNING FOR ASSESSMENT

In order to obtain the most relevant information in an efficient manner, assessments must be carefully planned. When preparing, it is helpful to organize yourself by asking the following questions:

1. What is the presenting problem or concern? What questions are being asked of the assessment? It is important to know, from the referrer's point of view, how the problem is viewed.

2. What do you already know? This includes obtaining and reviewing pertinent case information such as medical records, school records, previous evaluations, and past therapy reports.

3. What do you want to find out during the assessment? Identify the missing data that you need in order to answer the presenting questions. What communication and collateral areas do you need to assess?

4. How will you find out what you want to know? This includes not only the particular tests you will use but also the contexts in which you want to observe the client and how you will sequence the assessment activities to maximize your productivity and efficiency.

Answering these questions will provide you with a preliminary plan for the assessment session. Remember that you will need to remain flexible enough to make changes in your plan if necessary. Figure 3.6 shows what planning for Darrell's assessment might look like.

STEPS IN THE ASSESSMENT PROCESS

The flowchart in Figure 3.7 details the typical sequence and problem-solving process involved in communication assessment from the point of referral to the completion of the assessment report. We can summarize the main steps in the diagnostic sequence, keeping in mind that the activities are not always quite as linear as they look. Data gathering, or the preassessment phase as it is sometimes called, is your first major task. This will include getting appropriate releases of information and obtaining and reviewing relevant records as described previously. In addition to written case history information, you (or another team member) will interview the client and/or family members and possibly consult with other professionals involved in the case. Although many agencies have written case history questionnaires, it is helpful to have a face-to-face discussion with the client and family even if they have filled out a form. This will give you an opportunity to follow up on topics of interest. Interviewing techniques and areas to be covered in a diagnostic interview will be discussed further in Chapter 7. The next phase consists of the administration of the tests, other assessment procedures, and stimulability activities in the communication and collateral areas that you have identified in your assessment plan.

The final phase of the assessment involves the scoring and interpretation of the various pieces of data you have obtained. The information gathered about the

---

Assessment Planning Worksheet

Name: _Darrell Thompson_   Age: _4 years, 6 months_

Presenting problems or concerns, reasons for the assessment:

Speech is difficult to understand. Child seems frustrated when not understood. Speech seems immature.

What do we know?

- Developmental milestones within normal limits (by parent report)
- Attends preschool
- Youngest of three children; older brother had speech-language therapy
- History of asthma, hay fever, croup, and ear infections
- Failed audiological evaluation; being treated with antibiotics for ear infection

What do we need to find out?	How will we get the information?
Are speech and language (vocabulary, syntax, morphology, phonology) developmentally appropriate?	Norm-referenced language test (TOLD-P:3); articulation and phonological testing (Goldman-Fristoe/ Khan-Lewis)
What percentage of speech is intelligible? What are typical language production skills?	Spontaneous communication sampling
What is status of other speech and communication areas (pragmatics, oral motor, fluency, voice)?	Screening, observation
What are skills in collateral areas (play, readiness, social, motor)?	Observation, informal tasks, parent report
What is stimulability for speech sounds and more advanced language forms?	Informal tasks, imitation

Figure 3.6.   Assessment planning worksheet for Darrell.

client's performance during the assessment must now be included with other information gathered during the process. This information is considered in light of other potential issues including particular life circumstances, cultural and linguistic differences, and developmental history.

Once you have analyzed and synthesized the data, you will need to make a statement about the severity of the person's communication problems. Severity is usually described as mild, moderate, severe, or profound. Although these judgments are somewhat subjective, there are some guidelines to follow as shown in Table 3.6. You will also make a statement of **prognosis**. Prognosis is a prediction about the course and outcome of the communication problem. This is based on all of the information that you have accumulated during the assessment and consideration of the research literature on the specific problem with which you are dealing. Paul (1995) cautioned that, in the case of young children, making short-

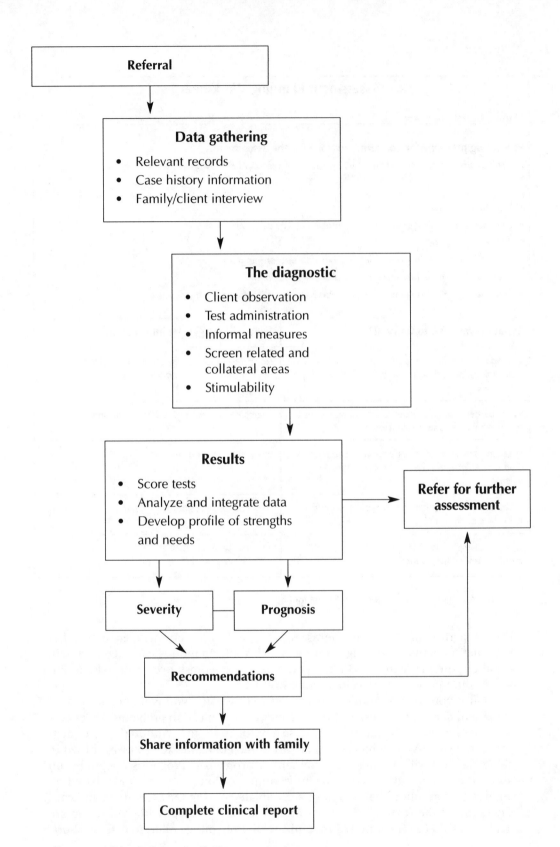

Figure 3.7. Steps in the communication assessment process.

Table 3.6.　Classifications of severity of mental retardation

Classification	Description
Mild	Some impact on academic and social performance but does not preclude participation in age-appropriate activities Able to function independently with minimal assistance
Moderate	Significant degree of impairment that requires accommodations to function in mainstream school setting Able to function in a supervised setting
Severe	Extensive support services required to function in typical setting May demonstrate some functional skills with supervision
Profound	Few functional skills Requires maximum assistance with basic activities

Sources: Accardo & Whitman, 1996, and American Association on Mental Retardation, 1992.

term prognoses and stating them positively is the best route. In the case of adults with neurogenic impairments, a variety of variables including general health, neurologic status, and severity of impairment must be considered in arriving at a prognosis (Brookshire, 1997). Stating your recommendations comes next. The recommendations must include a statement of whether therapy is indicated. If it is, it is important to include appropriate goals for intervention and specific techniques or strategies that you have observed to be successful with the client during the assessment process.

All of this information must now be shared with the client and family. The feedback should be provided in an empathic, family-friendly, culturally sensitive manner (see Chapter 7). Finally, all of this information has to be put into a clinical report. Diagnostic reports follow a fairly standard format and are discussed in Chapter 7. When preparing your report, keep in mind the intended audience. Foremost, remember that your report will be read by parents and other professionals who may have little knowledge of the field. Therefore, your report must be professionally written, but without using jargon. If the report will be sent to a funding agency, such as an insurance company or school district, it is important to include the information that the agency will use to make decisions regarding funding. An outline for an assessment report can be found in Chapter 7, and a sample report is included in the appendix at the end of this chapter.

CHALLENGES IN ASSESSMENT

During your career, you will be asked to evaluate clients who, for various reasons, may be difficult to assess. Clients may be extremely passive and withdrawn or they may be overly active, impulsive, and noncompliant. Clients may present with severe physical disabilities, be medically fragile, or easily fatigued. Despite these challenges, no client should be considered untestable. It may be necessary, however, to make adaptations in the environment and in your interactions with the client in order to gather useful information. Paul (1995) pointed out that usually when a client is labeled "untestable," the clinician means that the client was not cooperative or responsive to standardized testing. As we discussed previously, many other types of instruments are available to the clinician. Strategies to elicit information in these less than optimal circumstances include the use of observational data and informal tasks rather than direct testing. Caregivers may be interviewed regarding typical communication behaviors for the client. Giving frequent breaks and providing small snacks may be necessary for the client who is weak or easily fatigued. For clients with behavioral compliance issues, reinforcement, including food, may be necessary to complete testing. Multiple sessions and multiple contexts are also helpful in getting representative behavior from such clients. The important thing to remember is that, even for the most difficult client, there are methods and strategies for gathering enough evidence to determine the existence of a problem, determine eligibility for services, and develop some initial goals for intervention.

CONCLUSION

Before ending the discussion on assessment, a final point must be made. No matter how skilled the examiner and how thorough the assessment protocol, it is important to remember that the assessment represents the client's performance in a limited number of situations during a limited time period, and under limited circumstances. The examiner can only observe what the client *does*, not necessarily what the client is capable of doing. The latter is inferred from the former. A skilled examiner who obtains a representative sample of the client's relevant behaviors and who uses reliable and valid accurately administered, scored, and interpreted assessment instruments will make the most accurate prognoses and appropriate recommendations.

You will discover that assessment and diagnosis are fascinating processes in their own right, but remember that they are only means to an end—the development of effective intervention plans to meet the individual needs of clients. Good assessment forms the beginning of effective intervention, and conversely, good intervention is characterized by regular assessment of its effectiveness. Communication assessment is an integral component of the chain of events resulting in effective management of communication disorders.

REFERENCES

Accardo, P.J., & Whitman, B.Y. (1996). *Dictionary of developmental disabilities terminology.* Baltimore: Paul H. Brookes Publishing Co.

American Association on Mental Retardation. (1997). *Mental retardation: Definition, classification, and systems of supports* (9th ed.). Washington, DC: Author.

American Speech-Language-Hearing Association. (1996, Spring). Scope of practice in audiology. *ASHA, 38* (Suppl. 16), 12–15.

American Speech-Language-Hearing Association. (1996, Spring). Scope of practice in speech-language pathology. *ASHA, 38* (Suppl. 16), 16–20.

American Speech-Language-Hearing Association. (1998). The role of otolaryngologist and speech-language pathologist in the performance and interpretation of strobovideolaryngoscopy. *ASHA, 40* (Suppl. 18), 32.

American Speech-Language-Hearing Association Audiologic Assessment Panel 1996. (1997). *Guidelines for audiologic screening.* Rockville, MD: Author.

Andrews, G., & Cutler, J. (1974). Stuttering therapy: The relation between changes in symptom level and attitudes. *Journal of Speech and Hearing Disorders, 39,* 318–319.

Bankson, N.W., & Bernthal, J.E. (1990). *Quick Screen of Phonology.* Chicago: Riverside.

Bates, E., Bretherton, I., & Snyder, L. (1988). *From first words to grammar: Individual differences and dissociable mechanisms.* Cambridge, NY: Cambridge University.

Bayles, K., & Tomoeda, C. (1991). *Arizona Battery for Communication Disorders of Dementia.* Tucson, AZ: Canyonlands.

Bernthal, J.E., & Bankson, N.W. (1998). *Articulation and phonological disorders* (4th ed.). Needham Heights, MA: Allyn & Bacon.

Blakeley, R. (1980). *Screening Test for Developmental Apraxia of Speech.* Austin, TX: PRO-ED.

Blank, M., Rose, S., & Berlin, L. (1978). *Preschool Language Assessment Instrument.* New York: Grune & Stratton.

Bloom, L., & Lahey, M. (1978). *Language development and language disorders.* New York: John Wiley & Sons.

Boone, D. (1993). *The Boone voice program for children.* Austin, TX: PRO-ED.

Boone, D.R., & McFarlene, S.C. (2000). *The voice and voice treatment.* Needham Heights, MA: Allyn & Bacon.

Brookshire, R.H. (1997). *Introduction to neurogenic communication disorders* (5th ed.). St. Louis: Mosby.

Carrow-Woolfolk, E. (1996). *Oral and Written Language Scales.* Circle Pines, MN: American Guidance Service.

Carrow-Woolfolk, E. (1999). *Test of Auditory Comprehension of Language* (3rd ed.). Austin, TX: PRO-ED.

Case, J.L. (1996). *Clinical management of voice disorders.* Austin, TX: PRO-ED.

Chapman, R.S. (1978). Comprehension strategies in children. In J.F. Kavanagh & W. Strange (Eds.), *Speech and language in the laboratory, school, and clinic* (pp. 308–327). Cambridge, MA: The MIT Press.

Coplan, J. (1993). *Early Language Milestones Scale* (2nd ed.). Austin, TX: PRO-ED.

Crago, M.B., & Cole, E. (1991). Using ethnography to bring children's communicative and cultural worlds into focus. In T.M. Gallagher (Ed.), *Pragmatics of language: Clinical practice issues* (pp. 99–131). San Diego: Singular Publishing Group.

Dabul, B. (2000). *Apraxia Battery for Adults* (2nd ed.). Austin, TX: PRO-ED.

Damico, J.S., Oelschlaeger, M., & Simmons-Mackie, N. (1999). Qualitative methods in aphasia research: Conversation analysis. *Aphasiology, 13,* 667–679.

Darley, F.L., & Spriestersbach, D.C. (1978). *Diagnostic methods in speech pathology* (2nd ed.). New York: Harper & Row.

Deem, J.F., & Miller, L. (2000). *Manual of voice therapy* (2nd ed.). Austin, TX: PRO-ED.

Duffy, J.R. (1995). *Motor speech disorders: Substrates, differential diagnosis, and management.* St. Louis: Mosby.

Dunn, L.M., & Dunn, L.M. (1997). *Peabody Picture Vocabulary Test-III.* Circle Pines, MN: American Guidance Service.

Emerick, L.L., & Hatten, J.T. (1974). *Diagnosis and evaluation in speech pathology.* Upper Saddle River, NJ: Prentice Hall.

Enderby, P.M. (1983). *Frenchay Dysarthria Assessment.* Austin, TX: PRO-ED.

Fenson, L., Dale, P., Reznick, J., Thal, D., Bates, E., Hartung, J., Pethick, S., & Reilly, J. (1993). *MacArthur Communicative Development Inventories.* San Diego: Singular Publishing Group.

Fluharty, N. (1978). *Fluharty Preschool Speech and Language Screening Test.* Chicago: Riverside.

Folstein, M.F., Folstein, S.E., & McHugh, P.R. (1975). "Mini Mental State": A practical method of grading the cognitive state of patients for the clinician. *Journal of Psychiatric Research, 12,* 189–198.

Gardner, M. (2000). *Expressive One Word Picture Vocabulary Test.* Novato, CA: Academic Therapy Publications.

Gauthier, S., & Madison, C. (1998). *Kindergarten Language Screening Scale* (2nd ed.). Austin, TX: PRO-ED.

Goldman, R., & Fristoe, M. (2000). *Goldman-Fristoe Test of Articulation*(2nd ed.). Circle Pines, MN: American Guidance Service.

Goldsworthy, C. (1982). *Multilevel Informal Language Inventory.* Columbus, OH: Merrill.

Goodglass, H., & Kaplan, E. (1983). *Boston Diagnostic Aphasia Examination.* Philadelphia: Lea & Febiger.

Guitar, B. (1998). *Stuttering: An integrated approach to its nature and treatment* (2nd ed.). Baltimore: Lippincott Williams & Wilkins.

Hammer, C.S. (1998). Toward a "thick description" of families: Using ethnography to overcome the obstacles to providing family-centered early intervention services. *American Journal of Speech-Language Pathology, 7,* 5–22.

Hammill, D., Brown, V., Larsen, S., & Wiederholt, J. (1994). *Test of Adolescent and Adult Language* (3rd ed.). Austin, TX: PRO-ED.

Hammill, D., & Newcomer, P. (1997). *Test of Language Development—Intermediate.* Austin, TX: PRO-ED.

Hedrick, D.L., Prather, E.M., & Tobin, A.R. (1984). *Sequenced Inventory of Communication Development—Revised.* Seattle: University of Washington.

Helm-Estabrooks, N., & Hotz, G. (1991). *Brief Test of Head Injury.* Chicago: Riverside.

Hirsh-Pasek, K., & Golinkoff, R.M. (1996). The intermodal preferential looking paradigm: A window onto emerging language comprehension. In D. McDaniel, C. McKee, & H.S. Cairns (Eds.), *Methods for assessing children's syntax* (pp. 105–124). Cambridge: The MIT Press.

Hiskey, M.S. (1966). *Hiskey-Nebraska Test of Learning Aptitude.* Lincoln, NE: Union College Press.

Hodson, B. (1986). *Assessment of Phonological Processes—Revised.* Austin, TX: PRO-ED.

Holland, A., Frattali, C., & Fromm, D. (1999). *Communication Abilities in Daily Living* (2nd ed.). Austin, TX: PRO-ED.

Individuals with Disabilities Education Act (IDEA) of 1990, PL 101-476, 20 U.S.C. §§ 1400 *et seq.*

Kent, R.D. (1994). The clinical science of motor speech disorders. In J.A. Till, K.M. Yorkston, & D.R. Beukelman (Eds.), *Motor speech disorders: Advances in assessment and treatment* (pp. 3–18). Baltimore: Paul H. Brookes Publishing Co.

Kertesz, A. (1982). *Western Aphasia Battery.* San Antonio, TX: Psychological Corporation..

Khan, L., & Lewis, N. (1986). *Khan-Lewis Phonological Analysis.* Circle Pines, MN: American Guidance Service.

Lahey, M. (1988). *Language disorders and language development.* New York: Macmillan.

Lidz, C.S. (Ed.). (1987). *Dynamic assessment: An interactional approach to evaluating learning potential.* New York: The Guilford Press.

Marshall, C., & Rossman, G.B. (1995). *Designing qualitative research* (2nd ed.). Thousand Oaks, CA: Sage Publications.

McCauley, R.J., & Swisher, L. (1984). Psychometric review of language and articulation tests for preschool children. *Journal of Speech and Hearing Disorders, 49,* 34–42.

McDonald, E. (1964). *Deep Test of Articulation.* Tucson, AZ: Communication Skill Builders.

Miller, J. (1978). Assessing children's language behavior: A developmental process approach. In R.L. Schiefelbusch (Ed.), *Bases of language intervention* (pp. 269–318). Baltimore: University Park Press.

Miller, J. (1983). Identifying children with language disorders and describing language performance. In J. Miller, D. Yoder, & R. Schiefelbusch (Eds.), *Contemporary issues in language intervention* (pp. 61–74). Baltimore: University Park Press.

Miller, J., & Chapman, R. (1983–2000). *Systematic Analysis of Language Transcripts (SALT), V6.1 [Computer software].* Madison: Language Analysis Laboratory, Waisman Center, University of Wisconsin.

Miller, J.F., Leddy, M., & Leavitt, L.A. (1999). *Improving the communication of people with Down syndrome.* Baltimore: Paul H. Brookes Publishing Co.

Miller, J.F., & Paul, R. (1995). *The clinical assessment of language comprehension.* Baltimore: Paul H. Brookes Publishing Co.

Newcomer, P., & Hammill, D. (1997). *Test of Language Development: Primary* (3rd ed.). Austin, TX: PRO-ED.

Paul, R. (1990). Comprehension strategies: Interactions between word knowledge and the development of sentence comprehension. *Topics in Language Disorders, 10*(3), 63–75.

Paul, R. (1995). *Language disorders from infancy through adolescence.* St. Louis: Mosby.

Peterson, H.A., & Marquardt, T.P. (1994). *Appraisal and diagnosis of speech and language disorders* (3rd ed.). Upper Saddle River, NJ: Prentice Hall.

Phelps-Terasaki, D., & Phelps-Gunn, T. (1992). *Test of Pragmatic Language*. Austin, TX: PRO-ED.

Pindzola, R. (1987). *Voice Assessment Protocol for Children and Adults*. Austin, TX: PRO-ED.

Prather, E.M., Beecher, S., Stafford, M.L., & Wallace, E. (1980). *Screening Test of Adolescent Language*. Seattle: University of Washington.

Prutting, C., Gallagher, T., & Mulac, A. (1975). The expressive portion of the N.S.S.T. compared to a spontaneous language sample. *Journal of Speech and Hearing Disorders, 40*, 40–49.

Reynell, J., & Gruber, C. (1990). *Reynell Developmental Language Scales—U.S. Edition*. Los Angeles: Western Psychological Services.

Riley, G. (1994). *Stuttering Severity Instrument for Children and Adults* (3rd ed.). Austin, TX: PRO-ED.

Rossetti, L. (1990). *Rossetti Infant-Toddler Language Scale*. East Moline, IL: LinguiSystems.

Salvia, J., & Ysseldyke, J.E. (1995). *Assessment in special and remedial education* (6th ed.). Boston: Houghton Mifflin.

Schuell, H. (1973). *Minnesota Test for Differential Diagnosis of Aphasia*. Minneapolis: University of Minnesota.

Semel, E., Wiig, E., & Secord, W. (1995). *Clinical Evaluation of Language Fundamentals—3*. San Antonio, TX: Psychological Corporation.

Semel, E., Wiig, E., & Secord, W. (1996). *Clinical Evaluation of Language Fundamentals—3 Screening Test*. San Antonio, TX: Psychological Corporation.

Semel, E., Wiig, E., & Secord, W. (1998). *CELF—3 Clinical Assistant [Computer software]*. San Antonio, TX: Psychological Corporation.

Siegel, G.M., Winitz, H., & Conkey, H. (1963). The influence of testing instruments on articulation responses of children. *Journal of Speech and Hearing Disorders, 28*, 67–76.

Sparrow, S.S., Balla, D.A., & Cicchetti, D.V. (1984). *Vineland Adaptive Behavior Scales*. Circle Pines, MN: American Guidance Service.

St. Louis, K., & Ruscello, D. (2000). *Oral Speech Mechanism Screening Exam* (3rd ed.). Austin, TX: PRO-ED.

Tomblin, J. B. (2000). Perspectives on diagnosis. In J.B. Tomblin & D.C. Spriestersbach (Eds.), *Diagnosis in speech-language pathology* (2nd ed.) (pp. 2–33). San Diego: Singular Publishing Group.

West, J., Sands, E., & Ross-Swain, D. (1998). *Bedside Evaluation Screening Test* (2nd ed.). Austin, TX: PRO-ED.

Wiig, E.H. (1990). *Wiig Criterion Referenced Inventory of Language*. San Antonio, TX: Psychological Corporation.

Williams, K. (1997). *Expressive Vocabulary Test*. Circle Pines, MN: American Guidance Service.

Witt, J.C., Elliott, S.N., Gresham, F.M., & Kramer, J.J. (1988). *Assessment of special children*. Glenview, IL: Scott Foresman.

Woodcock, R. (1991). *Woodcock Language Proficiency Battery—Revised*. Allen, TX: DLM Teaching Resources.

World Health Organization. (1980). *International classification of impairments, disabilities, and handicaps*. Geneva: Author.

Yairi, E., Ambrose, N., Paden, E.P., & Throneburg, R.N. (1996). Predictive factors of persistence and recovery: Pathways of childhood stuttering. *Journal of Communication Disorders, 29*, 51–77.

Zebrowski, P. (2000). Stuttering. In J.B. Tomblin & D.C. Spriestersbach (Eds.), *Diagnosis in speech-language pathology* (2nd ed.) (pp. 199–231). San Diego: Singular Publishing Group.

Zimmerman, I., Steiner, V., & Pond, R. (1992). *Preschool Language Scale—3*. San Antonio, TX: Psychological Corporation.

1. Describe three different models of assessment. How would you decide which model to use?

2. List six purposes of assessment. Give an example of each.

3. Discuss the relative advantages and disadvantages of using norm-referenced tests.

4. List and define five important characteristics of norm-referenced tests.

5. Discuss the relative advantages and disadvantages of using criterion-referenced tests.

6. Discuss the relative advantages and disadvantages of using behavioral observations in assessment.

7. Name and describe the major communication and collateral areas to be covered during a communication assessment.

8. What are some key questions to ask when preparing for an assessment?

9. Describe the main steps in the assessment process.

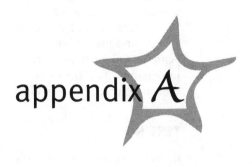

Sample Communication
Evaluation Report

COMMUNICATION EVALUATION

Name: Darrell Thompson

Parents: Margaret and Daniel Thompson

Date of birth: 4/3/97

Age: 4 years, 6 months

Dates of evaluation: 9/29/01, 10/6/01

Home language: English

BACKGROUND

Darrell was referred for a speech and language evaluation by his parents, Margaret and Daniel Thompson. They are concerned that Darrell's speech is very difficult to understand. Mrs. Thompson reports becoming concerned about Darrell's speech about a year ago when he started nursery school and she noted that the other children were more intelligible than Darrell. Darrell has not had any previous developmental or speech and language evaluations.

An audiological evaluation was recently completed on 9/12/01. Results revealed a mild bilateral conductive hearing loss and restricted eardrum mobility. It was noted that speech discrimination was very good in the right ear, but only fair in the left ear. Recommendations included medical consultation regarding middle ear pathology and a re-evaluation in 1 year. It was further recommended that Darrell's middle ear status be monitored. The Thompsons have followed these recommendations and Darrell has just completed a course of antibiotics for an ear infection.

Mrs. Thompson reported that her pregnancy and Darrell's birth history were normal. She does not recall specific ages at which developmental milestones were achieved. Darrell has a history of asthma and hay fever. He has had six episodes of croup and five ear infections since birth. Darrell has no known food allergies and is described by his mother as a good eater who enjoys a variety of food types and textures (e.g., raw vegetables, yogurt, granola bars, peanut butter). Mrs. Thompson described Darrell as a "very neat" eater who uses a fork and a knife.

Darrell lives with his parents and siblings (Jennifer, age 7, and Robert, age 13). Darrell spends much of his free time playing with his sister and a 5-year-old neighbor. Darrell's older brother had a history of speech difficulties and received therapy until third grade.

Darrell currently attends nursery school twice a week. Darrell seems to love school, and his teachers report that his speech has improved somewhat since last year. He enjoys playing with other children but gets easily frustrated if he is not understood. The Thompsons are most interested in helping Darrell to improve his speech before he enters kindergarten next year.

TESTING

Darrell was seen at the clinic for two 1-hour sessions. Mrs. Thompson was present during both sessions. Darrell was initially shy and needed some encouragement to participate in the assessment activities during the first session. During the second session, Darrell was cooperative and actively participated in all tasks.

Results

The following is a summary of tests administered and Darrell's performance.

Test	Standard Score	Percentile Rank
Peabody Picture Vocabulary Test-III (PPVT; Form A)	83[a]	13
Expressive One Word Picture Vocabulary Test (EOWPVT)	90[a]	25
Test of Language Development (TOLD-P:3) Composite	80[a]	9
Subtests		
Picture vocabulary	7[b]	16
Relational vocabulary	7[b]	16
Oral vocabulary	7[b]	16
Grammatic understanding	9[b]	37
Sentence imitation	5[b]	5
Grammatic completion	8[b]	25
Supplemental subtests		
Word discrimination	7[b]	16
Phonemic analysis	6[b]	9
Word articulation	5[b]	5

[a]These tests have a mean of 100 with a standard deviation of 15.
[b]These subtests have a mean of 10 with a standard deviation of 3.

Mean Length of Utterance (MLU): 3.50 (expected mean for age is 5.02; range is 3.96–6.08)

Goldman-Fristoe Test of Articulation: 36/73 (49%) correct; 3rd percentile for age

Khan-Lewis Phonological Analysis: Age equivalent score of 2 years, 11 months; demonstrated excessive speech simplification and use of phonological processes

Oral Speech Mechanism Screening: Structures adequate for speech production; difficulty with sequencing movements and speech sounds noted

Interpretation

Receptive Language and Comprehension   Darrell's single-word vocabulary recognition skills appear to be in the low average to below average range as demonstrated by his performance on the PPVT-III and picture vocabulary subtest of the TOLD. He scored in the average range on the grammatic understanding subtest of the TOLD. This subtest requires comprehension of syntactic differences at the sentence level (e.g., *he* versus *she* versus *they*).

Mrs. Thompson reported that Darrell's comprehension of language appears to be adequate and that he has a good memory for past events. During this evaluation, Darrell was able to follow two- and three-step directions during play and informal tasks, although he was unable to maintain the correct sequences. For example, given an array of up to 10 small objects, he was able to follow two- to three-step commands involving their manipulation, although out of sequence, about 70% of the time (e.g., put the *dog* on the *bed*, put the *baby* on the *chair*, put the *cup* on the *table*).

During informal testing and conversation, it was noted that Darrell had difficulty demonstrating comprehension of some basic concepts such as body parts (e.g., knee, elbow), shapes (e.g., square, triangle), and colors (e.g., yellow, orange). Mrs. Thompson reported that Darrell is usually able to identify colors correctly.

Expressive Language   Darrell scored in the average range on the EOWPVT, a test of expressive naming. Despite this, in his spontaneous speech and during other testing, Darrell demonstrated several instances of word-finding difficulties. He used some immature labels; for example, Darrell called a drum *boom-boom* and a train *choo-choo*. He also used associative words; for example, calling a Christmas tree *Santa Claus tree*. In another instance, he was unable to come up with the label for *scissors*. First he called it a *knife*, then *paper*. Finally, when given a sentence frame, "You cut paper with _____" he was able to come up with the correct word.

On the relational vocabulary and oral vocabulary subtests of the TOLD, which require the child to tell how two words are related and to define words respectively, Darrell scored in the low average range. He used many gestures to supplement his explanations (e.g., pretending to fly when trying to define *bird*).

Darrell's usage of grammatical forms appears to be somewhat below average to low average for his age, as shown in the results of the grammatic completion subtest of the TOLD and spontaneous language sampling. Darrell's MLU of 3.50 is somewhat below the range typically seen in children of his age (3.96–6.08). Darrell showed evidence of using different sentence types (e.g., statements, questions); however, his usage of grammatical markers such as pronouns and verb tenses was variable. He inconsistently omitted word endings that mark plurals, third person singular, and past tense. These errors may be related to phonological difficulties discussed later in the evaluation. He also substituted immature forms (e.g., "me see horsie in there"). Darrell's spontaneous speech was very difficult to understand; therefore, these results may be a minimal estimate of his actual level of grammatical knowledge. Darrell had significant difficulty imitating sentences.

Darrell used language for a variety of communicative intentions including requesting, protesting, commenting, and greeting. Several times, he attempted to clarify a message when the examiner said that she did not understand. He turned to his mother for help in getting the examiner to understand him. Darrell was able to maintain a simple conversation about his toys over several turns with the examiner. Mrs. Thompson reported that Darrell is talking much more recently. She commented on the fact that his utterances are more elaborate when he initiates the topic than when he is asked to respond to a direct question or request. This was also confirmed during the evaluation.

Speech Production and Phonological Skills   Darrell demonstrated below average word discrimination, phonemic analysis, and significantly below average word articulation skills (TOLD word discrimination, phonemic analysis, and word articulation subtests, Goldman-Fristoe). On the Goldman-Fristoe, Darrell correctly produced 49% of the test items. His errors were further analyzed using the Khan-Lewis Phonological Analysis system. Darrell demonstrated difficulties in the following areas: initial voicing (i.e., substituting voiced sounds for voiceless, as in *d*up for *c*up), syllable reduction (i.e., omitting unstressed syllables in multisyllabic words, as in *jamas* for *pajamas*), fronting (i.e., substituting sounds made more forward in the mouth, as in *bu*s for *bru*sh), stopping and stridency deletion (i.e., substituting stop sounds for most fricatives, as in *d*iken for *ch*icken), and cluster simplification (i.e., omitting portions of consonant clusters, as in *d*um for *dr*um).

Darrell's connected speech is very difficult to understand, particularly if the context is not clear. Approximately 50% of Darrell's utterances during this evaluation contained unintelligible elements.

Darrell's pitch, loudness, voice quality, and fluency were judged to be within normal limits for his age and gender.

An oral-mechanism examination revealed oral structures to be adequate for speech production. Darrell was able to demonstrate tongue protrusion, tip elevation outside of the mouth, and lateral movements. He had difficulty puffing out his cheeks and biting his lower lip on command. He also had difficulty sequencing oral motor movements (e.g., stick out tongue, blow, then wag tongue from side to side). Darrell had difficulty performing rapid speech movements and sequencing syllables (e.g., say *pa* as fast as you can).

SUMMARY AND IMPRESSIONS

Darrell demonstrates a range of speech, language, and communication skills from significantly below average to within the average range for his age. Areas of relative strength include single-word vocabulary recognition, adequate comprehension of grammatical structures, and many appropriate pragmatic skills, including conversational skills when he initiates and controls the topic. Areas of weakness include poor intelligibility of speech, difficulties with oral motor sequencing, usage of immature grammatical forms, and possible word retrieval problems. At this time, Darrell exhibits a mild-moderate expressive language disorder and a moderate phonological disorder. With intensive intervention to address his speech and language problems, Darrell's high level of motivation to communicate and the strong involvement and support of his family are seen as positive indicators for growth.

RECOMMENDATIONS

1. Darrell would benefit from intensive speech and language intervention. Therapy on an individual or small group basis is recommended to address difficulties in speech production and expressive usage of grammar. A phonological process approach to therapy appears warranted for Darrell. Specific activities designed to improve oral motor skills may be helpful as well. Specific long-term goals for therapy might include the following:

   - To increase intelligibility of speech

   - To increase age-appropriate usage of grammatical forms

2. Periodic monitoring of Darrell's middle ear status as well as audiological re-evaluation in 6 months is warranted given the air–bone gap seen in his audiogram.

3. A developmental/educational evaluation is recommended to assess Darrell's skills in other areas, such as readiness concepts.

4. Darrell would benefit from a preschool group involvement on a more regular and frequent schedule (four to five times per week). This group should contain some peers who could be age-appropriate speech and language models.

_____   _____
Clinician's signature   Date

Speech-Mechanism Assessment

G. Robert Buckendorf
Candace J. Gordon

When issues of speech production, intelligibility, or dysphagia are present, it is important to assess the speech mechanism in all of your clients, from children through adults. This assessment provides both valuable diagnostic information about the role of structural and functional differences in speech production and swallowing. It also offers a baseline measure by which you can evaluate progress. It is important to assess the *structure* of the mouth, which includes lips, tongue, palate, teeth, throat, and jaw, as well as the symmetry and shape of the client's face. *Function* is assessed through range of motion, strength, rate of movement, and accuracy of hitting the speech target. It is important to remember that other factors, besides structure and movement of the oral mechanism, also have a bearing on intelligibility and the viability of speech as a mode of communication. For example, breath support, posture, and general physical condition also impact speech production. Physical structure at times has a direct bearing on speech abilities, such as when a child has a cleft lip and palate or when neuromotor difficulties, such as cerebral palsy, are present. At other times, the cause of the disorder is linguistically based and relates to a specific phonological impairment (e.g., final consonant deletion). In these cases, the speech disorders are not likely to be related to structure or function (Ingram, 1997). Still, you need to be sure that there are no significant structural or functional limitations to speech production or swallowing. For this reason, oral-mechanism assessment is an important part of the evaluation.

Norm-based assessments of performance, including rate of tongue and lip movement, can provide initial assessment information as well as data about treatment effectiveness (Fletcher, 1972). It is important to remember, however, that the normal range of function and structure is very broad and that, despite a good deal of variety, most people produce speech that is easily understood. Students and clinicians often assume that just because a client is missing some teeth or seems to be unable to move his or her tongue as quickly as the norms indicate, any speech problem present is associated with structural or functional impairments. You will see many clients who have marked structural deviations but are perfectly understandable. You will also see clients whose structure and function appear intact but whose speech is very difficult to understand.

In the adolescent and adult population, measures of speech function also allow the clinician to obtain information regarding cranial nerve function. The information from this examination could also lead to referrals to other professionals such as **neurologists, otolaryngologists,** or dentists. Jack, a 68-year-old man who was referred for an evaluation by his general practitioner, complained that his "speech was not as strong as it used to be." During the speech evaluation, Jack's speech was 100% intelligible and the sound level meter readings suggested that his volume was within normal limits. It was during the speech-mechanism examination that tongue tremors were noted. This information was communicated to Jack's physician and a referral to a neurologist was recommended. The neurologist who saw Jack diagnosed *Parkinson's disease* and was able to prescribe medication that was helpful to his condition.

Tiffany, a 4-year-old girl, came to the clinic with a parental complaint that her speech was very difficult to understand. During the oral-mechanism examination, Tiffany's oral structure appeared to be within normal limits but she was extremely hypernasal with no soft-palate movement noted during the functional examination. She also had a significant medical history, including heart surgery at 3 weeks of age. After the examination, she was referred to an otolaryngologist for further evaluation. It was eventually determined that she fit the diagnostic profile of velocardiofacial syndrome (Shprintzen, 2000), and she was referred for a pharyngeal flap to manage her **velopharyngeal** incompetence. Following surgery, Tiffany still needed extensive articulation treatment to learn new speech behaviors to complement her new structures.

BEFORE YOUR FIRST SPEECH-MECHANISM EXAMINATION

Before you see your first client for a speech-mechanism examination, take the time to observe at least 10 typical people during speech production to help you focus on normal tone and structure of the speech mechanism. Complete the speech-mechanism examination on yourself while looking into a mirror to be able to easily identify the structures and use one of the standard forms available for recording the assessment (see Figure 4.1). Next, complete the examination on at least three people before you try the speech-mechanism examination on a client. The more experience that you have assessing normal structure and function, the better you are able to identify problems when they exist.

Preparation for the Speech-Mechansism Examination

It is important to follow **universal precautions** when performing a speech-mechanism examination. This means that it is necessary to protect yourself and the client from contact with any bodily fluids. You will want to have rubber gloves, a pen flashlight, a tongue depressor, a stopwatch, and facial tissue. In addi-

Oral Mechanism Evaluation Form

Name: _____ Date: _____

1. Lips

a. Structure

Touch when teeth are in occlusion: yes _____ no _____

Upper lip length: normal _____ short _____ long _____
(describe)

Evidence of cleft lip or other structural impairment: yes _____ no _____

b. Function

Can retract unilaterally

Left: yes _____ no _____

Right: yes _____ no _____

Equal retraction bilaterally: yes _____ no _____

Number of times can produce /pʌ/ in 5 seconds:

trial 1 _____ trial 2 _____ trial 3 _____

Does stabilizing the jaw facilitate the activity? yes _____ no _____

c. Adequacy for speech: 1 ____ 2 ____ 3 ____ 4 ____

2. Teeth

a. Structure

Occlusion: normal _____ neutroclusion _____

distoclusion _____ mesioclusion _____

Anteroposterior relationship of incisors: normal _____

Mixed (some in labioversion, some in liguaversion) but all upper and lower teeth contact; all upper incisors lingual to lower incisors but in contact ____ not in contact ____

Vertical relationship of incisors: normal ____ openbite ____ closebite ____

Continuity of cutting edge of incisors: normal ____ rotated ____ jumbled ____

missing teeth ____ supernumerary teeth ____

If lack of continuity, identify teeth involved and describe nature of deviation.

Figure 4.1. Oral mechanism evaluation form. (From *Diagnosis in Speech-Language Pathology, 2nd edition,* by Tomblin, Morris, and Spriestersbach ©2000. Reprinted with permission of Delmar, a division of Thomson Learning. Fax: 800-730-2215.)

Figure 4.1. *(continued)*

b. Dental appliance or prosthesis: yes _____ (describe)   no _____

c. Adequacy for speech: 1 _____   2 _____   3 _____   4 _____

3. Tongue

  a. Structure

  Size in relation to dental arches: too large _____   appropriate _____   too small _____

  symmetrical _____ asymmetrical _____

  b. Function

  Can curl tongue up and back: yes _____ no _____

  Number of times can touch anterior alveolar ridge with tongue tip without sound in 5 seconds:

   trial 1 _____   trial 2 _____   trial 3 _____

   above average _____   average _____   below average _____

  Number of time can touch the corners of mouth with tongue tip in 5 seconds:

   trial 1 _____   trial 2 _____   trial 3 _____

   above average _____   average _____   below average _____

  Number of times can produce /tʌ/ in 5 seconds:

   trial 1 _____   trial 2 _____   trial 3 _____

   above average _____   average _____   below average _____

  Number of times can produce /kʌ/ in 5 seconds:

   trial 1 _____   trial 2 _____   trial 3 _____

   above average _____   average _____   below average _____

  Restrictiveness of lingual frenum:

   not restrictive _____   somewhat restrictive _____ markedly restrictive _____

  c. Adequacy for speech: 1 _____   2 _____   3 _____   4 _____

4. Hard palate

  a. Structure

  Intactness: normal _____ cleft, repaired _____ cleft, unrepaired _____

Palatal fistula: yes _____ (describe)   no _____

Alveolar cleft: yes _____ (describe)   no _____

Palatal contour:

    normal configuration _____ flat contour _____ deep and narrow contour_____

b. Adequacy for speech: 1 _____   2 _____   3 _____   4 _____

5. Palatopharyngeal mechanism

  a. Structure

  Soft palate

  Intactness: normal _____ cleft, repaired _____ cleft, unrepaired _____

                symmetrical _____   asymmetrical _____

  Length: satisfactory _____   short _____   very short _____

  Uvula

    normal _____   bifid _____   deviated from midline to right _____

    to left _____   absent _____

  Oropharynx

    Depth: shallow _____   normal _____   deep _____

    Width: narrow _____   normal _____   wide _____

  b. Function

  Soft palate

    Movement during prolonged phonation of /ɑ/:

      none _____   some _____   marked _____

    Movement during short, repeated phonations of /ɑ/:

      none _____   some _____   marked _____

    Movement during gag reflex:

      none _____   some _____   marked _____

    If some movement, then amount:

      same for both halves _____ more for right half _____ more for left half _____

Figure 4.1. *(continued)*

Oropharynx

Mesial movement of lateral pharyngeal walls during phonation of /ɑ/:

none _____   some _____   marked _____

Mesial movement of lateral pharyngeal walls during gag reflex:

none _____   some _____   marked _____

Audible nasal emission while blowing out a match:

yes _____ (describe) no _____

Inconsistency in nasal emission during speech or blowing tasks:

yes _____ (describe) no _____

Patient stimulable to oral productions of pressure consonants:

yes _____ (describe) no _____

Nares construction during speech or blowing tasks:

yes _____ (describe) no _____

Oral manometer ratio (instrument _____)

trial 1: nostrils open_____   nostrils closed_____   ratio_____

trial 2: nostrils open_____   nostrils closed_____   ratio_____

trial 3: nostrils open_____   nostrils closed_____   ratio_____

c. Adequacy for speech: 1 _____   2 _____   3 _____   4 _____

6. Fauces

a. Structure

Tonsils: normal _____   enlarged _____   atrophied_____   absent _____

Pillars: normal _____   scarred _____   inflamed _____   absent _____

Area of faucial isthmus: above average_____   average_____   below average_____

b. Function

Posterior movement during phonation of /ɑ/: none_____   some_____   marked_____

Mesial movement during phonation of /ɑ/:   none_____   some_____   marked_____

Restriction of velar activity by pillars: none_____   some_____   marked_____

c. Adequacy for speech: 1 _____   2 _____   3 _____   4 _____

tion, a small dental mirror and gauze pads may be necessary. Before putting the gloves on, clean the table with disinfectant and wash your hands thoroughly with antibacterial soap. You will need to select an appropriate form to rate your client's performance on the speech-mechanism assessment (see Figure 4.1). Always explain to the client what you will be doing and why you are doing it during the evaluation.

INITIAL IMPRESSIONS

The speech-mechanism assessment should begin as soon as you see the client. Generally speaking, the assessment moves from broad to specific. First, observe whether there is anything unusual, for example, on the face or asymmetry of features. This is also when you will want to be aware of the client's breathing. It should be noted if the client has a mouth-open posture and adequate breath support for connected speech. Again, strong observational skills will allow you to notice asymmetry of oral movement during connected speech and control of saliva when speaking. Be aware of the client's overall voice quality because that could be suggestive of possible speech-mechanism problems such as nasality due to inadequate velopharyngeal closure. Engaging the client in a brief conversation or in play will also allow you to have an idea of overall speech patterns. Some of your most valuable diagnostic information can be noted in functional situations. These initial impressions will guide you in the diagnostic process, directing you to the areas that may require additional attention when completing the speech-mechanism assessment. Remember, too, that accurate results, in any testing situation, are best obtained when you and the client are actively engaged. So, try to maintain a light, conversational tone throughout, in order to help the client relax and give the most valid performance.

EXTERIOR FACE

Facial structure is a clue to the presence of certain syndromes. In fragile X syndrome in adult males, for example, the face tends to be long and narrow. Low set, rotated ears are characteristic of Noonan syndrome. Facial asymmetry is common in velocardiofacial syndrome. It is important, then, to examine the external face for any indication that some syndrome might be present. When there is indication of syndromic features, referral to a geneticist is appropriate.

The first step in the formal assessment is the evaluation of the facial symmetry. It is important to watch for any tremors, spasms, or tics, especially in the adult population. Is there any abnormal tension or lack of normal muscle tone in the oral musculature? Is there any drooping on either side of the face?

Next, observe if the client is able to maintain good lip approximation. Is there any scarring or evidence of a cleft? A mask-like appearance with minimal facial expression could be suggestive of Parkinson's disease. Observing overall facial expression, such as symmetrical smiles and frowns, suggests normal facial enervation, whereas slight drooping on one side of the lips or face could suggest nerve damage. Table 4.1 provides information about using some information from the examination of the external face to assess function of cranial nerves V, VII, X, and

Table 4.1. Summary of physical examination results and patient complaints for cranial nerves V, VII, X, and XII

Cranial Nerve	Function	Technique of examination	Patient complaints	Changes in structure
V—Trigeminal	Motor—masticatory muscles; Sensory—face and mucosal surfaces of the eyes, tongue, and parts of the nasopharyngeal space	Opening the mouth, clenching the teeth for palpation of the masseter and temporalis muscles	Motor—chewing difficulty, drooling, jaw difficult to close; Sensory—decreased sensation in face, cheek, tongue, teeth, or palate	Jaw may hang open
VII—Facial	Muscles of expression	Furrowing the brow, screwing up the eyes, sniffling, whistling, pursing the lips	Drooling, biting the cheek or lip when chewing or speaking, difficulty keeping food in the mouth	Affected side sags at rest; nasolabial fold is often flattened
X—Vagus (recurrent branch only)		Vocal characteristics; laryngoscopic examination		
XII—Hypoglossal	Innervation of tongue muscles	Tongue protrusion	Problem with oral articulation and chewing; difficulty handling saliva; tongue feels "thick"	Atrophy on the weak side
X—Vagus (above the pharyngeal branch)	Motor and sensory —innervation of the muscles of the soft palate, pharynx, and larynx	Gag reflex symmetry; vocal characteristics; laryngoscopic examination	Changes in voice and resonance; nasal regurgitation during swallowing	Soft palate hangs lower on the side of the lesion
X—Vagus (superior branch only)		Vocal characteristics; laryngoscopic examination	Voice changes	

From Yorkston, K., Beukelman, D., Strand, E., & Bell, K. (1999). *Management of motor-speech disorders in children and adults* (pp. 222–224). Austin, TX: PRO-ED; adapted by permission.

Changes in function		Changes in speech	
Unilateral	Bilateral	Unilateral	Bilateral
Jaw deviates to weak side, partly opened jaw may be pushed easily to the weak side by the examiner; decreased contraction on palpation on weak side	Individual may be unable to open or close jaw	None	Imprecise consonants, distorted vowels, slow rate
During lip retraction, face will retract toward the intact side; facial symmetry during movement	Decreased ability to retract, purse, or puff the cheeks	Mild distortion of bilabial and labiodental sounds	Distortion of bilabial and labiodental sounds, slow rate
Affected vocal fold fixed in paramedian position; dysphagia may be present; cough weak; may be airway compromise	Both folds in the paramedian position; airway compromise; inhalatory stridor	Reduced loudness; diplophonia	Reduced loudness
Tongue deviates to weak side; decreased lateral strength may be fasciculations	Atrophy and fasciculations on both sides; protrusion limited but symmetrical	Mild consonant imprecision	Mild to severe consonant imprecision; vowel distortion
Soft palate pulls to the paralyzed side on phonation; gag reflex diminished on weak side	Minimal palatal movement on phonation; nasal regurgitation	Breathiness; decreased loudness and pitch; short phrases; hoarseness; diplophonia; mild hypernasality; nasal emission; mildly weak plosing	Breathiness; aphonia; short phrases; inhalatory strider; moderate hypernasality; nasal emission; weak plosing
Affected vocal fold appears shorter than normal; epiglottis and anterior larynx shifted toward the intact side	Both cords appear short and are bowed; epiglottis will overhang and obscure the anterior portion	Breathy hoarseness; short phrases	Breathy, hoarse voice; decreased loudness and pitch range

XII. Look at spacing, shape, and symmetry of the eyes and ears. If there are any facial abnormalities, determine through medical history whether they are acquired (secondary to injury or disease) or congenital (cleft palate or related to a syndrome).

Perceptual skills, including tactile sensitivity, give you clues to symmetry, tactile acuity, and localization abilities of the individual. An inability to discriminate two points separated by an inch or more may provide clues as to the patient's diagnosis and areas that you may need to be aware of in treatment. Assess sensation on the upper and lower lips and cheeks by having your client close his or her eyes and see if he or she can identify a soft touch (Q-tip) and hard touch (tongue depressor). Assess two-point discrimination (with two tongue blades separated about an inch) and sensitivity to the temperature contrasts of hot (spoon warmed in hot water) and cold (spoon cooled in cold water).

LIPS

The lips are very important for nutrition, facial expression, and speech production. Lip approximation is an integral part of many speech sounds, and lip closure is a part of the swallowing process. If a person is unable to easily approximate his or her lips or the movement appears effortful, then there may be an impact on speech production.

The initial observation allows you to determine if the lips are symmetrical in a resting posture and during speech. Many times, observing a natural smile is a good way to assess lip retraction. Scars on the upper lip could suggest a repaired cleft lip or an accident. This is a good time to assess overall facial tone. To assess lip seal, ask clients to fill their cheeks with air and hold that air for 10–15 seconds. Did you notice any air leaking from the lips? Are your client's lips sealed at rest? Can the client lateralize, protrude, and retract lips bilaterally and sustain a rapid series of bilabial sounds? Can the client rapidly open and close the lips several times a second? Push against the protruded lips with a tongue blade or gloved finger. Is there good resistance? Ask the client to grimace or pucker rapidly several times in a second. Count how many repetitions the client can make in 10 seconds. Do you notice groping behaviors during these tasks or does the client repeat these lip movements easily and quickly?

Because lip protrusion (lip rounding) is especially important in the production of vowels, it is a good idea to count the number of times the client can pucker and then smile or open and close his or her mouth. Then ask the client to repeat "o-e" as many times as possible and count the number of complete repetitions of "o-e." During the production of bilabial sounds (m,p,b), you can observe whether the person uses both lips or makes compensatory movements to achieve closure. You can also observe speed of alternating movements and look for any drooping of the client's mouth. In the Dworkin-Culatta Oral Mechanism Examination and Treatment System (Dworkin & Culatta, 1996), the client is asked to perform many of these activities as well as repeat "puppy" as rapidly as possible for 5 seconds. Again, these observations help you determine whether there are functional impediments that occur in both speech and nonspeech situations or whether articulation errors are confined to speech contexts alone.

JAW

Jaw movement, including opening and closing, as well as freedom of movement and stability of the **temporo-mandibular joint (TMJ),** is important to speech production and chewing. If freedom of movement is impaired, rate of movement is slowed, or the client has habituated a clenched-jaw posture that may affect speech production and needs to be addressed during the evaluation.

The jaw opens and closes many times during speech, and limited movement secondary to injury or neurological disorder can have a significant effect on speech intelligibility. Does the client have adequate movement of the jaw or present with more of a clenched-jaw posture, like a ventriloquist? This is also a good time to listen for any TMJ noise, such as grinding or popping sounds during wide-mouth opening. Some clients may not be able to open their mouths fully because of TMJ problems and a referral to a dentist may be in order. Jaw lateralization is important for chewing and provides information about cranial nerve function, so you want to observe whether the client can move the jaw from side to side.

NOSE

Breathing irregularities can lead to decreased respiratory support for speech, so it is important to assess whether there are any obstructions in the nasal cavity that could affect breath intake. You can ask the client to move his or her head back and assess the nasal area for any abnormalities such as a **deviated** septum or obstruction of the nasal cavity. This is especially important if you have observed that the client is a mouth breather. Also note any **nasal air emission** during speech. That is best observed by either placing a small dental mirror under the client's nose and asking him or her to repeat words with no nasal phonemes, or placing a small strip of paper under his or her nose and observing movement of the paper during those same words. When a client uses words with no nasal phonemes, there should be no clouding of the mirror or movement of the paper.

Many clients are unable to breathe comfortably through their nose because of allergies or swollen adenoids. This should be noted both during the examination and in the case history, and clients should be referred for medical management of this issue. Nighttime snoring and chronically red upper gums are additional clues to this condition. If the client is unable to breathe comfortably through the nose, then the adoption of an unhealthy mouth-open breathing posture becomes more likely.

INTRAORAL EXAMINATION

Looking inside the client's mouth gives you a view of the structures and functions of the articulators. This is necessary in order to determine if there is any obstruction or inadequacy that might contribute to a speech problem. In preparation for the **intraoral** examination, you will need to glove and review the characteristics of tissue indicating structural abnormalities in Table 4.2. Also, you will want to be familiar with terminology such as *tremors, tics,* and *spasms* to describe any invol-

Table 4.2.   Characteristics of tissue indicating structural abnormalities

Characteristic	Example
Unusual color	Red (inflammation); blush tint (absence of underlying tissue, as with submucousal cleft; cyanosis)
Rough, fissured, or furrowed texture	Ulceration; atrophy of muscular structure
Unexpected discontinuities in surface or underlying structure (especially at sites of midline union of structures)	Pits or notches in lips, clefts, fistulas, bifid uvula
Absence of structure	Velar musculature inserts anteriorly into hard palate (i.e., no palatal aponeurosis, missing teeth)
Disproportionate size in relation to surrounding structures	Short velum in relation to depth of oropharynx; enlarged palatine tonsils occlude oropharynx
Asymmetry in shape or size of bilateral structures	Unilaterally reduced muscle bulk or wasting on tongue; depressed nasal ala
Misalignment of adjacent or functionally related structures	Mandibular retrusion; dental malocclusion
Unusual contour (elevations or depressions in tissue where not expected)	Peaked hard palate; torus on hard palate
Constrained range of muscular structures	Lingual or labial frenum attached over extended area of structure

From Hodge, M. (1988). Speech mechanism assessment. In D. Yoder & R. Kent (Eds.), *Decision making in speech-language pathology* (p. 106). St. Louis: Mosby; reprinted by permission.

untary movements that you may observe. When working with children, you may want to help them become accustomed to the procedure by letting them look in your mouth first, letting them hold the flashlight or tongue blade, or performing the assessment on a doll or stuffed animal. You can increase their willingness to open their mouths by telling them that you want to see what they had for lunch or see if there are any elephants (or dinosaurs or giraffes) in there. Maintaining a playful tone may help to relieve the natural anxiety that children often feel about this procedure.

It is important to note the color of the oral cavity because, according to Shipley (1992), a gray color might be a result of **paresis,** whereas a translucent color could be a result of a cleft. If dark spots are noted, then they should be highlighted in the evaluation write-up and brought to the attention of the referring physician.

When evaluating the size and shape of the oral cavity, it is important to remember that there is a great deal of normal variation. Still, anything that seems out of the ordinary should be noted. As we have said, it is important to get a good deal of practice in this assessment so that you become familiar with the normal range of variation in mouths and faces.

PALATE

The hard and soft palate provide the division between the oral and nasal cavities as well as resonating and directing the voice. The hard palate must be intact in order for oral sounds to be produced. The soft palate must be able to close off the nasal cavity quickly and repeatedly during running speech and when swallowing.

Assessment of those structures is a very important part of the oral-mechanism assessment.

With your flashlight, you will be able to assess the hard and soft palate. Does the hard palate have a normal arch and healthy looking tissue (uniformly pink, moist, and free from signs of disease) with no growths? Observe the palate for its height and arch. Are the **rugae** (the ridges on the alveolar ridge) smooth and rounded or sharp and angular? In some children, excessively prominent ridges may be associated with an abnormal swallow or indicate habitual mouth-breathing. With your gloved hand, you can ask the client to open his or her mouth, then palpate from front to back and side to side. Here you will be feeling to detect indentations or depressions that might signal a submucosal cleft of the palate (i.e., a cleft in the layer of tissue or bone beneath the surface epithelial tissue of the hard palate). Does the length of the soft palate appear adequate (i.e., long enough to easily reach the posterior pharyngeal wall)? Even though adequate soft palate length and elevation itself does not ensure velopharyngeal closure, a short palate is a risk factor for velopharyngeal insufficiency. By asking the client to say "ahhh," you will be able to observe soft palate elevation and assess the quality of the phonation. Do you note any weakness on one side of the soft palate or the other during phonation? Is there any nasal air emission during production of the low-back "ahhh" or the high-front "eee?" Certainly note if the client has a prosthesis, such as a palatal lift or **obturator.** Observe the tonsils (see Figure 4.2). If they are excessively large or almost make contact with each other, a medical referral may be indicated. Sometimes tonsils interfere with movement of the back of the client's tongue or cause problems breathing. Usually the tonsils decrease in size as a child matures.

Look at overall structural intactness. Note whether there are any openings (**fistulas**) through the palate into the nasal cavity. Those openings often occur as a result of cleft palate surgery. They are usually small enough that they do not

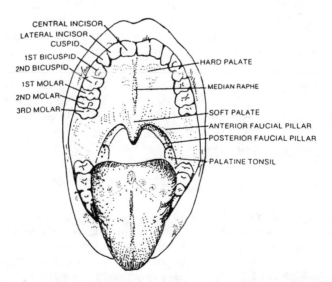

Figure 4.2.   Schematic of oral cavity and adjacent structures. (From Meitus, I., & Weinberg, B., *Diagnosis in speech-language pathology* [p. 43]. 1984. Reprinted by permission by Allyn & Bacon.)

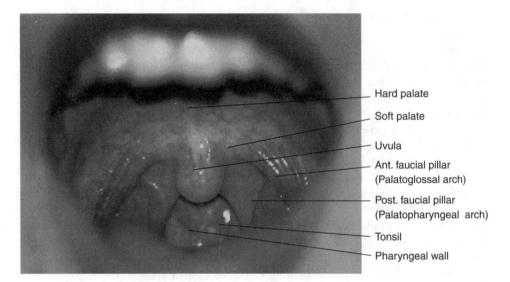

Figure 4.3.   Photograph of an oral cavity.

have any direct effect on speech production but may cause difficulties in some individuals. Look at the uvula and decide if its shape is uniform and is a single, unbroken structure or if it is split (**bifid**). It is possible to have a bifid uvula without any other problems but it might be suggestive of a submucosal cleft and/or of velopharyngeal insufficiency (i.e., the inability of the soft palate to adequately close off the nasal cavity during production of oral sounds). Figure 4.3 provides an illustration of a normal palatal structure for reference. A test used to assess **hyper-nasality** in the speech of children with possible **velopharyngeal insufficiency** is the Iowa Pressure Articulation Test (Morris, Spriestersbach, & Darley, 1961; see Figure 4.4). Children are asked to pronounce a set of words chosen for their sensitivity to problems with nasality. Children who produce nasal emissions or other nasal errors on this test require further evaluation for velopharyngeal problems.

Oral-mechanism assessment also involves evaluating the client's **gag reflex.** Absence of a gag reflex or presence of a hyper-sensitive reflex has an impact on types and consistency of foods tolerated and also provides the clinician with information about tongue position during a swallow. Evaluating the gag reflex is done by asking your client to open his or her mouth wide while you stimulate the soft and hard palate gently with a tongue blade until a gag occurs. This procedure may not be appropriate for all clients and needs to be done with care.

DENTITION

Although most people compensate quite easily for missing teeth, the overall condition of the client's dentition may affect his or her speech production. Some speech sounds require approximation between teeth and lip or tongue. If those teeth are missing, then distortions may occur. You will want to note the condition of the teeth as well as the gums. Assess dental alignment by asking your clients to bite their teeth together and smile. Note that a client's teeth can occlude

Iowa Pressure Articulation Test

Name: _____ Date of birth: _____ Age: _____

Date of test: _____ Score: _____

Number correct:_____ Percentage correct:_____

tongue	_____	sheep	_____	fork	_____
kiss	_____	dishes	_____	planting	_____
pocket	_____	fish	_____	clown	_____
duck	_____	jar	_____	glass	_____
girl	_____	bread	_____	block	_____
wagon	_____	tree	_____	wolf	_____
dog	_____	dress	_____	smoke	_____
telephone	_____	crayons	_____	snake	_____
knife	_____	grass	_____	spider	_____
soap	_____	paper	_____	possum	_____
bicycle	_____	cracker	_____	stairs	_____
mouse	_____	tiger	_____	sky	_____
scissors	_____	washer	_____	books	_____

Figure 4.4. Iowa Pressure Articulation Test. (From Morris, H., Spriestersbach, D., & Darley, F. [1961]. An articulation test for assessing competency of velopharyngeal closure. *Journal of Speech and Hearing Research, 4*, 48. © 1961 American Speech-Language-Hearing Association; reprinted by permission.)

or close in several ways: a normal occlusion (Class I), where the dental arches close normally but there are crooked or misaligned teeth; a Class II condition, where the lower dental arch is too far back; and Class III, where the jaw is too far forward in relation to the upper arch (see Figure 4.5). You should also note other dental abnormalities including **crossbites** and **openbites.**

TONGUE

The tongue is probably the single most important articulator and also is critical for moving solids and liquids around in the mouth during chewing and swallowing. Tongue mobility and speed of movement are both very important to these two functions and need to be addressed.

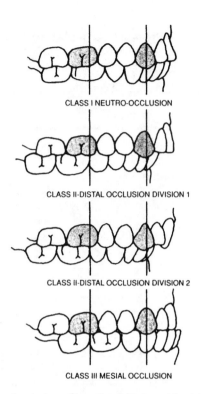

CLASS I NEUTRO-OCCLUSION

CLASS II-DISTAL OCCLUSION DIVISION 1

CLASS II-DISTAL OCCLUSION DIVISION 2

CLASS III MESIAL OCCLUSION

Figure 4.5.   Examples of types of occlusions. (From *Head, Neck, and Dental Anatomy, 2nd edition,* by M.J. Short and D.L. Goldstein © 1994. Reprinted with permission of Delmar, a division of Thomson Learning. Fax: 800-730-2215.)

The areas that you will want to assess will be the size, color, symmetry, and mobility of the tongue. Observe the tongue in a resting position on the floor of the mouth to assess the size. A healthy tongue is a velvety-pink muscular organ. According to Mayo Clinic Healthoasis (http://www.mayohealth.org), tongue disorders, such as red and white patches or what appears to be black hair, result from nutritional deficiencies, poor oral hygiene, or use of some medications. **Atrophy** of one side of the tongue can be seen in clients following damage to the XII cranial nerve. Also, bite marks on the tongue can be noted in stroke clients due to decreased sensation on the paralyzed side of the tongue. Again, it is important to look for any tremors, spasms, or tics. Ask the client to protrude the tongue and look for any deviation to one side or the other that could suggest tongue weakness. Some speech-mechanism assessments suggest that the clinician hold the tongue with gauze and lift the tongue to evaluate the floor of the mouth and the **frenulum** (i.e., the thin piece of tissue that connects the underside of the tongue with the floor of the mouth; see Figure 4.6).

This is usually the time to try a variety of nonspeech tasks to assess the client's tongue mobility. These tasks may include moving the tongue from left to right repetitively, elevating the tongue to the alveolar ridge, and licking the lips. For young clients, lollipops can be used for the tongue protrusion tasks. The client can be asked to move his or her tongue up, down, and laterally, following the lollipop. We have seen several children with a history of severe speech disorder who were unable to touch their hard palates or their frontal incisors with their tongue tips. That information, which we gathered during the oral-motor evaluation, helped us focus a small part of each session on some brief activities that gradually helped the children gain greater tongue mobility. It is a good idea to do these activities at the *end* of the evaluation, so that the child can be given the lollipop to keep.

A few years ago, Kristin, a young woman in her twenties, had most of her tongue removed due to cancer. Her oral-mechanism examination revealed that she had only a short, narrow piece of tongue remaining. If a clinical decision based on structure alone had been made, then the prognosis would probably have been that this client would not be able to communicate verbally. Fortunately, the oral-mechanism examination includes both structural and functional portions. An evaluation of speech behaviors showed that Kristin's speech was indeed distorted, but she was able to engage successfully in verbal communication despite her structural deficiency. This finding impresses, again, the resilience of the speech mechanism and the need for comprehensive structural and functional evaluations when treating clients with speech problems.

DIADOCHOKINESIS

One of the classic evaluations of the speech mechanism is the diadochokinetic rate. Slowed rates and imprecise movements are sometimes associated with dysarthria in adults following neurological insult. You have norms for this task to provide some measure of oral-motor sequencing and this, at least, provides a comparison to normal functioning. The client is timed during the repetition of 20 /pʌ/ productions. The same procedure is completed with /tʌ/ and /kʌ/. Finally, the client is asked to say /pʌtʌkʌ/ 10 times and the length of time required for

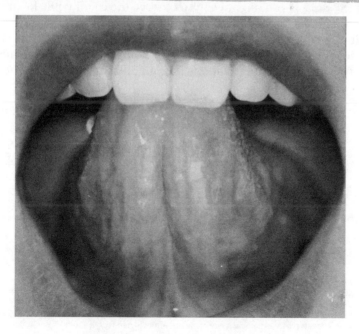

Figure 4.6.   Intraoral view of the lingual frenulum.

that production is noted. The norms for this task are listed in Table 4.3. If a client's productions are very slow, labored, or erratic, then some oral-motor strengthening tasks might be helpful. These norms may provide some measure of change over time to assess progress and to help isolate the nature of the problem.

RESPIRATION

Again, impressions derived from the initial interactive observation provide important information on respiration, as to whether, for example, the client's breathing is easy and smooth, or labored. In order to evaluate respiration further, you can ask your clients to take a breath in through their nose and slowly let the air out through their mouth. That task allows you to observe posture, tension, and evenness of exhalation. You should note whether the client appears to run out of air during speech or if speaking occurs on inhalation. Watch and listen for shallow breathing that requires the person to take a breath after only a few words. You should also listen for **stridor** (breath noise on inhalation) or hoarseness and look for neck or chest tension that may indicate poor breathing habits. Have clients place their hand on their abdomen and then place your hand on top of their hand. When they inhale, observe whether they push out against your hand. If their abdomen goes in instead, they may be inhaling by lifting their shoulders or chest instead of using their diaphragm properly. This may be compensating for some respiratory difficulty and needs further evaluation.

CHEWING AND SWALLOWING

Part of the oral-motor assessment will often include information gained as your client eats and drinks. You might want to observe the client while he or she is eating two or three textures of substances (i.e., pudding, cracker, gummy bears) as well as drinking thin and thick textures from a spoon and from a cup. Observing how the client eats with both a spoon and with finger foods can provide valuable information. During such observations, it is important to note lip and jaw pos-

Table 4.3.   Normative data on mean rate of response (MRR) in syllables/second for various syllable patterns

Age (years)	pʌ	tʌ	kʌ	fʌ	lʌ	pʌtə	pʌkə	tʌkə	pʌtəkə
6	4.2	4.1	3.6	3.6	3.8	2.0	1.9	1.9	1.0
7	4.7	4.1	3.8	3.7	3.8	2.0	1.9	1.9	1.0
8	4.8	4.6	4.2	4.1	4.4	2.4	2.1	2.1	1.2
9	5.0	4.9	4.4	4.4	4.4	2.5	2.3	2.3	1.3
10	5.4	5.3	4.6	4.8	4.8	2.7	2.3	2.3	1.4
11	5.6	5.6	5.0	5.0	5.3	3.1	2.6	2.6	1.5
12	5.9	5.7	5.1	5.4	5.4	3.2	2.6	2.7	1.6
14	6.1	6.1	5.4	5.6	5.7	3.6	2.9	2.9	1.8
Adults	6.0–7.0[a]	6.0–7.0[a]	5.5–6.5[a]	6.4[b]	6.5[b]	4.6[c]	—	—	2.5[c]

Data for children are Fletcher's (1972) and Kent, Kent, & Rosenbeck's (1987) time-by-count values converted to count-by-time values; MRR data for adults are shown for comparison. © 1987 American Speech-Language-Hearing Association; reprinted with permission. (Key: [a]Approximate range of means; [b]from Sigurd [1973]; [c]from Tiffany [1980]).

tures as well as the efficiency of the chew itself. Overflow behaviors, such as associated upper body tension or tremors, during chewing and swallowing should be observed, as should any excessive drooling.

CONCLUSION

As we discussed previously, the purpose of the oral-mechanism assessment is to provide both diagnostic information as well as ongoing information regarding treatment effectiveness. The coordinated movements of tongue, lips, palate, and jaw are critical for speech production and effective swallowing. In order for an accurate prognosis or to determine appropriate steps in treatment, you must be aware of normal structure and function and provide referrals to appropriate professionals when necessary. You also use the information from the oral-mechanism evaluation to direct you to the appropriate level at which to start treatment. For instance, children with a diagnosis of hypernasality secondary to velopharyngeal incompetence often have a trial period of intense speech treatment (1–2 months) to look at their ability to achieve oral air pressure. Re-assessment provides important feedback regarding need for continuing treatment or referral for surgery or a speech appliance. The oral-mechanism assessment is an important part of an initial assessment and your findings are critical to providing treatment direction and overall prognosis. It is important to summarize the results of the oral-mechanism examination and share that information with the client, family, and other professionals, both for treatment planning and to provide information to the professionals to whom you are referring the client.

REFERENCES

Dirckx, J. (Ed.). (1997). *Stedman's concise medical dictionary* (3rd ed.). Baltimore: Lippincott Williams & Wilkins.

Duffy, J. (1995). *Motor speech disorders: Substrates, differential diagnosis, and management.* St. Louis: Mosby.

Dworkin, J., & Culatta, P. (1996). *Dworkin-Culatta Oral Mechanism Examination.* Nicholasville, KY: Edgewood Press.

Fletcher, S. (1972). Time-by-count measurement of diadochokinetic syllable rate. *Journal of Speech and Hearing Research, 15,* 763–770.

Hall, P.K. (1994). The oral mechanism. In J.B. Tomblin, H.L. Morris, & D.C. Spriestersbach (Eds.), Diagnosis in speech-language pathology (pp. 95–97). San Diego: Singular Publishing Group.

Hodge, M. (1988). Speech mechanism assessment. In D. Yoder & R. Kent (Eds.), *Decision making in speech-language pathology* (p. 106). Toronto: Decker.

Ingram, D. (1997). The categorization of phonological impairment. In B. Hodson, & M. Edward (Eds.), *Perspectives in applied phonology* (pp. 19–41). Gaithersburg, MD: Aspen Publishers.

Kent, R., Kent, J., & Rosenbeck, J. (1987). Maximum performance tests of speech production. *Journal of Speech and Hearing Disorders, 52,* 367–387.

Morris, H., Spriestersbach, D., & Darley, F. (1961). An articulation test for assessing competency of velopharyngeal closure. *Journal of Speech and Hearing Research, 4,* 48.

Prather, E., Hedrick, D., & Kern, C. (1975). Articulation development in children aged two to four years. *Journal of Speech and Hearing Research, 40,* 179–191.

Sander, E. (1972). When are speech sounds learned? *Journal of Speech and Hearing Disorders, 37,* 55–63.

Shipley, K., & McAfee, J. (1992). *Assessment in speech-language pathology*. San Diego: Singular Publishing Group.

Shprintzen, R. (2000). *Syndrome identification for speech-language pathology*. San Diego: Singular Publishing Group.

Sigurd, B. (1973). Maximum rate and minimal duration of repeated syllables. *Language and Speech, 16*, 373–395.

Tiffany, W. (1980). The effects of syllable structure on diadochokinetic and reading rates. *Journal of Speech and Hearing Disorders, 23*, 894–908.

Yorkston, K., Buekelman, D., Stand, E., & Bell, K. (1999). *Management of motor speech disorders in children and adults* (2nd ed.). Austin, TX: PRO-ED.

Zemlin, W. (1998). *Speech and hearing science* (4th ed.). Needham Heights, MA: Allyn & Bacon.

STUDY QUESTIONS

1. Why do we do an oral-peripheral exam?

2. Why is it important to look at function as well as structure when assessing clients?

3. What are some other factors influencing speech intelligibility besides structure and function?

4. What are some important precautions to take before you actually perform the oral-peripheral examination?

5. What are some important parts of the structural and functional evaluation of the hard and soft palate?

6. Describe the overall contribution of the lips, tongue, jaw, and palate to speech production.

7. Why do we measure diadochokinetic rate?

Communication
Sampling Procedures

Rhea Paul
John A. Tetnowski
Ellen S. Reuler

One of the earliest means of studying children's language was the diary study. Parents who were deeply interested in language development—Charles Darwin was among them—kept detailed recordings of their children's early speech productions (Bar-Adon & Leopold, 1971). This method not only yielded a great deal of quantitative information about what children said at which point in development but also introduced the idea of carefully observing, recording, and analyzing natural behavior as a means to understand language use. These early studies were focused on a small number of children, on a small range of questions concerning single-word use and the beginning of two-word combinations, on a narrow age range, on production only, and on typical development only. None-the-less, the studies set the stage for the development of a broader use of language sampling procedures to address a range of issues in clinical work with people with communication disorders.

There is a simple reason why language sampling became an important part of the assessment of communication problems: It provides a key piece of information about a person's ability to communicate. As you saw in Chapter 3, one of the purposes of assessment is to identify baseline function and target goals for intervention. In order to achieve these purposes, communication sampling is essential. Although standardized tests can tell us whether a person is significantly different from his or her peers, the test cannot tell you how that person uses the communication skills that he or she has to interact in real-life situations. And it is this ability to interact in day-to-day encounters that we need to address in our interventions. So, to know what we need to work on, we need to see how the client really communicates—what difficulties he or she has, what strengths he or she shows, and what communicative situations need to be addressed. This is where communication sampling comes in. Communication sampling provides us with our most valid assessment of a client's communicative skill because it examines communication behavior itself, in a naturalistic environment that is closely related to the kinds of settings the client needs to communicate in every day.

An important issue in communication sampling, then, is to establish that the sample bears a strong resemblance to the kinds of interactions in which clients really engage. This issue is known as the *representativeness* of the sample. Because you may be seeing clients in a clinic setting with which they are unfamiliar or in an interaction with an unfamiliar partner (the clinician, whom they may not know well yet), the communication that you observe for your sample may not be quite like the client's communication in everyday settings. It is part of your job to ensure that the sample is as representative as possible. We will address some methods for maximizing sample representativeness as we go along.

Communication sampling can be used with clients of all ages to investigate a broad range of speech, language, and hearing problems. You can use samples of communication to examine the understanding and use of words and sentences (**semantics** and **syntax**); the appropriateness of communication in context (pragmatics); the sound system and its intelligibility (**phonology**); fluency, the use of **paralinguistics** or **prosody** in speech; and the quality and resonance of the speaking voice. We can divide these kinds of analyses into three broad categories:

1. Nonverbal communication, which includes the range of functions or communicative intentions expressed; the rate or frequency of communication; and the form in which communication is produced, whether with gestures, vocalizations, body movements, and so forth

2. Language, which includes semantics, syntax, and pragmatics

3. Speech, which includes phonology, prosody, fluency, and voice

In discussing communication sampling, we will look first at sampling procedures for *nonverbal* communication. *Language* across a range of developmental levels will be discussed next. Then, we will examine sampling for aspects of *speech* production.

NONVERBAL COMMUNICATION

Clients who are at preverbal levels of development, when symbolic language has not yet been acquired, do still communicate, of course; so do clients who have lost previously acquired skills through injury or illness and those whose long-standing level of functioning has precluded symbolic language learning. The issue of collecting a representative sample for clients with nonverbal functioning is particularly difficult. Often, these individuals are hard to engage. If they are very young children, then they may be unwilling to interact with an unfamiliar examiner. If they are older, then they may be exceedingly passive or withdrawn after years of inability to communicate. If they have lost communicative ability after a stroke or accident, then they may be deeply frustrated with the mismatch between the intents that they have to express and the means available to them for expression.

The purpose of communicative sampling for nonverbal individuals varies with their developmental level. For young children who are not talking, you may want to determine whether speech or some other form of symbolic communication, such as signs of **American Sign Language** (ASL) or **Blissymbols** (see Figures 5.1 and 5.2), would be appropriate, based on the child's current means and rate of communication. You may also use communication sampling in this population to assist in differential diagnosis. For example, we expect children with developmental disorders, such as mental retardation, specific language impairments, or hearing impairments, to show fairly typical skills in nonverbal communication, even when language in absent. But for children with more pervasive developmental disorders, such as autism, nonverbal communication is also affected.

For older clients who have developmental delays, you may be considering a new form of augmentative or alternative communication and you need to determine what kinds of ideas the client is attempting to communicate so that you can match the assistive system to the client's needs. When working with clients who have acquired losses, you may need to determine what kinds of communication skills have been spared so that you can identify the best intervention strategies for making use of the communicative functions the client has. For all of these clients, communication sampling is used to answer the following questions:

- What can the client respond to in a linguistic interaction; or, what are functional comprehension skills like?

- What types of communicative intentions can the client express; are a range of intentions available, or is the range very limited?

- How frequently does the client attempt to communicate?

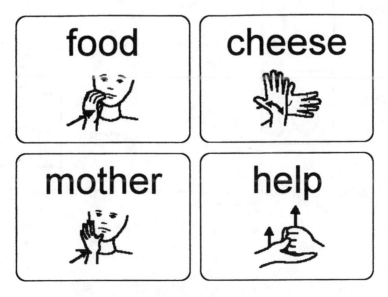

Figure 5.1. Examples of signs from American Sign Language.

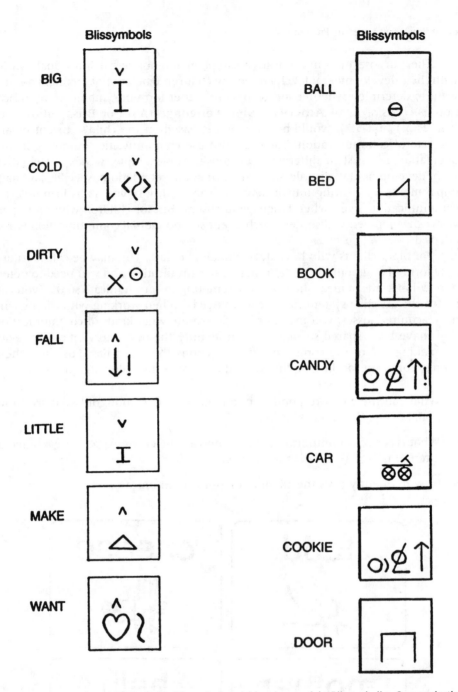

Figure 5.2. Examples of Blissymbols. Blissymbols used herein copyright Blissymbolics Communication International, Toronto, Canada. Exclusive licensee 1982.

- By what means does the client attempt to get messages across? Does he or she use gestures, gaze, vocalizations, words, or some combination of these?

COLLECTING THE SAMPLE

Collecting a representative sample from a nonspeaking client necessitates using a sampling context that is as much like a typical interaction as possible. For very young clients, this will usually mean a play session with developmentally appropriate toys and a familiar interlocutor, such as a parent. For children with motor impairments, you need to be especially careful to provide opportunities for the child to express wants, needs, and intents because many of these children get used to having everyone around them anticipate their desires and become somewhat passive communicators (Calculator, 1997). For older clients with more severe impairments and for those with acquired disorders, it will be important, too, to use developmentally appropriate materials in collecting the sample and to choose a context in which communication will be an important part of the activity. This may mean observing the client in a daily living setting, such as choosing food items from a menu for the next day's meal or doing vocational activities that involve interaction. It will also be important to check in with those who know the client well and to ask whether the interaction observed is typical of the client's current communication. The sample that you collect should be long enough to contain a broad range of communicative behaviors. For active communicators, 15–20 minutes is usually long enough. For clients who communicate less frequently, you may need to collect a longer sample. Generally, you would want to continue collecting data until you have at least 20 purposeful acts of communication from the client.

RECORDING THE SAMPLE

For nonverbal clients, of course, much of the communicative interaction will take place in visual modalities. For this reason, it is usually a good idea to record the communication sample on videotape so that it can be analyzed at a later time. Videotaping also allows you to watch the interaction several times and to score one aspect of communication during each pass. This makes it possible to answer all of the questions that you have posed for the assessment with only one sample of communication.

ANALYZING THE SAMPLE

One issue that you address in your analysis of nonverbal communication is the degree to which the client's behavior suggests an understanding of language. You will want to make some inferences about how the language spoken to the client influences his or her behavior in a natural setting. This information will be an important adjunct to your more formal testing of language comprehension because it will allow you to see whether the client uses what Chapman (1978) called *comprehension strategies*. The use of these strategies allows a client to act as if language comprehension has occurred, even though linguistic knowledge of specific words and grammatical forms may be lacking. You see these strategies operating in typically developing children, for example, when a mother looks at a ball, points to it, and says, "See the ball?" to a 12-month-old. The infant does not have to understand the word *ball* in order to appear to understand; he or she only has to look at what mother points to. This strategic looking gives the impression that the child "knows" the word, even though the child might not be able to identify *ball* in an array of several objects without the mother's gaze cue. If clients do better in these natural interactions than they do on standardized testing of language comprehension, then you have gathered an important piece of information: The child takes advantage of interactive cues in the environment. This performance would contrast with a client who did poorly on formal receptive testing and did not look much better in natural situations.

Figure 5.3 presents an observation form that might be used to examine a nonverbal client's receptive behaviors in a naturalistic communication sample. The form can be used to record the frequency and context for behaviors that appear to suggest language comprehension. An assessment such as this can be helpful for clinicians working with young children who have hearing impairments in order to assess the degree to which residual hearing is used to support natural communication.

The other questions that we posed about nonverbal clients concern the range, frequency, and means of communication expressed. Again, using a video-taped representative communication sample, you can assess how often, in what form, and for what purpose the client communicates. In assessing communication in nonspeakers, it is important to be conservative about attributing intention to the client's actions. You do not want to call every act of the client's an act of communication. In order to count as communicative, a client's action should meet more than one of the following criteria:

- It should be directed by means of gaze, body orientation, or gesture toward the interlocutor

- It should have an effect on the interlocutor

- It should convey a recognizable message that could be "translated" into words

- It should be persistent; if the act does not immediately gain its objective, it should be repeated or revised

An observation form like the one in Figure 5.4 can be used to summarize this assessment.

Some more formal procedures have been developed to assess preverbal communication skills. One example is the *Communication and Symbolic Behavior Scales* (Wetherby & Prizant, 1993). This procedure involves a structured play session that can be used to assess behaviors similar to the ones that we have been discussing for children at early stages of communicative development.

When assessing nonverbal communication in older clients who have not developed or who have lost speech, a clinician will examine the communication that is present, using methods such as the ones discussed here. You will also need to investigate the means of communication that can be used or expanded to

Client response			
	Responds appropriately	Responds inappropriately (describe)	Does not respond
Context Partner gives verbal instruction			
Partner asks question			
Partner offers choice verbally			
Partner suggests joint activity			
Partner remarks on object/event			

Figure 5.3.   Assessing comprehension in natural contexts.

Form					
	Gaze	Body movement	Gesture	Vocalization	Word/ approximation
Communicative function Request object/action					
Protest					
Comment (joint attention)					
Greeting/ social interaction					
Request information					
Give new information					
Acknowledge partner's remark					

Figure 5.4.   Assessment of nonverbal communication behaviors.

increase the client's communicative capacity, often using augmentative or alternative modes of communication. Although this assessment is beyond the scope of this text, readers will find many useful resources in Beukelman and Mirenda (1998) and Glennen and DeCoste (1997).

LANGUAGE SAMPLING

We sample client language in order to observe the meanings expressed (semantics), the forms used for expression (syntax), and the appropriateness of communication in a social context (pragmatics). Because language changes and develops over the life span, we use somewhat different methods at each level of development. We discuss language sampling, then, in terms of the broad developmental periods: the preschool level (3–5 years), the school-age level (5–16 years), and the adult level (16 years and older).

Sampling Language in Preschoolers

Children between 3 and 5 years of age are typically in the phase of language development when the basic words and sentence structures of the language are being acquired. Communication sampling in this period often focuses on the syntactic structures and morphological markers that are significant indicators of growth during this developmental phase, but you can look at other aspects of language as well.

Collecting the Sample   Language samples from preschoolers are usually collected in play interactions. The choice of materials for these play sessions has been shown to make a difference in the kinds of language that children produce. The best samples are collected when toys are used that represent familiar, domestic objects that lend themselves to pretending (even with little boys!). Toy vehicles or objects that are too exciting or novel tend to elicit more exploratory play and vocalization ("Vroom! Vroom!") than verbalization (O'Brien & Nagle, 1987).

Even the most appropriate materials will not necessarily get a preschooler to talk, though. Miller (1981) suggested some strategies to help establish rapport and elicit talk from young children. The first is to say nothing except for "Hi" for the first few minutes. Then, the clinician may begin parallel play with intermittent comments about ongoing actions ("You're stacking the blocks; I'll stack mine, too!"). Next, the clinician can initiate some interactive play while maintaining a low frequency of talking for the first few minutes. When the child appears "warmed up," the clinician may begin trying to get some verbal responses from the child.

The clinician's own use of language is critical in obtaining a representative sample. In a study looking at parental questions and topic continuations, Yoder and Davies (1990) found that adult topic continuations elicited the most responses of any length from children. Multiword replies from children were most likely to occur after explicit prompts that continued the child's topic (Child: "Baby cry." Examiner: "Oh! That's sad! What can we do?"). Questions can be used effectively to break the ice early in the session and to determine interest in a specific topic, but it is unwise to ask many yes–no or **closed questions** ("What is that?" "Where is the dog?" "Who is this?") because these typically elicit one-word responses. The technique of parallel talk, in which the clinician describes what the child is doing, is often more effective for eliciting language. Clinicians can narrate child actions and then lead into an **open-ended comment** or question. Repetition of a child's utterance, perhaps with a change of inflection, can also be used effectively to increase the child's output. (It also helps to repeat a child's utterance when he or she has reduced intelligibility.) Another effective technique is a one-word response followed by silence. An example is *"Really?"* because it shows interest and implies wanting to know more. Playful statements that are obviously false can be useful in eliciting more elaborated forms as well (Examiner: "My doggy is green!" Child: "No it not!").

How long a sample do you need from a preschooler? Most authorities (Miller, 1981; Nelson, 1998) suggest 50–100 utterances. If it is possible to collect two 50-utterance samples in two different settings, this is ideal. For children functioning at the 3- to 5-year level, a sample of this length can generally be collected from a 15-minute interaction. If language or developmental level is delayed, however, a somewhat longer sample of 20–30 minutes may be needed to get enough speech to analyze.

Recording the Sample   You normally will not need to videotape a communication sample with a preschool-age child. Because you are interested in only the spoken language, audiorecording will usually be sufficient. The only exceptions would be for children who are using a visual communication system such as ASL or who are so unintelligible that you will need the nonverbal context to help decide what they are saying. When you plan to analyze a sample from an audiorecording, it is important that the setting be conducive to tape recording. This means that background noise should be at a minimum and that the tape recorder and microphone be carefully chosen and situated in the room. An external, unidirectional microphone is recommended, as are high-quality audiotapes. It is critical that a clinician test the tape recorder and microphone. There is nothing more frustrating than spending 15–20 minutes of time obtaining a language sample only to find that the tape recorder was not working!

Transcribing the Sample   Transcribing a speech sample puts it into a tangible form that you can examine in a variety of ways. It is important to retain in transcription all of the errors that the child produces so that you can examine these errors for patterns that you will want to address in intervention. Many clinicians are surprised to find that although they understood what a client was saying during the interaction, it is much harder to do so when they listen later to the audiotape. For this reason, some clinicians find it helpful to repeat the child's utterances, often with a rising intonation that invites the child to say some more. Others make written notes as they collect the sample to remind them of what was happening.

Another challenging aspect of transcribing the sample is how to separate the child's speech into utterances. This is important because you often calculate the average of particular structures *per utterance*. Generally, clinicians use syntactic, intonational, contextual, and pausing features to make decisions regarding utterance separation. For preschoolers, Leadholm and Miller (1992) suggested using either a falling or rising intonation contour or a pause of more than 2 seconds to indicate the end of one utterance and the start of another. Lund and Duchan (1993) also presented rules that can be used at this language phase. These included using intonational, syntactic, and contextual information to make decisions regarding utterance separation.

There are a variety of formats for transcribing language samples. The one suggested by Retherford (1993) appears with a sample transcript in Table 5.1.

Analyzing the Sample   When you look closely at a language sample to discover patterns of error and areas of strength, you cannot truly separate form, meaning, and use. When you do analyses of speech samples, you often artificially divide these aspects of language, but, it is wise to remember that in real communication, they are integrated. We will examine several analysis procedures for each of these areas of language, but you should remember that, in fact, they all work together to express the clients' intents.

Semantics and Syntax   Analyzing language samples is one of the most time-consuming aspects of your practice. For this reason, it is important to use language sampling judiciously. You should only collect a language sample after you have already established that the client has an impairment in expressive language, as documented by a standardized test (see Chapter 3). Your goal in language sampling is NOT to get a score but to answer questions about the client's communication and to identify appropriate intervention goals. As you complete a language sample analysis, some questions to ask include

- How does the language sample compare with other aspects of the child's language performance, both receptively and expressively?

- Is the child using language structures consistently at one developmental level or stage?

Table 5.1.   Sample transcription format

Adult		Child		Context
1.	What have you got there?			Child plays with toy dog and bone.
2.	Is it a doggy?	1.	Uh-huh.	
3.	I have a dog at home.			
4.	Tell me about who's at your house.	2.	We have kitty.	Child leaves toy and looks up at examiner.
5.	Oh, cool!			
6.	I like cats.			
7.	Tell me about yours.	3.	Black.	
		4.	It have white foots.	
8.	I'll bet it's pretty!			Child returns to playing with toy dog.

Source: Retherford, 1993.

- Is there variety in the structures that the child uses, or does he or she use the same constructions over and over?

- Are there consistent error patterns, or are errors inconsistent and erratic?

Usually when you collect a language sample, in addition to thinking generally about questions such as these, you will want to do some formalized analysis to help you understand the sample more fully. There are two basic methods of analyzing language samples: manual methods and computer-assisted procedures.

Manual Methods   There are a variety of paper-and-pencil methods that have been developed to examine language form during the preschool period. Some examples are given in Table 5.2. Perhaps the most widely used of all language sample analysis procedures is the computation of the mean length of utterance in morphemes (**MLU**). Roger Brown (1973) first used this measure to index the stages of syntactic development in young children in his pioneering research on child language acquisition. A **morpheme** is a minimal meaningful unit of language. Computing the MLU involves counting the total number of morphemes in the language sample and dividing by the total number of utterances. A client's MLU can be compared with normative values reported by Leadholm and Miller (1992) or Paul (2001) to decide if the client's performance represents a significant delay. MLU is also a useful tool to measure a child's growth in the use of syntax. Clinicians who compute an MLU as part of the initial assessment battery have a baseline to which subsequent MLU's can be compared.

RULES FOR COUNTING MORPHEMES AND COMPUTING MLU

Counting rules

1. Use only completely intelligible utterances.

2. Count morphemes in the first 50 consecutive utterances.

3. Repetitions or false starts within an utterance are assigned morphemes only in the most complete form (In "My my mom is pretty," count only "my mom is pretty"). If repetition is for emphasis, count each word (In "My dad is big BIG," count all words, including repetition for emphasis).

4. Fillers (um, well, oh) are not counted. *Hi, no, and yeah* are counted.

5. Compound words (*birthday, somebody*), proper names (*Mickey Mouse*), and ritualized reduplications (*choo-choo, night-night*) are counted as one morpheme.

6. Diminutive forms (*doggie, daddy, toesie*) are counted as one morpheme.

7. Auxiliary verbs are counted as one morpheme, even if they are contracted ("He is running" = three morphemes; "He's running" = three morphemes).

8. Catenatives (*gonna, wanna, gotta, hafta*) count as just one morpheme.

9. All inflections (possessive 's, plural s, regular past -ed, etc.) are counted as one morpheme (shoes = two morphemes; baby's = two morphemes).

10. Negative contractions such as *can't, don't,* and *won't* are assigned two morphemes only if there is evidence elsewhere in the transcript that the child uses each part of the contraction separately.

Computing MLU

Count the total number of morphemes produced by the speaker.

Divide by the number of utterances counted (usually 50).

Source: Brown, 1973.

Additional analysis of the sample beyond MLU can give more in-depth syntactic and semantic information while still using the framework of Brown's stages (Miller, 1981). Miller's Assigning of Structural Stage Procedure (ASSP) includes counting the occurrences of the 14 grammatical morphemes originally studied by Brown (1973) and deVilliers and deVilliers (1973) and charting the use of various simple sentence constructions, both of which correspond to Brown's stages. This procedure looks at use of noun and verb phrase elaborations, negations, questions, and the use of complex sentences. Assigning stages to these aspects of language production gives more detailed information about the strengths and weaknesses in the child's use of syntax. It does, though, require a detailed knowledge of the sequence of normal syntactic acquisition. Miller (1981), Owens (2001), and Retherford (1993) provided information on this sequence that will be important for clinicians working in this developmental phase to know.

The ASSP is qualitative in nature and allows you to look at patterns in the child's use of language. Table 5.3 presents a worksheet as it might be used to record and summarize information about syntactic development using the ASSP.

Table 5.2.   Examples of language sampling procedures

Procedure	Reference
Mean Length of Utterance (MLU)	Brown, 1973
Language Assessment, Remediation, and Screening Procedure (LARSP)	Crystal, Fletcher, and Garman, 1991
Assigning of Structural Stage Procedure (ASSP)	Miller, 1981
Developmental Sentence Score (DSS)	Lee, 1974
Language Sampling, Analysis, & Training (LSAT)	Tyack and Gottsleban, 1974
Index of Productive Syntax (IPSyn)	Scarborough, 1990

Table 5.3.   Sample Assigning of Structural Stage Procedure (ASSP) worksheet

Stage	Grammatical morphemes	Noun phrase	Verb phrase	Negation	Yes–No Qs	Wh-Qs	Complex sentences
I							
II	*-ing* 100% *in* 100% plural 100%		‖‖‖				
III	*on* 100% Possessive 100%	‖‖‖ ‖‖‖ ‖‖‖	‖‖‖ ‖‖‖	‖‖‖ ‖	‖‖	‖	
IV		‖‖‖ ‖‖‖	‖‖‖ ‖‖	‖‖			‖‖
V	Copula *be* 33% Regular past 45% Irregular past 50% Regular third person singular 25%						
V+	Auxilliary *be* 33% Irregular third person singular						
V++							

Source: Miller, 1981.

Scarborough (1990) presented an extension of Miller's (1981) procedure. The Index of Productive Syntax (IPSyn) includes structures from the ASSP, plus additional forms that Scarborough found to be diagnostic in a child's speech. Use of the IPSyn involves counting the first two correct occurrences of each of these structures to determine whether each is part of the child's repertoire. The IPSyn provides both norm-referenced and criterion-referenced information that can be useful in selecting treatment goals and in measuring progress in language usage.

Another language sample analysis procedure that has been used widely for more than 25 years is Lee's (1974) Developmental Sentence Analysis (DSA). This procedure has two components—Developmental Sentence Types (DST) and Developmental Sentence Scoring (DSS). DST is a criterion-referenced analysis for young children whose language is primarily at the one- and two-word phrase level. The child's presentence utterances are sorted into the following five categories:

1.   Nouns and noun phrases

2.   Designators

3.   One-word descriptors and predicative phrases

4.   Verbs and verb phrases

5.   Vocabulary items

The distribution of utterances across these categories is used to determine which types are frequent in the child's speech, which should be used as a basis for developing longer utterances, and which are infrequent and should be elicited first in one- to two-word utterance form.

The more widely used part of the DSA is DSS, which provides both norm-referenced and criterion-referenced information. This analysis procedure was designed for use with children using subject–verb sentences consistently. It analyzes eight syntactic categories that were selected based on their appearance in the speech of young children and because of the developmental characteristics of their acquisition:

1.   Indefinite pronouns: *it, that, this,* and so forth

2.   Personal pronouns: *I, you, he,* and so forth

3.   Main verbs: *-ed, is+[verb]-ing,* use of auxiliary verbs, and so forth

4.   Secondary verbs: infinitives, gerunds, and so forth

5.   Negatives: *can't, don't, isn't, won't,* and so forth

6.   Conjunctions: *and, but, so, or,* and so forth

7.   Interrogative reversals: *Isn't it...?*

8.   Wh- questions: *What...?, Where...?, Who...?* and so forth

DSS scoring assigns forms in each category to one of eight developmentally ordered levels of complexity, with one "DSS point" assigned for the least complex level and eight "points" for the most complex. An additional "sentence point" is awarded for a fully grammatical sentence by adult standards. A DSS score is computed by adding the total number of points per sentence in the 50-sentence sample and dividing by 50. The child's score can be compared with his or her same-age peers using the DSS normative data. Norms were established from 2-0 years to 6-6 years. If a child is below the 10th percentile for his or her age, he or she is considered to have a language impairment. Figure 5.5 presents a sample worksheet for analyzing and computing DSS. Like the ASSP and IPSyn, the qualitative information obtained from a DSS analysis can provide useful information in understanding an individual child's language usage, determining treatment goals, and measuring progress in intervention.

Utterance #	Indefinite pronouns	Personal pronouns	Main verbs	Secondary verbs	Negatives	Conjunctions	Interrogative reversals	Wh-Qs	Sentence point
1									
2									
3									
4									
5									
6									
7									
8									
9									
10									
11									
12									
13									
14									
15									
16									
17									
18									
19									
20									
21									
22									
23									
24									
25									
26									
27									
28									
29									
30									
31									
32									
33									
34									
35									
36									
37									
38									
39									
40									
41									
42									
43									
44									
45									
46									
47									
48									
49									
50									

Figure 5.5. Sample worksheet for analyzing and computing Developmental Sentence Scoring.

Computer-Assisted Procedures   Computers assist you in much of the work that you do and can be used to assist in language sampling as well. There are several computerized forms of language sample analysis available. Miller, Freiberg, Rolland, and Reeves (1992) described the benefits of computer technology for language sampling in the areas of transcription, analysis, accuracy, and interpretation. The ability to perform multiple analyses on the same transcript is perhaps the biggest advantage in using a computer program. Larson and McKinley (1995) cautioned that it is still up to the clinician to obtain a reliable and representative language sample and to transcribe it accurately.

The widely used Systematic Analysis of Language Transcripts (SALT) was developed by Miller and Chapman (1985, 2000) and provides some standard pre-configured analysis. These include MLU and several lexical analyses: Type-Token Ratio (TTR), Number of Different Words (NDW), and Number of Total Words (NTW). Miller et al. (1992) showed that both MLU and NDW are sensitive to language development and delay during the preschool and school-age periods. SALT also allows users to design their own analyses. The SALT program provides a reference database (RDB; Leadholm & Miller, 1992) that allows a client's performance to be compared with that of children in the reference sample from Wisconsin and discusses the issues that you need to consider when comparing samples of children from culturally or linguistically different backgrounds. Some additional computer-assisted forms of language analysis are as follows.

COMPUTER-ASSISTED LANGUAGE ANALYSIS PROCEDURES

Child Language Analysis and Transcription (CLAN, CHAT; McWhinney, 1996): includes programs for doing automatic DSS and IPSyn analyses on entered transcripts

Lingquest (Mordecai & Palin, 1982)

Computerized profiling (Long & Fey, 1993)

Pragmatics   *Pragmatics* is defined as the study of how language is used in the context of communication. Evaluating the child's pragmatic skills is a natural extension of evaluating a language sample because pragmatic skills must be assessed in a naturalistic context. The goal of assessment in this area is to compare a child's pragmatic skills with his or her skills in the areas of syntax, semantics, and phonology to help determine the communicative basis the client has for learning language.

There are several organizing schemes that can be used to evaluate pragmatic skills as observed in the language sample. One that is widely used is Prutting and Kirchner's (1983) Pragmatic Protocol. This allows a clinician to look at pragmatic behaviors as they occur within the context of the language sample and to make an overall judgment as to whether they are generally *appropriate* or *inappropriate*. An adaptation of this coding scheme appears in Figure 5.6. Roth and Spekman (1984) provided additional guidelines for analyzing communication intentions

Communicative act	Appropriate	Inappropriate	No opportunity to observe
Utterance acts			
A. Verbal/paralinguistic			
1. Voice quality			
2. Vocal intensity			
3. Prosody			
4. Fluency			
B. Nonverbal			
1. Proximity			
2. Posture			
3. Gestures			
4. Gaze			
5. Facial expression			
Expression of meaning			
A. Word use			
1. Specificity			
2. Accuracy			
B. Relations between words			
1. Word order			
2. Given/new information			
C. Register variation			
1. To adults			
2. To peers			
Communicative functions			
A. Speech acts			
1. Remarks are relevant to previous speakers'			
2. Uses broad range of communicative functions[a]			
B. Topics			
1. Selection			
2. Introduction			
3. Maintenance			
4. Change			
C. Turn-taking			
1. Initiation			
2. Response			
3. Repair/revise			
4. Pause time			
5. Interrupts			
6. Gives feedback			
7. Quantity and conciseness			

Figure 5.6.   A form for recording pragmatic behaviors in communication samples. *Note:* [a]such as requests, pretend, reasoning, predictions, planning, giving new information, narrations, explanation, and commenting. (From Prutting, C., & Kirchner, D. [1983]. Applied pragmatics. In T.M. Gallagher & C.A. Prutting [Eds.], *Pragmatic assessment and intervention issues in language* [pp. 29–64]. San Diego: College-Hill Press; adapted by permission.)

and discourse organization from a conversational language interaction between the child and an adult.

Language Sampling in School-Age Children and Adolescents

In this developmental period, basic sentence structures, vocabulary, and conversational rules have been learned. Analysis focuses on the refinement and elaboration of communication skill.

Collecting the Sample   In collecting a spontaneous speech sample from an older, school-age child, Evans and Craig (1992) found that use of an interview format elicited more representative language behaviors than free play with toys and games. They suggested using the following three open-ended questions to elicit 15 minutes of speech from children in the 7 to 12-year age range:

1.   Tell me about your family.

2.   Tell me about your school.

3.   What do you do when you aren't in school?

For school-age students, it may be especially useful to have at least part of the language sample collected during interaction with a peer. Peer conversation tends to contain more complex language than conversation with adults during this period because children tend to take a relatively passive role in interacting with authority figures and communicate more assertively with those their own age. If a peer interaction can be arranged, information from this portion can be combined with the interview sample for analysis. Suggested topics for a peer conversation would include shared interests, such as sports or entertainment figures, or the explanation of a game or activity by the client.

Recording and Transcribing the Sample   In general, you will continue to use primarily audiorecording for students at this developmental level. The computer-assisted methods of transcription listed on page 126 can be used with both school-age and preschool children. There are some modifications that are typically used in transcribing speech samples from school-age children, however, which have to do with how utterances are segmented.

Hunt (1965) developed a system called a **T-unit,** or Terminal unit, segmentation for use with samples of language from school-age children. Hunt observed that school-age children sometimes produced run-on sentences such as this:

Well, last weekend I went skiing with my buddies from school and it was gonna be a long trip so I packed a sandwich and a bottle of pop and I put them on my seat on the bus so I would have them for later and I wouldn't get too hungry before we stopped at McDonald's and had some dinner on the way home from the trip but then I got hungry and ate half the sandwich before we got to the mountain so...

Hunt reasoned that to count such a long utterance as just one sentence was not really representative of how complex the student's language was. He devised the

T-unit to compensate for these run-ons. A *T-unit* is defined as one main clause with all of the subordinate clauses and nonclausal phrases attached to it. We would divide the sentence above into T-units as follows:

Well, last weekend I went skiing with my buddies from school
and it was gonna be a long trip
and I packed a sandwich and a bottle of pop
and I put them on my seat on the bus so I would have them for later
and I wouldn't get too hungry before we stopped at McDonald's to have some
*   dinner on the way home from the trip*
but then I got hungry and ate half the sandwich before we got to the mountain...

Once the sample is segmented into the T-units, various analyses can be completed, including MLU per T-unit.

Analyzing the Sample   At this developmental period, language sample analysis focuses not so much on missing forms but on the degree to which communication is complex and flexible.

Semantics and Syntax   There are fewer procedures developed to analyze the expressive language of children in the school-age period. Most clients at this developmental level have mastered the basic syntax, semantics, pragmatics, and phonology of communication. The difficulties that they have tend to be in contexts that demand more specific, complex language skills related to literacy and school success. Some of the analyses that we discussed for preschoolers can be used with younger school-age clients. The DSS can be used up to age 7, which usually corresponds to second grade. The SALT reference database contains information on MLU, NDW, and NTW, as well as use of **bound morphemes,** personal pronouns, question words, negative markers, **conjunctions,** and **modal verbs** (*can, will, shall, may, could, would, should, must,* and *might*) for children from 3 to 13 years.

Another analysis adapted from those used for preschoolers is also informative for school-age clients: their use of **complex sentences.** Paul (2001) argued that complex sentences are particularly sensitive to development and delay in the school-age period because they reflect the ability to combine ideas within a sentence, an important aspect of literary language. Paul recommended reviewing a transcript for the complex sentences it contains and analyzing it for:

- The proportion of complex sentences to total sentences in the sample

- The types of complex sentences used (such as infinitive clauses, relative clauses, etc.)

- The number and type of conjunctions (such as *and, if, because, when, so,* etc.)

This analysis will reveal whether the student is using appropriately complex language and, if not, what aspects of complex language ought to be addressed in the intervention program. A sample worksheet for this analysis appears in Figure 5.7.

Additional aspects of language form that are frequently problematic for students with language disabilities were noted by Miller et al. (1992). Clinicians may want to look for the presence of the following difficulties in language samples as well:

- Utterance formulation difficulties, including false starts, repetitions, and reformulations

- Word-finding problems as evidenced by single-word reformulations and/or circumlocutions

- Semantic impairments as evidenced by limited vocabulary and use of general words as opposed to specific names (*thingy, stuff, whatchamacallit*)

Pragmatics   Larson and McKinley (1995) developed the Adolescent Conversational Analysis, a format that looks at the student's role as both a listener and a speaker. Here, as in Prutting and Kirchner's (1983) procedure for younger children, the clinician evaluates the student's conversational behaviors as *appropriate, inappropriate,* or *not observed* in a 10-minute sample of conversation with each of several partners, including a peer. As a listener, the student's ability to understand the vocabulary and main ideas of the speaker is evaluated, in addition to how he or she responds to nonverbal feedback. As a speaker, the student is evaluated for specific language and paralinguistic features. The student is also evaluated on communication functions and conversational rules. A sample worksheet for this analysis appears in Figure 5.8.

Brinton and Fujiki (1992) found that using probes in interaction increases the efficiency of the sample and can also be effective in identifying various pragmatic behaviors. Some probes that they have found to be effective are:

- Initiating new topics in the midst of conversation (e.g., "By the way, I went skiing last weekend.") to look for responsiveness, maintenance of the new topic, and relevance of the student's comment

- Requesting repairs in the context of ongoing conversation (e.g., "What kind of music was it?") to look for responsiveness, adjustment to listener needs, and appropriateness of repair strategies

- Inserting sources of communication breakdown (e.g., "Can you get me the scissors?" when no scissors are available) to look for assertiveness, ability to monitor the interaction, and requests for clarification

Narrative   **Narrative** skills are a second type of discourse that you may need to evaluate in students with communication disorders. According to Westby (1998), narratives serve as a crucial bridge from the more informal styles of communication that children learn at home to the more formal, literate types of language that they will need to succeed in school. For this reason, examining students' narrative skills will help a clinician evaluate their higher-level language ability and assess the degree to which impairments in these skills may have a negative effect on school performance. Larson and McKinley (1995) recommended

Student name: A. J. Nevarow Date of birth: 11/20/89

Teacher: R. Paul Grade: 6

Clinician: E. Reuler Date of examination: 10/10/01

School: Ruttles Sampling context: Interview

Number of T-units in sample: 50

Number of complex sentences in sample: 22

Percentage of complex sentences in sample (b/a): 44%

Complex sentence type	T-unit	Conjunction used
S-conjunction-S	5. He plays soccer, and I play baseball. 9. I like ice cream, but I don't want yours.	and but
Simple infinitive	14. I need to go home right after school. 34. He wants to beat me at Myst.	
Adverbial clause	16. After I get home, I watch television. 46. If my mom isn't home, I get a snack.	after if
Propositional clause	11. I know I can still beat him, though. 27. I wish that I had the new 'Nsync CD.	that
Wh- clause	3. Mom knows where I am. 41. I don't know who that is.	where who
Sentences with three or more VPs	18. I want to go see it, but my mom won't take me. 23. After we go to the circus, we like to stop for ice cream.	but after
Relative clause	25. That's the kind I like. 30. They're the kids that I play ball with.	that
Infinitive clause with different subject	15. He wants me to go with him. 20. My teacher wants you to teach me.	
Infinitive with wh-	19. I know how to do that. 28. Did you tell me when to stop?	how when
Passive infinitive	7. He doesn't want to get hit by the truck. 10. Do you want to be picked by the teacher?	
Gerund clause	26. Snowboarding is fun. 49. My favorite thing is playing computer games.	

Figure 5.7. Sample worksheet for complex sentence analysis (with example utterances).

Conversational skill	Appropriate	Inappropriate	No opportunity to observe
Listening skills			
1. Understands partner's vocabulary and syntax			
2. Follows conversational topics introduced by others			
3. Indicates understanding or misunderstanding with verbal feedback			
Speaking skills			
A. Linguistic features			
1. Produces a variety of forms			
2. Uses some figurative language, slang			
3. Uses precise vocabulary			
4. Produces few mazes or false starts			
B. Paralinguistic features			
1. Inflection			
2. Pausing			
3. Rate			
4. Fluency			
5. Intelligibility			
C. Communicative functions			
1. Give information			
2. Request information			
3. Describe objects and events			
4. Express beliefs, intentions, feelings			
5. Persuade listener to do, believe, feel			
6. Solve problems with language			
D. Discourse management			
1. Initiate conversation			
2. Choose topics			
3. Maintain topics			
4. Shift topics			
5. Repair/revise when necessary			
6. Yield floor			
7. Interrupt			
E. Conversational rules			
1. Quantity (doesn't talk too much or too little)			
2. Makes sincere comments			
3. Makes relevant comments			
4. Expresses thoughts clearly and concisely			
5. Uses tact, politeness			
F. Nonverbal behaviors			
1. Gestures and facial expressions			
2. Eye contact and gaze			
3. Maintains proximity			

Figure 5.8. Sample worksheet for adolescent conversational analysis. (*Source:* Larson & McKinley, 1995.)

that the clinician obtain two narrative samples, one a reformulation task in which the student retells a story and the other a formulated task in which the student relates a personal experience. Many of the analyses used to evaluate narratives are based on Applebee's (1978) discussion of the stages that characterize the development of narrative skills in children. These stages were later modified by Klecan-Aker and Kelty (1990) and augmented by Hughes, McGillivray, and Schmidek (1997). An overview of these stages is presented in Table 5.4.

Clinicians may want to examine narrative samples gathered from students in order to assign them to one of these levels of development. If students' narratives are less mature than would be expected for their grade level, then intervention can be aimed at advancing narrative production to the next level in this sequence, with the long-term goal of developing grade-appropriate narrative skills.

Table 5.4. Stages of narrative development

Approximate age (in typical development)	Narrative type	Description of type
2 years	Heap	Labels and descriptions of events or actions using simple declarative sentences
3 years	Sequence story	Events are related around a central theme, character, or setting; however, one event does not necessarily follow temporally or causally from another
3–4 years	Primitive narrative	Contains a core or a central person, object, or event and contains three elements: an initiating event, an action or attempted action, and a consequence of that action or attempt; there are no definitive endings to these stories and no evidence in the telling of why characters act as they do (psychological motivation)
4–5 years	Chain	Show some cause–effect and temporal relationships; the three elements listed previously are present, in addition to some elements of character motivation
5–6 years	True narrative	Express a theme or moral; have a plot with a central theme and characters; there are logical and temporally ordered sequences and the ending represents a resolution to the story
7–8 years	Narrative summary	Stories have complete episodes, contain multiple episodes; students at this level can provide summaries of stories heard
11–12 years	Complex narrative	Contains complex, embedded, and interactive episodes
13 years	Narrative analysis skills	Can describe narrative style; compare or contrast stories

Sources: Applebee, 1978; Hughes, McGillivray, & Schmidek, 1997; Klecan-Aker & Kelty, 1990; and Paul, 2001.

Language Sampling in Adults with Acquired Disorders

Adults who acquire language disorders through accidents or illness are said to have **aphasia.** These disorders can affect the ability to retrieve and understand words, to formulate and comprehend sentences, and to imitate language. Clinicians sample language from adults with aphasia for the same reasons that they do for younger clients: to examine the functional use of language in real communicative situations and to supplement standardized evaluation procedures with information from these more naturalistic assessments.

Collecting the Sample   Shadden (1998) suggested several contexts for eliciting language samples from adults:

- Conversing about a familiar topic

- Describing the picture of a common scene, such as people watching television in a living room; a well-known picture, such as a Normal Rockwell painting; or a commonly used clinical stimulus, such as the "cookie theft" picture from the *Boston Diagnostic Aphasia Examination* (Goodglass & Kaplan, 1983)

- Retelling a story heard verbally

- Generating a story from a set of pictures

- Listing procedures involved in a well-known event, such as shopping in a grocery store

She emphasized the importance of collecting samples in more than one of these contexts in order to assess the client's ability to deal with several levels of difficulty in discourse situations.

Recording and Transcribing the Sample   Most of the recording and transcription conventions used for younger clients are appropriate for transcribing adult language as well. T-unit segmentation is often used in adult samples for the same reasons that you use it in younger populations. Likewise, the same computer-assisted procedures, such as the SALT and CHAT programs, are available to be used to transcribe adult discourse.

Analyzing the Sample   In analyzing speech from adults with aphasia, we look for disruptions of well-learned language processes and for situations in which frustration occurs due to an inability to find forms for intentions that the adult has in mind.

Semantics and Syntax   According to Shadden (1998), the primary areas of interest in analyzing language form in adult clients with aphasia include the following:

- Sentence length

- Syntactic complexity, diversity, and completeness

- Semantic diversity and accuracy

- Use of morphological forms

Because these are many of the same issues that we look at in school-age children, we can apply some of the same analysis procedures, including MLU per T-unit and percentage of complex sentences. Shadden (1998) suggested some additional analyses that can be helpful for adults:

- Words/clauses: total number of words divided by total number of clauses

- Clauses/T-units: total number of clauses (both independent and subordinate) divided by total number of T-units

- The percentage of 1-, 2-, and 3+-clause sentences

All of these analyses can be used as baseline measures, against which to monitor progress in increasing syntactic complexity during the course of a therapy program.

   As an index of syntactic accuracy and completeness, Shadden (1998) suggested assigning each T-unit in a sample a "+" if it is fully grammatical and a "−" if it contains errors such as

- Verb marking errors

- Obligatory word omissions

- Additions of extra elements

- Incomplete forms

- Morphological errors

- Pronoun errors

- Word order errors

A clinician can then calculate the percentage of syntactically accurate and complete T-units and compare this percentage across discourse tasks or over time in intervention. A similar procedure can be used to assess semantic accuracy and completeness, with "−" scores given for errors such as

- Empty or vague word use

- Given/new information errors

- **Neologisms** or **paraphasias**

- Inaccurate information

- Ambiguous or contentless information

- Inappropriate word use

- Incompleteness

An additional semantic analysis that is frequently of interest for adult clients concerns the amount, efficiency, conciseness, accuracy, and completeness of the information conveyed. Shadden (1998) suggested that many patients with acquired disorders have specific difficulty with the **informativeness** of their discourse; that is, with conveying the appropriate amount of information and with conveying information of sufficient quality without irrelevancies, redundancies, off-topic interjections, or overly personalized content. Efficiency and conciseness are also problematic for these clients, who may produce discourse that is unfocused and prone to delay, errors, excessive detail, and effortful production. Several approaches have been developed to provide data on these kinds of discourse problems.

Content unit analysis involves developing a list of content units for a particular stimulus and comparing a client's response to that stimulus to the list generated by the clinician or a panel of typical controls. The following information provides an example of a content unit analysis that might be developed for a picture description task, using a picture created by Nicholas and Brookshire (1993), which appears in Figure 5.9.

CONTENT UNIT ANALYSIS FOR
NICHOLAS AND BROOKSHIRE'S (1993) "BIRTHDAY PARTY" PICTURE IN FIGURE 5.9

woman	little	women coming in	dog
mother[a]	boy	with children	under couch/sofa
standing	crying	to living room	hiding[a]
with broom	sad[a]	mothers[a]	afraid to come
looking	standing beside	guests[a]	out[a]
at dog	mother[a]	carrying boxes	left footprints
angry[a]	upset about	birthday gifts[a]	after eating cake[a]
for stealing cake[a]	cake[a]	surprised[a]	ruined party[a]

Sources: Myers, 1979; Nicholas & Brookshire, 1993; Shadden, 1998.

Note: [a]interpretive units.

These units can be derived for a variety of discourse tasks, including procedural descriptions such as "going shopping" or "eating in a restaurant." The number of content units included within a retelling can be tabulated, as well as the number of units that are irrelevant, redundant, or inaccurate. Figure 5.10 presents such an analysis for the "Birthday Party" picture as it might be produced at two points in time by a client. Nicholas and Brookshire (1995) reported that this analysis allows a clinician to look for increases in quantity of appropriate information and decreases in inappropriate information as an index of progress in therapy.

Informational content analysis is used to assess the efficiency of communication. Here, the ratio of meaningful to nonmeaningful units of information can be tracked across several discourse contexts, as well as over time. Cheney and Canter

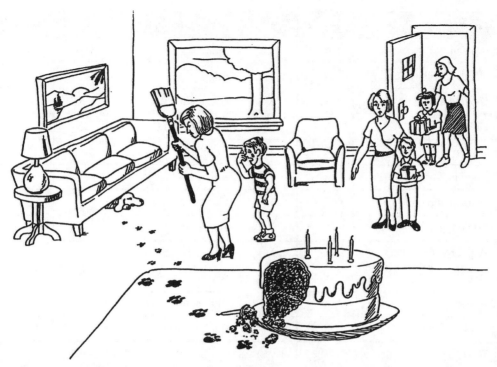

Figure 5.9.   Sample picture used in a content unit analysis. (From Nicholas, L., & Brookshire, R. [1993]. A system for quantifying the informativeness and efficiency of the connected speech of adults with aphasia. *Journal of Speech and Hearing Research, 36,* 346. © American Speech-Language-Hearing Association; reprinted by permission.)

(1993) have provided data on normal range for this analysis. Figure 5.11 provides a sample worksheet for the information content analysis that can be used to examine production across several discourse tasks.

Verbosity, or excessive talking, is often seen in acquired aphasias and can be measured in a variety of ways:

- Calculating the number of information units per minute (Yorkston & Beukelman, 1980)

- Calculating the number of words per story or discourse unit (Gleason et al., 1980)

- Calculating the number of content units in the first 50 words in a discourse task (Arbuckle, Gold, Frank, & Motard, 1989)

Gold, Andres, Arbuckle, and Schwartzman (1988) suggested distinguishing two kinds of verbosity: off-target verbosity or irrelevant speech, in which clients speak about topics not relevant to the current one; and digressive speech, in which clients remain on the topic but say too much about it.

Pragmatic Analysis   As you did for older children, you will want to look at both conversational and narrative samples from adult clients. To analyze conver-

Content units	Time 1	Time 2	Interpretive units	Time 1	Time 2
Woman	X	X	Mother	X	X
Standing with broom	X	X	Angry		X
Looking at dog	X	X	For stealing cake	X	X
Little boy	X	X	Birthday child		
Crying	X	X	Upset		X
Standing beside	X	X	About cake	X	X
Women and children	X	X	Guests and mothers		
Coming into living room	X	X	Surprised		X
With boxes	X	X	With birthday gifts		X
Dog	X	X	Afraid to come out	X	X
Under sofa	X	X	After eating cake		X
Left footprints	X	X	Ruined party		
TOTALS	12/12	12/12		4/12	9/12
Irrelevant/incorrect/ inaccurate units	3	1			

Figure 5.10.   Content unit analysis for the "Birthday Party" picture.

sation, formats that were looked at for younger clients, such as Prutting and Kirchner's (1983) Pragmatic Protocol and Larson and McKinley's (1995) Adolescent Conversational Analysis, can be used. Halper, Cherney, Burns, and Mogil (1996) developed a rating scale specifically for assessing adult communication skills (see Figure 5.12).

For narrative analysis, too, many of the forms that you used for older children can likewise be used with adult clients (Coehlo, 1998). Hughes et al. (1997) outlined a wide variety of narrative assessments designed for school-age clients that can be used effectively with adults as well. One analysis that can be particularly informative for adult narrative samples is the analysis of **cohesive ties,** the structural coherence among parts of a text (Halliday & Hasan, 1976). Liles and Coehlo (1998) identified a set of linguistic markers of cohesion that can be examined in stories produced by clients. These markers can be identified within a discourse sample and rated as to whether they are:

Complete: information referred to by the tie is easily found and defined without ambiguity

Example: *Alice* was hungry. *She* ate some cake.

Student name: _____ Date of birth: _____

Teacher: _____ Grade: _____

Clinician: _____ Date of examination: _____

School: _____ Sampling context: _____

Task/sample date	Meaningful units		Nonmeaningful units				Efficiency (number of meaningful/nonmeaningful)
	Essential	Elaborations	Irrelevant	Redundant	Inaccurate	Off-topic	
Cookie theft picture description Date:							
How to make scrambled eggs procedure description Date:							
Story retelling Date:							
Conversation Date:							
Normal range (from Cheney & Canter, 1993)	40%–78%	10%–33%	7%–38%	0%–6%	0%–1%	0%	4%–14%

Figure 5.11. Sample worksheet for informational content analysis. (*Source:* Shadden, 1998.)

139

	1 Markedly abnormal	2 Limited or inconsistent	3 Appropriate most of the time	4 Consistently appropriate
Nonverbal communication				
Intonation				
Facial expression				
Eye contact				
Gestures				
Proxemics				
Verbal communication				
Conversational initiation				
Turn-taking				
Topic maintenance				
Referencing				
Response length				
Repair and revision				
Quantity of information				

Figure 5.12.   A rating scale for adult conversation skills. (*Source:* Halper, Cherney, Burns, & Mogil, 1996.)

Incomplete: information referred to by the tie is not provided in the text

Example: James walked home from school. He saw them at the bus stop.

Erroneous: the tie guides a listener to ambiguous information

Example: Tom and Dick were at the video arcade. He had lots of quarters.

Figure 5.13 presents a summary of the cohesive ties identified by Liles and Coehlo (1998) in a format that can be used to assess cohesive adequacy in client discourse samples.

SPEECH SAMPLING

One way in which communication sampling is efficient is that the same sample can be analyzed on a variety of dimensions. Just as you can look at both syntax and pragmatics in the same sample, you can, in addition, look at the same sample in terms of its articulation, intelligibility, fluency, prosody, quality, and resonance. We will look again at our three developmental periods (preschool, school-

Cohesive market type	Examples	Cohesive element in client discourse (word)	Found in T-unit #:	Cohesive adequacy		
				Complete	Incomplete	Error
Reference						
Personal	*He, she, mine, it*					
Demonstrative	*This, that, these, those*					
Conjunction						
Causal	*Because, to that end, otherwise*					
Adversative	*Yet, although, instead, but*					
Temporal	*Then, afterward, subsequently*					
Additive	*Likewise, furthermore, incidentally*					
Lexical						
Reiteration						
•repetition	*I have a <u>house</u> on the beach. It is a tiny <u>house</u>.*					
•synonym	*He's a good <u>boy</u>. One of the finest <u>lads</u>...*					
•superordinate	*You can have the <u>carrot</u>. I don't like <u>vegetables</u>.*					
•general word	*I gave <u>John</u> the money. The <u>doofus</u> lost it.*					
Collocation	*I'll get the <u>doctor</u>. You look <u>sick</u>.*					
Ellipsis						
Nominal	*What do you want to <u>drink</u>? <u>Coke</u>.*					
Verbal	*Who's <u>coming to the store</u>? We <u>are</u>.*					
Clausal	*Has <u>he done it all</u>? He <u>has</u>.*					
Substitution						
Nominal	*I need a <u>coat</u>. Would you get me <u>one</u>?*					
Verbal	*I don't know <u>how to fix this</u>, and I don't think you <u>do</u> either.*					
Clausal	*They <u>won, didn't they</u>? Unfortunately <u>not</u>.*					

Figure 5.13.   Worksheet for assessing cohesive adequacy. (*Source:* Liles & Coehlo, 1998.)

age, and adult) to see what aspects of speech production can be analyzed through samples of communication.

Preschool Speech Sampling

When sampling speech in the preschool period, you generally have two goals:

1. Assessing the occurrence of phonological errors in continuous speech

2. Assessing **intelligibility,** or the degree to which speech is understandable by listeners

Phonological Analysis   Analysis of running speech is often advocated as a way of looking at the types of articulation errors made in naturalistic situations (Lund & Duchan, 1993; Shriberg & Kwiatkowski, 1980). Just as the types of syntactic errors made in imitation activities often differ from the types made in natural speech (Prutting, Gallagher, & Mulac, 1975), so the types of errors made on articulation tests are not always the same ones that you hear children make in real conversation (Morrison & Shriberg, 1992). That is why many clinicians supplement articulation testing with an analysis of articulation in conversation. One procedure often used is to collect a **phonetic inventory,** a list of all of the sounds that the client produces in a sample of speech. Shriberg (1993) divided the consonant phonemes of English into three groups, based on their order of acquisition. Table 5.5 provides a worksheet for recording the appearance of these sounds in a spontaneous language sample in order to assess the range of phonemes in the repertoire, as well as whether the client is following a typical pattern of acquisition.

The preschool period is the time during which phonological errors are most prevalent. There are a variety of published methods that can be used to structure the coding and analysis of phonological errors in continuous speech samples. Shriberg and Kwiatkowski (1980), for example, suggested one analysis method that is based on the first 100 different words in a continuous speech sample. This method looks at the eight most commonly used **phonological processes** or systematic changes in sound production:

Table 5.5.   Worksheet for recording the appearance of developmentally ordered speech sounds

Early sounds	/m/	/b/	/j/	/n/	/w/	/d/	/p/	/h/
Middle sounds	/t/	/ŋ/	/k/	/g/	/f/	/v/	/tʃ/	/dʒ/
Late sounds	/ʃ/	/θ/	/s/	/z/	/ð/	/l/	/r/	/ʒ/

Source: Shriberg, 1993.

1. *Final consonant deletion* (FCD): leaving off the last sound in a word

2. *Velar fronting* (VF): changing /k/ to /t/ and /g/ to /d/

3. *Palatal fronting* (PF): changing /ʃ/ and /tʃ/ to /s/; changing /ʒ/ and /dʒ/ to /z/

4. *Stopping* (S): changing fricatives (e.g., /s/, /z/, /f/, /v/) to their corresponding stops (/t/, /d/, /p/, /b/, respectively)

5. *Liquid simplification* (LS): Mispronouncing or omitting /l/ or /r/

6. *Assimilation* (A): making the sounds in a word more alike (e.g., pronouncing *doggie* as *doddie*)

7. *Cluster reduction* (CR): leaving out or changing sounds in consonant blends (e.g., pronouncing *play* as *pway,* or *lamp* as *lam*)

8. *Unstressed syllable deletion* (USD): leaving out the weakest syllable in a word (e.g., pronouncing *tomato* as *mato,* or *banana* as *nana*)

Figure 5.14 provides a worksheet for scoring the appearance of these processes in a 100-word sample.

Intelligibility   For young children, the degree to which speech is intelligible is often a concern. Special considerations arise when collecting a sample of speech from unintelligible clients. You cannot analyze speech that you did not understand! For highly unintelligible children, it may be necessary to use a more structured sampling format in order to have a better chance of understanding what they mean to say. Activities such as having the child make up a story about a set of sequence pictures or telling the story depicted in a picture book, although less ideal than interactive conversation, may be the best bet for obtaining a sample that can be deciphered and analyzed.

Traditionally, clinicians have used subjective measures in which judgments of intelligibility are made. Probably the most common subjective measure is percentage estimation in which the clinician assigns a percentage of intelligibility to the speech sample based on an "educated guestimate" of the proportion of words understood by the clinician in running speech. There are more objective measurements that lead to quantifiable judgments, though. One method of assessing intelligibility is to transcribe the sample, using Xs for any unintelligible words, and to compute the percentage of intelligible words per 100-word sample. Another procedure is described by Weiss (1982) in the *Weiss Intelligibility Test.* Using this method, the clinician listens to an interaction between the client and a familiar listener. While listening, the clinician records a dot (.) for each word understood and a slash (/) for each one not understood on a 10 x 10 grid, until each box of the grid is filled in. Then, the percentage of unintelligible words is computed by dividing the number of slashes by 100. The advantage of this procedure is that it does not require transcription but can be scored during an interaction. Shriberg and Kwiatkowsi (1982) advocated using the percent consonants correct (PCC) as a measure of intelligibility. This measure requires phonemic transcription of a 100-word sample. The clinician transcribes all of the consonants

Target word	Realization	Opportunities (O)/occurrences (Ø) of phonological processes							
		FCD	VF	PF	S	LS	A	CR	USD
Play	/pwe/					Ø		Ø	
Trees	/twiz/	O			O	Ø	O	Ø	
Sheep	/dip/	O		Ø	Ø		Ø		
Chicken	/dIkIn/	O	O	Ø	Ø		Ø		O
a. Number of opportunities									
b. Number of occurrences									
Percentage use (b/a)									

Figure 5.14. Worksheet for coding eight common phonological processes in 100 words from a continuous speech sample. Instructions: record a circle for each opportunity for a process to occur in a target word; put a line through each circle in which the process is used in the word's realization. Compute the percentage usage of each process in the 100-word sample. (*Source:* Shriberg & Kwiatkowski, 1980.)

144

that the client produced and also transcribes a **gloss,** or the target consonant that the client intended to produce. For example, the client may say, "pway" and the clinician may gloss, or interpret, this utterance to mean "play." In this case, the clinician would record /pwe/ for the production and /ple/ for the gloss. PCC is derived by counting the number of consonants that agree with their gloss (or are pronounced correctly) and dividing this number by the number of glossed consonants transcribed in the 100-word sample. This number is the PCC.

School-Age Speech Sampling

Articulation and intelligibility can be issues at the school-age level. When older children present these problems, the same methods of speech sampling can be adapted for this age group that were used for younger children. Another issue that is often problematic for school-age children involves the smoothness or flow of speech, often referred to as **fluency.**

Fluency   There are two aspects of fluency that you need to think about in sampling communication for school-age children: **stuttering** and **maze** behavior, which often affects students with language and learning disorders. We will talk first about sampling for students who stutter and then about other types of **dysfluency.**

Stuttering   The most commonly used means of assessing stuttering through natural speech involves counting stuttering events (words or syllables) from samples of the speaker's talking and, if age appropriate, from reading as well. An example of a commonly used tool for accomplishing this assessment is the *Stuttering Severity Instrument-3* (SSI-3; Riley, 1994). The cover sheet is reproduced in Figure 5.15 and illustrates that a client's evaluation is completed through a combination of scores. These scores include: 1) stuttering frequency, 2) stuttering duration (which is measured by the average of the three longest stuttering events), and 3) physical concomitant behaviors (those behaviors that are associated with stuttering, such as head movements, facial grimaces, and distracting sounds). From these three scores, a total overall score is obtained. The total score is then assigned a percentile and a degree of severity (very mild, mild, moderate, severe, or very severe).

A common critique of many standard stuttering assessments is that they do not evaluate speech in a full range of natural settings (Conture, 1996; Ingham & Riley, 1998). In order to compensate for some of these criticisms, Tetnowski (1999) devised a protocol for evaluating stuttering that assesses speech in a variety of settings and at various levels of complexity. This protocol gathers information on percentage of stuttering, length of stuttering events, and physical concomitants, as does the SSI-3; however, it includes additional information about stuttering behaviors by:

- Sampling stuttering in a variety of situations

- Sampling stuttering at various levels of length and complexity

- Sampling **postponement and avoidance behaviors**

- Sampling data related to **adaptation** and **consistency**

- Including data related to other measures such as standardized testing, **qualitative assessment, fluency induction** tasks, **speech naturalness,** and speech attitude scales

- Sampling stuttering in a variety of situations (including both in-clinic and out-of-clinic settings, with familiar and unfamiliar conversational partners)

- Sampling stuttering at various levels of length and complexity (e.g., single-word tasks, multiple-word tasks, continuous monologue and dialogue tasks; as well as tasks at various levels of cognitive difficulty, such as reading, repetition, and spontaneous formulation tasks)

The results of speech sampling procedures such as these, along with other assessment methods, can help in the differential diagnosis among stuttering and other fluency disorders.

    Maze Behavior   Another type of dysfluency is often referred to as *maze behaviors.* These include the interruption in the smooth flow of speech that is characterized primarily by mazes, which are speech disruptions that include false starts, repetitions, and revisions. Maze behaviors are often very difficult to differentiate from stuttering, in practice. But because the management implications for these two types of dysfluency are so different (one is treated as a speech disorder, the other as a language disorder), it is especially important to be able to distinguish the two types reliably. A scheme for differentiating stuttering from maze behaviors, developed by Grinager Ambrose, and Yairi (1999), appears in Table 5.6.

    Dollaghan and Campbell (1992) discussed methods of assessing this kind of dysfluency in spontaneous speech. A description of the kinds of maze behaviors typically seen in the speech of school-age clients with language-learning disorders appears in Table 5.7. Dollaghan and Campbell suggested that if *eight or more* of

Table 5.6.   Stuttering-like dysfluencies and maze behaviors

Category	Type of dysfluency	Example
Part-word repetition	Stuttering-like dysfluency	"thi-thi-this"
Single-syllable word repetition	Stuttering-like dysfluency	"and-and-and"
Disrhythmic phonations		
1. Prolongations	1. Stuttering-like dysfluency	1. "cooooookie"
2. Blocks	2. Stuttering-like dysfluency	2. "#toy"
3. Broken words	3. Stuttering-like dysfluency	3. "o#pen"
Interjections	Maze behavior	"um"
Revision/abandoned utterance	Maze behavior	"Mom ate/Mom fixed dinner"
Multisyllable word/phrase repetition	Maze behavior	"because-because" "I want-I want to go"

Source: Grinager Ambrose & Yairi, 1999.
Note: # is a pause in phonation.

these maze behaviors occur per 100 words of spontaneous speech (with words that are part of mazes or dysfluent speech events *excluded* from the 100 words), then the speech can be considered significantly disrupted.

SSI-3

Stuttering Severity Instrument-3

TEST RECORD AND FREQUENCY COMPUTATION FORM

Name _____

Sex M F   Grade _____   Age _____

Date _____   Date of Birth _____

School _____

Examiner _____

Preschool ___ School Age ___ Adult ___ Reader ___ Nonreader ___

READERS TABLE

1. Speaking Task		2. Reading Task		NONREADERS TABLE 3. Speaking Task	
Percentage	Task Score	Percentage	Task Score	Percentage	Task Score
1	2	1	2	1	4
2	3			2	6
3	4	2	4	3	8
4–5	5	3–4	5	4–5	10
6–7	6	5–7	6	6–7	12
8–11	7	8–12	7	8–11	14
12–21	8	13–20	8	12–21	16
22 & up	9	21 & up	9	22 & up	18

Frequency Score (use 1 + 2 or 3) ☐

Average length of three longest stuttering events timed to the nearest 1/10th second		Scale Score
Fleeting	(.5 sec or less)	2
Half-second	(.5– .9 sec)	4
1 full second	(1.0– 1.9 secs)	6
2 seconds	(2.0– 2.9 secs)	8
3 seconds	(3.0– 4.9 secs)	10
5 seconds	(5.0– 9.9 secs)	12
10 seconds	(10.0–29.9 secs)	14
30 seconds	(30.0–59.9 secs)	16
1 minute	(60 secs or more)	18

Duration Score (2 – 18) ☐

Evaluating Scale

0 = none
1 = not noticeable unless looking for it
2 = barely noticeable to casual observer
3 = distracting
4 = very distracting
5 = severe and painful-looking

DISTRACTING SOUNDS	Noisy breathing, whistling, sniffing, blowing, clicking sounds	0 1 2 3 4 5
FACIAL GRIMACES	Jaw jerking, tongue protruding, lip pressing, jaw muscles tense	0 1 2 3 4 5
HEAD MOVEMENTS	Back, forward, turning away, poor eye contact, constant looking around	0 1 2 3 4 5
MOVEMENTS OF THE EXTREMITIES	Arm and hand movement, hands about face, torso movement, leg movements, foot-tapping or swinging	0 1 2 3 4 5

Physical Concomitants Score ☐

Frequency _____ + Duration _____ + Physical Concomitants _____ = ☐

Percentile _____

Severity _____

© 1994 by PRO-ED, Inc.

10 9 8 7 6   96

For additional copies of this form (#6722), contact PRO-ED, 8700 Shoal Creek Blvd., Austin, TX 78757

Figure 5.15.   The Stuttering Severity Instrument-3. (From Riley, G. [1994]. *Stuttering Severity Instrument-3* [p. 1]. Austin, TX: PRO-ED; reprinted by permission.)

Voice Quality and Resonance   Children's voice problems typically stem from three main sources:

1. **Vocal abuse,** or the straining of the voice due to prolonged periods of loud talking, yelling, or attempting to speak at an unnatural pitch

2. **Craniofacial anomalies,** such as a cleft palate or lip, which result in structural differences that affect voice quality and resonance

3. **Cerebral palsy,** a congenital neurological disorder that may lead to a difficulty in motoric aspects of speech production

Methods of assessment for these kinds of voice problems are similar for children and adults and will be discussed when we look at adult voice problems.

Speech Sampling in Adults

Like aphasias, speech problems are often acquired by adults as a result of illness or injury. In fact, aphasias are often accompanied by **dysarthrias** and **apraxias**, which affect speech intelligibility.

Articulation and Intelligibility   Disorders of articulation and intelligibility in adults are most frequently the result of acquired motor speech disorders that affect respiration, phonation, resonance, and articulation. These disorders of

Table 5.7. Maze behaviors

Maze behaviors	Description	Example
Pauses		
Filled	Nonword, one-syllable filler vocalization	*um, er*
Silent	Silent intervals of 2 seconds or more	
	More than one silent or filled pause in succession	*He, um, said [pause] I could leave early.*
Repetitions		
Forward	Repetition of an incomplete unit, which is then completed	*He, he said I could leave early.*
Exact	Repetition of a completed unit	*He said I could leave I could leave.*
Backward	Insertion of additional word(s) before the repeated unit, without changing it	*He said I guess he said I could leave.*
Revisions	Modifications to correct errors, add or delete information	*I have two puddies, puppies.* *My older brother my brother hates soccer.* *My sister, I means my brother, is late.* *I have a sister, two sisters.*
Orphans	Linguistic units without obvious relations to other parts of the utterance	*I saved up in all my money.* *And spuh that's her date.*

speech production are usually classified as dysarthrias and apraxias and are contrasted with acquired language disorders such as aphasia. Aphasia and related disorders affect language understanding and formulation; motor speech disorders, however, affect only the actual motor production of the speech signal. Motor speech disorders include the speech patterns associated with Parkinson's disease, multiple sclerosis, amyotrophic lateral sclerosis (ALS), cerebral palsy, tumor, trauma, and stroke, as well as other disorders that affect the speech-production mechanism.

Dysarthrias are motor speech impairments that are marked by consistent errors due to a neuromuscular impairment of the speech mechanism. Because the muscles used to control speech also control other functions, dysarthria affects speech movements as well as nonspeech movements such as chewing, smiling, swallowing, and so forth. Apraxias, however, are a disturbance of neuromotor programming. **Apraxia of speech** can exist without any apparent muscle weakness or paralysis, which are the defining characteristics of dysarthria. It should be noted that because dysarthria, apraxia, and aphasia can be a result of damage to the central nervous system, they can, and often do, exist in combination with each other. This can make differential diagnosis quite difficult.

Duffy (1995) has outlined principles for assessment of motor speech disorders, which should include complete oral mechanism and standardized motor speech evaluations, in addition to the assessment of intelligibility and the acoustic properties of speech that come out of the analyses of spontaneous speech samples. Many of the same procedures that we discussed for assessing intelligibility in speech samples from school-age children can be applied to those adults with motor speech disorders. A phonetic transcription of a speech sample could be used to study error patterns produced by the client. PCC or the *Weiss Intelligibility Test* can also be used to determine overall rate of intelligibility in adult speakers. In addition to analysis of spontaneous speech, standard reading passages are often used to gather information on adults with speech disorders. These passages are constructed to contain all of the phonemes of English so that a relatively short sample provides an example of the client's production of each sound in the language. The "Rainbow Passage" (Fairbanks, 1940) is an example of a reading task often used in this way.

Fluency   Fluency issues, particularly those related to stuttering, can be problems for adults as well as children. The speech sampling approaches that we talked about for school-age children can be used with adults as well. With adults, reading samples are an especially important part of the sampling procedure and are often contrasted to spontaneous speech.

Prosody   Much of the meaning conveyed through language comes not from the words themselves, but from the way they are said: the rate at which we speak, the intonation that we use, the pauses that we insert, and the stress that we place on parts of the utterance. All of these paralinguistic cues go into determining the prosody of speech—its rhythm and music. Prosodic function is affected in a variety of communication disorders. Certain kinds of brain damage result in **dysprosody.** Children with autism and some kinds of specific language disorders may show prosodic impairments. People with hearing impairments

THE RAINBOW PASSAGE

When the sunlight strikes raindrops in the air, they act like a prism and form a rainbow. The rainbow is a division of white light into many beautiful colors. These take the shape of a long round arch, with its path high above, and its two ends apparently beyond the horizon. There is, according to legend, a boiling pot of gold at one end. People look, but no one ever finds it. When a man looks for something beyond his reach, his friends say he is looking for the pot of gold at the end of the rainbow.

Throughout the centuries men have explained the rainbow in various ways. Some have accepted it as a miracle without physical explanation. To the Hebrews it was a token that there would be no more universal floods. The Greeks used to imagine that it was a sign from the gods to foretell war or heavy rain. The Norsemen considered the rainbow as a bridge over which the gods passed from earth to their home in the sky. Other men have tried to explain the phenomenon physically. Aristotle thought that the rainbow was caused by reflections of the sun's rays by the rain. Since then physicists have found that it is not reflection but refraction by the raindrops that causes the rainbow. Many complicated ideas about the rainbow have been formed. The difference in the rainbow depends considerably upon the size of the water drops, and the width of the colored band increases as the size of the drops increases. The actual primary rainbow observed is said to be the effect of superpositioning of a number of bows. If the red of the second bow falls on the green of the first, the result is to give a bow with an abnormally wide yellow band, because red and green lights when mixed form yellow. This is a very common type of bow, one showing mainly red and yellow, with little or no green or blue.

From Fairbanks, G. (1940). *Voice and articulation drillbook* (p. 127). New York: Harper & Brothers; reprinted by permission.

often produce abnormal prosody, as do people with apraxia of speech, either developmental or acquired. Prosody is usually evaluated in spontaneous speech by making a global judgment as to its overall acceptability in conversation. Several of the pragmatic rating scales that we looked at earlier include prosody as one element of their checklist. A more formal measure of prosodic production was developed by Shriberg, Kwiatkowski, and Rasmussen (1990). Their *Prosody Voice Screening Protocol* (PVSP) allows trained raters to assess three independent aspects of prosody (phrasing, rate, and stress)—as well as the pitch, quality, and resonance of the voice—in each utterance in a spontaneous speech sample. The proportion of utterances judged to contain inappropriate prosody in each of these areas can be computed and compared with a database of typical speakers. McSweeney and Shriberg (in press) have applied this analysis to several types of communication disorders and shown varying patterns of dysprosody across these disabilities.

Voice Quality and Resonance

Vocal Quality   A majority of assessment of voice in spontaneous speech relies on the clinician's "trained ear." That is, clinicians develop the experience and knowledge to judge when a voice is far enough away from the ideal for age, physique, health status, and gender that a difference or disorder exists. The following dimensions of the voice are usually evaluated, using the trained ear:

- Fundamental frequency: too high or too low

- Loudness: too loud or too soft

- Quality: breathy, hoarse, or harsh (see the following information)

Voice specialists also use direct **endoscopic observation** of the larynx, as well as instrumental acoustic and aerodynamic evaluations, to assist in an accurate diagnosis of the voice. More information on these formal analyses can be found in

---

PERCEPTUAL DESCRIPTIONS OF VOCAL PARAMETERS

Breathiness: the perception of expressive air leakage during voice production due to the vocal folds not completely closing. This can be due to vocal fold paralysis; irregularities along the edge of the vocal fold(s); or mass lesions such as **nodules, polyps,** or **cysts.**

Hoarseness: the perception of breathiness along with the perception of "noise" in phonation. This is caused by irregular vibration of the vocal folds and can be related to mass lesions, inflammation of the vocal folds (laryngitis), or **Reinke's edema.**

Harshness: the perception of excessive tension, tightness, or effort in the voice. This is also associated with hard glottal attacks and overadduction of the vocal folds. Harshness is often associated with many neurological abnormalities or structural abnormalities of the larynx. It can also be noted in learned abnormal behavior patterns or overcompensation for a learned behavior.

Hypernasality: the perception of too much nasality in the voice. It is commonly noted in structural abnormalities like clefting of the palate and with neurological impairments affecting cranial nerves IX, X, and XI.

Hyponasality: the perception of not enough nasality in the voice. This is the perceptual quality that you hear in clients with severe colds or allergies. The voice is marked by a lack of nasal quality in the voice where you would normally expect a nasal quality (i.e., /n/, /m/, /g/) and the vowels that surround them. In addition to these descriptive terms, you can also evaluate patients based on the appropriate use of pitch and loudness.

Baken (1996); Bless and Bacon (1992); Orlikioff and Bacon (1993); and Till, Yorkson, and Beukelman (1994). Computer-assisted methods are often used to make many of the relevant measurements of the voice without equipment that is invasive to the client. A review of these systems is provided by Bielamowicz, Kreiman, Gerratt, Dauer, and Berke (1996) and Read, Buder, and Kent (1992). Acoustic analysis tools such as these can provide information related to **fundamental frequency, spectral analysis, formant analysis, signal-to-noise ratio,** and **perturbation** of the speaking voice. Examples of these systems are shown in Figures 5.16 and 5.17.

    Resonance   An assessment for appropriate nasality, or **resonance** patterns, is often needed for children with cleft palates and patients who undergo **laryngectomy** surgery, as well as adults with motor speech disorders (Andrews, 1995; Deem & Miller, 2000; Prater & Swift, 1984). The clinician's trained ear is again the analysis tool used initially to determine the appropriateness of resonance in connected speech. The clinician's determination usually involves a judgment as to whether speech demonstrates

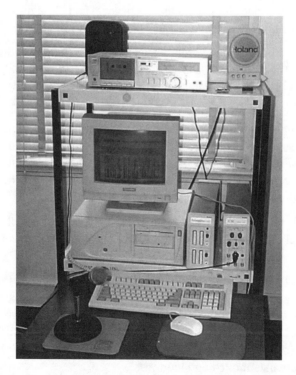

Figure 5.16. Example of a desktop computer speech analysis tool from Kay, Computerized Speech Laboratory.

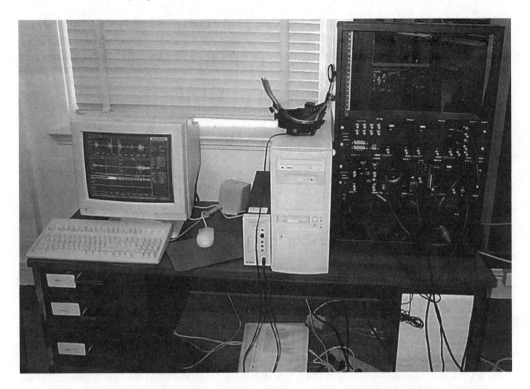

Figure 5.17.   Example of a desktop computer speech analysis tool from Tucker-Davis Technologies, System II with Computerized Speech Research Environment Software.

- Normally nasality

- Hypernasality (overly nasal speech)

- Hyponasality (denasal speech, which is produced when a person has "a *code* in the *dose*")

Again, when clinicians detect an abnormal degree of nasality, they will often follow up with more structured tasks, requiring the subject to repeat sentences with high loading of nasal consonants ("*Mary* has *nine new* stuffed a*nim*als.") and those without ("Ted has a dog with white feet."), in order to determine how the client is able to constrain nasality within an utterance. Instrumental evaluations of resonance may also be part of the assessment battery.

CONCLUSION

The sampling of spontaneous communication is an essential part of the assessment of any communication disorder. Only by observing and analyzing clients' real communication in natural settings can clinicians understand what clients are attempting to get across, where their communication breaks down, and what we can do to improve their communicative effectiveness. Communication sampling can be examined throughout all developmental levels for a wide range of speech and language domains, including syntax, pragmatics, semantics, phonology, and vocal presentation. The sampling and analysis of a client's spontaneous communicative behavior is one of the most fundamental of clinical methods and one in which every clinician needs to be competent.

REFERENCES

Andrews, M.L. (1995). *Manual of voice treatment.* San Diego: Singular Publishing Group.

Applebee, A. (1978). *The child's concept of a story: Ages 2 to 17.* Chicago: University of Chicago Press.

Arbuckle, T., Gold, D., Frank, I., & Motard, D. (1989, November). *Speech of verbose older adults: How is it different?* Paper presented at the Gerontological Society of America, Minneapolis, MN.

Baken, R. (1996). *Clinical measurement of speech and voice.* San Diego: Singular Publishing Group.

Bar-Adon, A., & Leopold, W. (1971). *Child language: A book of readings.* Upper Saddle River, NJ: Prentice Hall.

Beukelman, D., & Mirenda, P. (1998). *Augmentative and alternative communication: Management of severe communication disorders in children and adults* (2nd ed.). Baltimore: Paul H. Brookes Publishing Co.

Bielamowicz, S., Kreiman, J., Gerratt, B.R., Dauer, M.S., & Berke, G.S. (1996). Comparison of voice analysis systems for perturbation measurement. *Journal of Speech and Hearing Research, 39,* 126–134.

Bless, D., & Bacon, R. (1992). Introduction: Assessment of voice. *Journal of Voice, 6,* 95–97.

Brinton, B., & Fujiki, M. (1992). Setting the context for conversational language sampling. In W. Secord (Ed.), *Best practices in school speech language pathology* (Vol. II, pp. 9–19). San Antonio, TX: Psychological Corp: Harcourt, Brace, Jovanovich.

Brown, R. (1973). *A first language, the early stages.* Cambridge, MA: Harvard University Press.

Calculator, S. (1997). Fostering early language acquisition and AAC use: Exploring reciprocal influences between children and their environments. *Augmentative and Alternative Communication, 13,* 149–157.

Chapman, R. (1978). Comprehension strategies in children. In J.F. Kavanaugh & W. Strange (Eds.), *Speech and language in the laboratory, school and clinic* (pp. 308–327). Cambridge, MA: The MIT Press.

Cheney, L., & Canter, G. (1993). Informational content in the discourse of patients with probable Alzheimer's disease and patients with right brain damage. *Clinical Apasiology, 21,* 123–134.

Coehlo, C. (1998). Analysis of story grammar. In L. Cherney, B. Shadden, & C. Coehlo (Eds.), *Analyzing discourse in communicatively impaired adults* (pp. 115–122). Gaithersburg, MD: Aspen Publishers.

Conture, E.G. (1996). Treatment efficacy: Stuttering. *Journal of Speech and Hearing Research, 39,* s18–s26.

Crystal, D., Fletcher, P., & Garman, M. (1991). *The grammatical analysis of language disability: A procedure for assessment and remediation.* San Diego: Singular Publishing Group.

Deem, J.F., & Miller, L. (2000). *Manual of Voice Therapy.* Austin, TX: PRO-ED.

deVilliers, J., & deVilliers, P. (1973). A cross-sectional study of the acquisition of grammatical morphemes. *Journal of Psycholinguistic Research, 2,* 267–278.

Dollaghan, C., & Campbell, T. (1992). A procedure for classifying disruptions in spontaneous language samples. *Topics in Language Disorders, 12,* 56–68.

Duffy, J.R. (1995). *Motor speech disorders: Substrates, differential diagnosis, and management.* St. Louis: Mosby.

Evans, J., & Craig, H. (1992). Language sample collection and analysis: Interview compared to freeplay assessment contexts. *Journal of Speech and Hearing Research, 35,* 343–353.

Fairbanks, G. (1940). *Voice and articulation drillbook.* New York: Harper & Brothers.

Gleason, J., Goodglass, H., Obler, L., Green, E., Hyde, M., & Weintraub, S. (1980). Narrative strategies of aphasic and normal-speaking subjects. *Journal of Speech and Hearing Research, 23,* 370–382.

Glennen, S., & DeCoste, D. (1997). *Handbook of augmentative and alternative communication.* San Diego: Singular Publishing Group.

Gold, D., Andres, D., Arbuckle, T., & Schwartzman, A. (1988). Measurement and correlates of verbosity in older people. *Journal of Gerontology, 43,* 27–34.

Goodglass, H., & Kaplan, E. (1983). *Boston Diagnostic Aphasia Examination.* Boston: Lea & Febinger.

Grinager Ambrose, N., & Yairi, E. (1999). Normative disfluency data for early childhood stuttering. *Journal of Speech, Language, and Hearing Research, 42,* 895–909.

Halliday, M., & Hasan, R. (1976). *Cohesion in English.* London: Longmon.

Halper, A., Cherney, L., Burns, M., & Mogil, S. (1996). *Clinical management of right hemisphere dysfunction* (2nd ed.). Gaithersburg, MD: Aspen Publishers.

Hughes, D., McGillivray, L., & Schmidek, M. (1997). *Guide to narrative language.* Eau Claire, WI: Thinking Publications.

Hunt, K. (1965). *Grammatical structures written at three grade levels* (Research Report No. 3). Urbana, IL: National Council of Teachers of English.

Klecan-Aker, J., & Kelty, K. (1990). An investigation of the oral narratives of normal and language-learning disabled children. *Journal of Childhood Communication Disorders, 13,* 207–216.

Larson, V., & McKinley, N. (1995). *Language disorders in older students.* Eau Claire, WI: Thinking Publications.

Leadholm, B., & Miller, J. (1992). *Language sample analysis: The Wisconsin guide.* Madison, WI: Wisconsin Department of Public Instruction.

Lee, L. (1974). *Developmental sentence analysis.* Evanston, IL: Northwestern University Press.

Liles, B., & Coehlo, C. (1998). Cohesion analysis. In L. Cherney, B. Shadden, & C. Coehlo (Eds.), *Analyzing discourse in communicatively impaired adults* (pp. 65–84). Gaithersburg, MD: Aspen Publishers.

Long, S., & Fey, M. (1993). *Computerized profiling* (computer program; version 7.2). Ithaca, NY: Computerized Profiling.

Lund, N., & Duchan, J. (1993). *Assessing children's language in naturalistic contexts* (3rd ed.). Upper Saddle River, NJ: Prentice Hall.

McSweeney, J., & Shriberg, L. (in press). Clinical research with the Prosody Voice Screening Protocol. *Journal of Speech, Language, & Hearing Research.*

McWhinney, B. (1996). The CHILDES system. *American Journal of Speech-Language Pathology, 5,* 5–14.

Miller, J. (1981). *Assessing language production in children: Experimental procedures.* Needham Heights, MA: Allyn & Bacon.

Miller, J., & Chapman, R. (2000). *SALT: Systematic analysis of language transcripts* (computer programs to analyze language samples). Madison: University of Wisconsin. (Originally published in 1985.)

Miller, J., Freiberg, C., Rolland, M., & Reeves, M. (1992). Implementing computerized language sample analysis in the public school. *Topics in Language Disorders, 12*(2), 69–82.

Mordecai, D., & Palin, M. (1982). *Lingquest 1 & 2* (computer program). East Moline, IL: Lingquest Software.

Morrison, J., & Shriberg, L. (1992). Articulation testing versus conversational speech sampling. *Journal of Speech and Hearing Research, 35,* 259–273.

Myers, P. (1979). Profiles of communications deficits in patients with right cerebral hemisphere damage. In R. Brookshire (Ed.), *Clinical aphasiology: Conference proceedings* (pp. 38–46). Minneapolis, MN: BRK.

Nelson, N. (1998). *Childhood language disorders in context: Infancy through adolescence* (2nd ed.). Columbus, OH: Charles E. Merrill.

Nicholas, L., & Brookshire, R. (1993). A system for quantifying the informativeness and efficiency of the connected speech of adults with aphasia. *Journal of Speech and Hearing Research, 36,* 338–350.

Nicholas, L., & Brookshire, R. (1995). Presence, completeness, and accuracy of main concepts in the connected speech of non-brain-damaged adults and adults with aphasia. *Journal of Speech and Hearing Research, 38,* 145–156.

O'Brien, M., & Nagle, K. (1987). Parents' speech to toddlers: The effect of play context. *Journal of Child Language, 14,* 269–279.

Orlikioff, R., & Bacon, R. (1993). *Clinical speech and voice measurement: Laboratory exercises.* San Diego: Singular Publishing Group.

Owens, R. (2001). *Language development* (5th ed.). Needham Heights, MA: Allyn & Bacon.

Paul, R. (2001). *Language disorders from infancy through adolescence: Assessment and intervention* (2nd ed.). St. Louis: Mosby.

Prater, R.J., & Swift, R.W. (1984). *Manual of Voice Therapy.* Austin TX: PRO-ED.

Prutting, C., Gallagher, T., & Mulac, A. (1975). The expressive portion of the N.S.S.T. compared to a spontaneous language sample. *Journal of Speech and Hearing Disorders, 40,* 40–49.

Prutting, C., & Kirchner, D. (1983). Applied pragmatics. In T.M. Gallagher & C.A. Prutting (Eds.), *Pragmatic assessment and intervention issues in language* (pp. 29–64). San Diego: College-Hill Press.

Read, C., Buder, E.H., & Kent, R.D. (1992). Speech analysis systems: A survey. *Journal of Speech and Hearing Research, 33,* 363–374.

Retherford, K. (1993). *Guide to analysis of language transcripts* (2nd ed.). Eau Claire, WI: Thinking Publications.

Riley, G. (1994). *Stuttering Severity Instrument-3.* Austin, TX: PRO-ED.

Roth, F., & Spekman, N. (1984). Assessing the pragmatic abilities of children: Part 1. Organizational framework and assessment parameters. *Journal of Speech and Hearing Disorders, 49,* 2–11.

Scarborough, H. (1990). Index of productive syntax. *Applied Psycholinguistics, 11,* 1–22.

Shadden, B. (1998). Sentential/surface level analyses. In L. Cherney, B. Shadden, & C. Coehlo (Eds.), *Analyzing discourse in communicatively impaired adults* (pp. 35–64). Gaithersburg, MD: Aspen Publishers.

Shriberg, L. (1993). Four new speech and prosody-voice measures for genetics research and other studies in developmental phonological disorders. *Journal of Speech and Hearing Research, 36,* 105–140.

Shriberg, L., & Kwiatkowski, J. (1980). *Natural process analysis.* New York: Macmillan.

Shriberg, L., & Kwiatkowski, J. (1982). Phonological disorders III: A procedure for assessing severity of involvement. *Journal of Speech and Hearing Disorders, 47,* 256–270.

Shriberg, L., Kiwatkowski, J., & Rasmussen, N. (1990). *Prosody voice screening protocol.* Tuscon, AZ: Communication Skillbuilders.

Tetnowski, J.A. (1999). *A stuttering profile.* Unpublished manuscript.

Till, J., Yorkson, K., & Beukelman, D. (1994). *Motor speech disorders: Advances in assessment and treatment.* Baltimore: Paul H. Brookes Publishing Co.

Tyack, D., & Gottsleben, R. (1974). *Language sampling, analysis, and training* (Rev. ed.). Palo Alto, CA: Consulting Psychologists Press.

Ulatowska, H., Doyle, A., Freedman-Stern, R., Macaluso-Haynes, S., & North, A. (1983). Production of procedural discourse in aphasia. *Brain and Language, 18,* 306–316.

Weiss, C. (1982). *Weiss Intelligibility Test.* Tigard, OR: C.C. Publications.

Westby, C.E. (1998). Communicative refinement in school age and adolescence. In W. Hayes & B. Shulman (Eds.), *Communication development: Foundations, processes, and clinical applications* (pp. 311–360). Baltimore: Lippincott Williams & Wilkins.

Wetherby, A., & Prizant, B. (1993). *Communication and Symbolic Behavior Scales.* Baltimore: Paul H. Brookes Publishing Co.

Yoder, P., & Davies, B. (1990). Do parental questions and topic continuations elicit replies from developmentally delayed children: A sequential analysis. *Journal of Speech and Hearing Research, 33,* 563–573.

Yorkston, K., & Beukelman, D. (1980). An analysis of connected speech samples of aphasic and normal speakers. *Journal of Speech and Hearing Disorders, 45,* 27–35.

Yorkston, K., & Beukelman, D. (1981). *Assessment of intelligibility of dysarthric speech.* Tigard, OR: C.C. Publications.

1. *Why is communication sampling an important part of assessment?*

2. *What are the specific questions an assessment of nonverbal communication attempts to answer?*

3. *For what kind of samples is video recording needed? Audio recording?*

4. *What sampling contexts are appropriate for preschoolers? School-age children? Adults?*

5. *What are the advantages and disadvantages of computer-assisted analysis methods? Of manual methods?*

6. *How are utterances segmented in transcription of preschool language samples? School-age samples? Adult samples?*

7. *In addition to looking at syntax, what other areas need to be examined in communication samples of adults with acquired disorders?*

8. *Discuss two methods for assessing speech intelligibility.*

9. *Discuss the difference between stuttering and maze behavior dysfluencies. Why is this distinction important?*

10. *What is the "Rainbow Passage" and for what is it used?*

11. *How are voice quality, resonance, and prosody typically assessed using communication sampling?*

Principles
of Intervention

Froma P. Roth
Rhea Paul

Perhaps you will recall the six clients we talked about in Chapter 3:

1. Darrell, a preschooler with immature, unintelligible speech whose parents want him to improve his speech before he begins kindergarten next year

2. Jonah, a 7-year-old, with a severe bilateral sensorineural hearing loss. His school district referred him for re-evaluation of his hearing, speech, and language and to determine whether his amplification equipment continues to be appropriate for him

3. Anna, a seventh-grade student with significant learning disabilities

4. Marlene, a 50-year-old woman with communication difficulty since her stroke 8 months ago

5. Richard, age 62, who recently underwent a total laryngectomy and wants to use esophageal speech

6. Thomas, a 27-year-old with a history of severe stuttering, who feels that his speech disorder is interfering with his ability to advance in his career

We talked in some detail about assessment strategies for these and other clients. Once the assessment is completed, though, a clinician is faced with implementing the recommendations made in the assessment. This phase of clinical practice is called **intervention.** The purpose of intervention is to affect change in communicative behavior to maximize an individual's potential to communicate effectively. The way in which this purpose is achieved varies according to the nature of the disorder, the age and therapy history of the client, the family situation, and the client's learning style and preferences. Whatever methods of intervention are chosen, intervention is designed to teach strategies for improving overall communication, rather than teaching specific behaviors. Olswang and Bain (1991) discussed three basic purposes that intervention can serve.

1. In some cases, the purpose is to *eliminate the underlying cause* of the disorder. For example, the provision of amplification to a 9-month-old infant with a mild hearing impairment may prevent, or at least minimize, the emergence of developmental speech and language difficulties. For Jonah, audiological re-evaluation may determine that his current speech and language difficulties are due to a change in hearing status that requires a change in amplification. In this case, a new intervention program, involving new hearing aids, may eliminate the underlying disorder.

2. In other cases, the purpose may be to teach a client **compensatory strategies** to improve functional communication. This purpose may be appropriate for Marlene, who needs to learn new ways to get her ideas across when her speech is unintelligible due to motor neuron damage as a result of a stroke. Anna, too, may need to learn compensatory strategies to help her cope in the school setting. And Richard's desire to learn esophageal speech shows that he is eager to find a compensatory mechanism to allow him to communicate vocally despite the loss of his larynx.

3. A third form of intervention is to *modify the disorder* by teaching specific speech, language, or pragmatic behaviors that enable an individual to become a more mature communicator. Darrell, for example, may receive instruction on the correct production of his error sounds or sound classes to achieve improved speech production skills and better overall speech intelligibility. Thomas, our client with dysfluency, may not be able to entirely eliminate stuttering moments. If this is the case, he may need to learn to modify his stuttering so that it interferes less with his social communication.

There are a variety of philosophies for planning intervention. The common thread among all approaches, however, is that communication intervention is a dynamic process that proceeds in a systematic progression. Following the diagnosis of a communication disorder, the clinician selects appropriate target behaviors for therapy. Training procedures are then developed and implemented to promote the acquisition of the target behaviors. The intervention process is completed when the client demonstrates mastery of these target behaviors. Periodic monitoring is often performed to ensure the retention and stability of the newly acquired behaviors (Roth & Worthington, 2001).

When planning intervention, there are three aspects of a program that need to be considered: its products, its processes, and its contexts (Paul, 2001). This chapter discusses the products and processes of intervention. The contexts, or the circumstances under which intervention takes place, are discussed in Chapter 9.

INTERVENTION PRODUCTS

The first step in planning intervention is the identification of the communicative behaviors to be acquired in the program. These are drawn from assessment data and are usually called *long-term goals*. Long-term goals are the relatively broad changes in communicative behavior to be achieved during a course of therapy. The achievement of these goals will be justification for *terminating* therapy.

Marlene's stroke left her very limited in speech production, unable to verbalize her wants and needs, and depressed as a result of her frustration. Long-term goals for Marlene include

- Increasing the amount of intelligible speech

- Increasing the ability to communicate wants and needs

- Decreasing the frustration by providing alternative means of communication

Once general long-term goals have been identified, clinicians must decide how to help the client progress toward them. This is accomplished by formulating steps so that progress can be observed and measured and will lead the client toward the long-term goal. To facilitate this, therapy steps are stated in a specific form as **behavioral objectives.** There are three components of a behavioral objective:

1. The *do* statement identifies the action that the client is to perform. This statement should contain verbs that name observable actions, such as *point, label, repeat, say, match, write, name, ask*. Words to avoid in behavioral objectives are those that refer to processes that cannot be observed directly, such as *understand, know, learn, remember, comprehend,* or *discover.*

2. The *condition* identifies the situation in which the target behavior is to be performed; such as when it will occur, where, in whose presence, and with what materials or cues. Examples of condition statements are:

   Following a clinician's model
   In response to a question
   Given a list of written words
   In response to pictures
   In presence of other therapy group members

3. The *criterion* specifies how well the target must be performed for the objective to be achieved. Typically used criteria include:

   90% correct
   Eight correct trials of 10
   Fewer than four errors in three consecutive sessions
   Consistently over a 10-minute period

At this point, you might like to try writing a behavioral objective for one of Marlene's long-term goals. One example follows, to help you get started:

Do statement	Condition	Criterion
1. Marlene will produce the words *no* and *yes* appropriately	In response to clinician questions	With 8 of 10 intelligible responses
2. Marlene will ...		

Before beginning a therapy program, the clinician must be sure that the client cannot already perform the target behavior independently. This might seem obvious; but often a diagnosis is made on the basis of standardized tests that include only one item for a particular communication element, and a client may have missed that one item for a variety of reasons. This is an example of why potential therapy targets must undergo a **pretest** before an intervention program is initiated. The pretest allows a clinician to establish that the client has not already mastered a target behavior. When the clinician observes that the client is achieving target behaviors in most intervention activities, he or she administers a **posttest** to determine the client's consistency with target behavior. The pretest and posttest are usually the same; they consist of a set of 10–20 opportunities for the client to produce the target form when presented with minimal cues, prompts, or other supports from the clinician. Suppose one behavioral objective for Darrell was

Do statement	Condition	Criterion
Darrell will produce fricative sounds (/s/, /z/, /ʃ/) in final position	In imitation of clinician's model with picture cues	With 8 of 10 correct responses

Before beginning intervention, a pretest (such as the one that follows) would be administered to ensure that a reasonable goal has been set:

Stimulus	Response	Criterion
Show picture card. "Here's a fish. What is it?"	*"fish"*	9 of 10 correct productions of final fricatives

If the client failed to attain the criterion on the pretest, intervention on this target would be provided using the techniques that follow. When the client achieves criterion levels of correct production in the intervention situation, a posttest is given to determine whether the objective has been met, using the same stimuli, responses, and criterion that were used in the pretest.

Once long-term and short-term objectives have been established and pretested, it is necessary to determine how to move the client toward achieving these objectives. This process usually involves **task analysis.** In a task analysis, a larger goal is broken down into small steps that can be followed to achieve it. To accomplish this breakdown, a clinician examines the input and output prerequisites necessary for completing the task. Consider Marlene's first long-term goal: increasing the intelligibility of speech. The requirements of the goal can be analyzed this way:

• Sensory: She must hear the speech spoken to her

• Motor: She must be able to make oral articulatory movements

• Language: She must have some degree of semantic (word meaning) and syntactic (sentence structure) skill

• Cognitive: She must have some degree of conceptual and problem-solving ability; she must not be inordinately confused or demented

A clinician would then proceed, by means of informal assessment, to determine whether Marlene has the requisite skills. If not, the clinician might revise the goal or work on developing its prerequisites. If Marlene demonstrates the requisite abilities, then the clinician devises a series of steps, or a **task sequence,** through which Marlene will be guided in order to achieve the goal. The whole process, from establishing task prerequisites to sequencing steps to achieving goals, is what we refer to as *task analysis*. Figure 6.1 presents a sequence of difficulty for both verbal and nonverbal behaviors that is typically used in communication intervention. A task analysis encourages the clinician to move from the simplest forms of response to more complex forms in the course of the intervention program. Table 6.1 gives an example of the sequence of steps a clinician might choose for Marlene to increase her production of intelligible speech. In summary, identifying the products or targets of intervention requires a clinician to

• Establish long-term goals, using pretest probes

• Identify short-term objectives that build toward the long-term goals

• Use task analysis to create task sequences through which clients progress toward their goals

Once these steps have been accomplished, the next challenge is to find activities that facilitate this progress. To face this challenge, a clinician has a range of intervention processes.

INTERVENTION PROCESSES: THE CONTINUUM OF NATURALNESS

Intervention activities vary in their degree of naturalness (see Table 6.2). These variations have been described by Fey (1986) as falling along a "continuum of naturalness." This continuum represents the degree to which intervention contexts correspond to everyday communication situations and interactions.

	Nonverbal	Verbal
Simple	Manipulated movement/gesture (clinician moves client's hand to form a gesture)	Immediate imitation (client repeats immediately after clinician)
	Imitated movement/gesture (clinician provides a model and asks client to imitate it)	Delayed imitation (clinician gives verbal model, some intervening speech, then asks client to imitate)
	Elicited movement/gesture (clinician asks client to produce gesture or movement without a direct model)	Partial imitation (clinician produces part of the target; client is asked to produce the whole target)
	Spontaneous movement/gesture (client produces movement/gesture appropriately without model or request for it)	Elicitation with object cue (clinician asks client for verbal response with an object as a cue)
		Elicitation with picture cue (clinician asks client for verbal response with a picture as a cue)
		Elicitation with written cue (clinician asks client for verbal response with a written word as a cue)
		Elicitation with question (clinician asks client for verbal response with a conversational question as a cue)
Complex		Spontaneous response (client produces target appropriately without model or request for it)

Figure 6.1.   Task sequence.

This framework can be adapted for a broad range of communication disorders and ages.

According to Fey (1986), three factors affect naturalness: 1) the intervention activity itself, 2) the physical context in which the activity takes place, and 3) the individuals with whom the client interacts during intervention (see Table 6.3). Clinician-directed (CD) approaches and client-centered (CC) approaches represent the end points of this continuum.

Clinician-Directed (CD) Approaches

In CD approaches, the clinician controls all aspects of the intervention from determining therapy goals to selecting stimulus materials, choosing the type and fre-

Table 6.1. Task sequence for Marlene

1. Using sounds she can produce, have Marlene imitate simple words, such as *no, uh-huh, come, stop, hi.*

2. Have Marlene produce these words without a direct imitative model (using delayed imitation; e.g., "Hi, Marlene. Nice to see you.").

3. Have Marlene practice using the words in "scripts" designed around daily activities, using picture cues (e.g., with a series of pictures, tell Marlene a story about a woman's day, starting with greeting a friend, refusing a cigarette, or agreeing with a colleague. Then have her produce the target word at an appropriate point in the story, using prompts if necessary.).

4. Have Marlene "practice" using these words in conversations with family members as the clinician "coaches" with cues and prompts.

quency of reinforcement, determining the order of activities, and identifying the specific target responses to be elicited. Behavioral theorists refer to these kinds of activities with the acronym A-B-C:

A: Antecedent or stimulus: The clinician provides a model of the desired behavior, or a prompt to produce it.

B: Behavior: The client responds by producing a target behavior.

C: Consequence: The clinician provides reinforcement if the client's behavior was produced correctly. If not, the clinician provides feedback or correction or may ignore the incorrect behavior.

Behaviorist theory holds that all behavior occurs following some identifiable antecedent that prompts it and is maintained or discouraged by its consequence. What a clinician needs to do, in this view, is to manage the antecedents and consequences so that they facilitate the production of desired behaviors. To accomplish this management, behaviorists rely heavily on the operant procedures that follow. These approaches are not considered naturalistic because of the degree of clinician control and their lack of adherence to the conventions of genuine reciprocal communication.

Table 6.2. Continuum of naturalness for a broad spectrum of communication disorders

Least natural ←	→	Most natural
CD	**Hybrid**	**CC**
Drill	Organized activities	Daily activities
Drill play	Milieu teaching	Facilitative play
CD modeling	Focused stimulation	Daily routines
	Script therapy	Vocational activities
	Role playing	
	Conversational coaching	
More naturalistic modifications of CD activities (e.g., structured scripts)		

Source: Fey, 1986.

Table 6.3.   Factors affecting the degree of naturalness of intervention

Activity	Drill	Organized activities	Daily activities
Physical context	Clinic	School/place of work	Home
Social context	Clinician	Teacher/co-worker	Family members

Source: Fey, 1986.

The most common CD approaches are *drill* and *drill play.* Drill is considered the most highly structured format (Shriberg & Kwiatkowski, 1982). The clinician selects the training stimuli, explains the specific target response to the client, presents stimulus items in a predetermined order, and reinforces correct responses tangibly (e.g., with candy or a token), verbally (e.g., "Good job!"), or nonverbally (e.g., the client gets a "high five" from the clinician). In drill play, the drill is embedded in a game format so that the client is motivated by the activity itself to produce the target forms as well as by the reinforcement that follows the correct production. For example, Darrell's clinician might have him play a game in which five paper bags are labeled with target words. He is given a sponge ball to toss into one of the sacks (motivating activity), then he must say the word on the sack. He is only reinforced for correct production. Reinforcement may be tangible or the chance to take another turn at the game.

CD approaches are thought to be most effective during the initial stages of intervention to establish a new target behavior. Once established, transitional activities can be introduced to provide the client with more naturalistic contexts in which to practice and use the new communicative behavior to achieve carry-over or **generalization**—the use of target forms outside of the therapy situation without support from the clinician.

Client-Centered (CC) Approaches

CC approaches emphasize the provision of communication therapy in authentic settings. The assumption underlying these approaches is that individuals will achieve therapy goals more readily and generalize newly learned behaviors more spontaneously when taught in the context of familiar experiences and activities with supportive communication partners. In CC activities, the client directs the intervention and determines the content, timing, and sequence of therapy. The key steps in naturalistic, or CC, approaches involve *waiting* for the client to initiate a behavior, *interpreting* the behavior as communicative (whether communication was intended), and *responding* to the behavior in a way that places it in a communicative context (Fey, 1986). In contrast to CD approaches, the clinician does not attempt to elicit a predetermined set of responses from the client. Instead, the clinician follows the client's lead and offers consistent and meaningful responses that relate to the client's own actions or utterances. CC approaches are considered highly naturalistic because the client is engaged in enjoyable and meaningful daily activities with a responsive, communicative partner.

The most common CC activity used with children is **facilitative play,** which is an indirect stimulation technique (Hubbell, 1981; Shriberg & Kwiatkowski,

Procedures Used in Operant Conditioning

Cue: A signal (verbal or nonverbal) that tells the client when to produce the response; for example, clinician taps child on the hand to cue the response to each stimulus.

Delayed imitation: Client echoes clinician after some intervening material that follows the stimulus; for example, clinician says, "This is green. It's my favorite color. What color is it?"

Direct (immediate) imitation: Client echoes clinician immediately after stimulus is presented; for example, clinician says, "This is green. This is_____."

Fading: Systematic withdrawal of reinforcement after a behavior is established; can be accomplished by decreasing the amount of reinforcement or by requiring more instances of the target behavior before reinforcement is given. Fading, then, causes variation in the reinforcement schedule.

Prompt: A hint, directive, or minimal guidance (verbal or nonverbal) to assist a client in producing a behavior; for example, clinician strokes his or her neck with a finger to remind the client with dysfluency to use easy onset.

Reinforcement: Item or activity that increases the frequency of a correct response; for example, a favorite food, a turn with a toy, or a monetary payment.

Reinforcer: Item or activity provided following a behavior that results in the increase of the behavior. Reinforcers can be:

- **Primary:** Biologically necessary or important, such as food or water

- **Secondary:** Items or activities that become important because they are linked to primary reinforcers; for example, if a bell is rung when food is presented, then the bell becomes a secondary reinforcer

- **Social:** Praise, approval, or attention is given as a consequence for a behavior, rather than a tangible object; for example, "That was good talking!"

Reinforcement schedule: The frequency with which reinforcement is given. Schedules can be

- **Continuous:** A reinforcement is given for every response; usually used to establish a new behavior

- **Intermittent:** Reinforcement is not given for every behavior; instead behaviors are rewarded at certain intervals (e.g., after 2 minutes of successful responses; after a certain number of correct responses; given randomly for some correct responses and not others). Intermittent schedules are generally used to stabilize and maintain newly learned behaviors.

Shaping: Providing positive reinforcement contingent on successive approximations toward a target behavior; for example, when targeting the production of final consonants in words, the clinician can first reinforce the production of ANY consonant in the final position. When this behavior is consistent, it is no longer reinforced; only a behavior closer to the target will be, such as producing a consonant in the same class (e.g., sibilant, stop) as the target.

1982). The clinician arranges the physical environment to encourage a child to generate target responses spontaneously during the natural course of a play sequence. The clinician uses several techniques to promote the child's communicative participation, such as the following.

FACILITATIVE PLAY TECHNIQUES

Self-talk: Clinician observes the child's behavior and engages in the same behavior while simultaneously engaging in an animated monologue that describes the clinician's ongoing actions.

Context: Child is building a sand castle at the sand table.

Clinician is building a sand castle and says, "I'm making a castle. A big castle. See how big it is?"

Parallel talk: Clinician produces an ongoing commentary on the child's actions.

Context: Child is building a sand castle at the sand table. Clinician watches child's actions and says, "You're building a castle. It's really big. Look how big your castle is."
(In both self-talk and parallel talk, the clinician comments on the actions and events that are within the immediate attentional focus of the child.)

Expansions: Clinician reformulates a child's utterance into a grammatically more complete version.

Child: Kitty drink water.

Clinician: Yes, the kitty is drinking the water.

Extensions (Expatiations): Clinician enlarges on a child's utterance by adding new semantic information.

Child: Kitty drinking water.

Clinician: Yes, he's very thirsty today.

Recasts: Clinician expands a child's utterance into a different sentence type (e.g., declarative question form ["Kitty drink water." "Is the kitty drinking water?"]).

CC intervention also can be used with adult clients. Two primary forms of naturalistic intervention employed with adults are: *functional therapy* and *conversational group therapy.* Functional therapy involves communicative activities of daily living, which the client practices with support and scaffolding from the clinician. Thomas, our fluency client, for example, may work on talking on the telephone with his clinician. The clinician may first conduct some structured activities to encourage easy onset. Then, Thomas would be asked to use easy onset in a role-playing activity with a telephone. Finally, he would be asked to make a real telephone call, with prompts and cues from the clinician.

Conversational group therapy often is a form of treatment for adults with neurogenic disorders. Rather than (or in addition to) receiving individual, skill-focused therapy, group members engage in conversations with other clients and a clinician. As in all CC approaches, the clients determine the structure and topics of the conversation. They receive natural feedback on the relevance, intelligibility, and appropriateness of their turns from others in the group. The clinician takes advantage of a set of facilitative techniques, just as does the young child's clinician. These techniques have been summarized by Ewing (1999) and are as follows.

CONVERSATIONAL GROUP TECHNIQUES

Attending: Letting participants know that their message is being received (e.g., "I heard Marlene say..."). Facilitating questions: Encouraging clients to query each other (e.g., "Do you need to ask him what he means?")

Negotiating goals: Helping clients decide how to accomplish goals, integrate new members, and renew goals as the composition of the group and the level of disability changes (e.g., "Richard, our group has been working on decreasing frustration in communication situations. Do you have any personal goals along those lines?")

Rewarding: Providing verbal praise for participation (e.g., "Marlene, that's a very insightful thought.")

Responding to feelings: Letting clients know you understand how they feel (e.g., "I can see that it really upsets Richard to talk about his cancer.")

Focusing: Keeping group discussion on track; discouraging "side" conversations (e.g., "We were talking about using the telephone, though. Has anyone else had trouble with that?")

Summarizing: Reviewing what has been said and setting out the next steps toward the group's goal (e.g., "It sounds as if everyone has felt frustrated about using the telephone. Should we plan to talk about suggestions to help on this front next time?")

Gatekeeping: Balancing participation between members so a small group does not dominate (e.g., "Richard, do you have a thought about what Marlene said?")

Modeling: Using demonstration to teach conversational skills (e.g., "When I feel that way, I sometimes say, 'Hold on! I've got a thought on that!'")

Mediating: Resolving conflicts; encouraging conflict resolution among members (e.g., "Marlene and Richard have a difference of opinion here; does anyone see some middle ground?")

Hybrid Approaches

Hybrid approaches represent a midpoint between the two extremes of natural-ness. Hybrid approaches use intervention activities that are highly natural, but the clinician maintains control over the therapy environment to maximize learn-ing and generalization. There are three main characteristics of hybrid approaches:

1. Only one or a small set of goals are targeted for intervention.

2. The clinician selects therapy activities and materials, choosing those that pro-mote the client's spontaneous use of the target behaviors.

3. The clinician produces utterances that are contingent to the client's commu-nication but that also model and accentuate the target forms.

There are four main types of hybrid instruction:

1. Focused stimulation

2. Milieu teaching

3. Script therapy

4. Conversational coaching

Focused Stimulation   The clinician deliberately arranges the verbal and non-verbal environment to increase the likelihood that the client will spontaneously produce the target form. The clinician provides frequent models of the target behavior in meaningful and highly functional contexts to facilitate client success. Although a response is not required from the client, the environmental setup is conducive to the production of the target form. For example, the clinician can increase the salience of a target behavior by presenting it in sentence-final or stressed positions. To elicit the production of the copula *is*, the clinician may respond to the client utterance, *She tall* with "She *is*?" or "*Is* she tall?"

Two procedures that encourage client production of a target behavior are *false assertions* (Crystal, Fletcher, & Garman, 1976) and *forced alternatives* (Fey, Cleave, Long, & Hughes, 1993). In false assertions, the clinician purposely makes an inaccurate statement to urge the client to generate communicative messages that obligate the use of the target behavior (e.g., Clinician: "That's not your hat!" to elicit the copula, "Yes, it <u>is.</u>"). Forced alternatives are questions posed by the clinician that provide a model of the target behavior (e.g., Clinician: "You do like it or you don't like it?" to elicit the negative form, "I <u>don't</u> like it.").

Milieu Teaching   Milieu teaching stresses the use of ongoing activities as the basis for intervention and incorporates the operant conditioning principles of imi-tation, modeling, and reinforcement into naturalistic settings. Incidental Teaching and the Mand-Model method are two specific milieu teaching techniques. The steps involved in the Incidental Teaching approach are outlined as follows (Hart & Risley, 1975).

STEPS IN INCIDENTAL TEACHING

The clinician arranges the environment so that desired objects or items are visible to the client but out of reach (e.g., toy, newspaper).

The client initiates the interaction verbally or nonverbally, such as pointing to the desired item.

The clinician selects the target response to be evoked from the client (e.g., "I want the newspaper so I can read it.").

The clinician uses cues to obtain a more elaborated response; the first cue is focused attention, which involves physically approaching the client, making eye contact, or issuing an expectant look. If the client does not respond after a brief waiting period, the clinician then asks a general question (e.g., "What do you want?"). If the client's response to the question contains the target response, then the clinician provides confirmation that includes a model of the target form (e.g., "Yes, you want the newspaper so you can read it.").

If the question does not elicit the target response, then the clinician issues a prompt in the form of a general request (e.g., "You need to tell me."); request for partial imitation (e.g., "Say, I want the newspaper so I can read it."); or request for complete imitation (e.g., "Say, I want the newspaper so..."). If the client does not generate the target response even after the prompts, the clinician gives one additional prompt.

If the client achieves the target behavior, the clinician provides confirmation, and the communicative intent is achieved (e.g., the client is given the newspaper).

If the client does not produce the target response, then the clinician gives the client the desired item and determines the type of cue(s) that may be more effective for the next therapy session.

The Mand-Model method (Rogers-Warren & Warren, 1980) is similar to incidental teaching with two exceptions. First, it does not require the client to initiate communication before teaching begins. Rather, the clinician observes the client carefully, and when the client displays interest in an object or some aspect of the environment, the clinician *mands* a response. (e.g., "Tell me what you need."). Second, the goals are more general (e.g., elicit two-word utterances; elicit well-formed sentences), rather than specific (e.g., elicit agent–object utterances; elicit conjoined sentences). If the client produces an appropriate response, then the clinician presents verbal reinforcement and the desired item (e.g., "Great! You told me why you wanted the newspaper, and here it is."). If the client's response is inappropriate, then the clinician offers prompts such as those used in incidental teaching.

Both of these milieu approaches extend the operant procedures of imitation, prompts, and reinforcement to naturalistic activities in which the client accomplishes authentic communication goals with the behaviors being trained. In addition, the reinforcement received is a natural outcome of the communication interaction.

Script Therapy   Script therapy is an approach in which target behaviors are taught within the context of a familiar routine or script (Olswang & Bain, 1991). A *script* is an ordered sequence of events that depicts a familiar activity, such as making dinner, going to a birthday party, or ordering a meal in a restaurant (Nelson, 1985). The clinician and client enact the script, during which the clinician can violate the sequence of activities (e.g., birthday party script: clinician eats the cake before blowing out the candles), providing a natural opportunity for the client to communicate verbally or with gestures. Other violations may include hiding props necessary for the script and introducing broken or incomplete materials (e.g., unwrapped gifts). Once a script is overlearned, the clinician can use it to introduce more complex forms. For example, the client can be told to pretend that the birthday party was yesterday or will be tomorrow to encourage the production of past and future tense markers. The clinician also can have the client pretend that the birthday boy received at least two copies of every gift to promote the use of plural tense forms.

Conversational Coaching   Conversational coaching was developed by Holland (1995) to facilitate functional communication skills of adults with aphasia. This technique simulates conversational interaction in a structured context. The clinician prepares a short written script based on the client's interests, experiences, and level of communication skills. According to Holland (1995), the scripts should be written in a communicative style, consist of short sentences to promote successful communication, and emphasize target communication behaviors. An example script and a summary of the recommended procedures follow.

SAMPLE SCRIPT AND PROCEDURES FOR CONVERSATIONAL COACHING

1.   I have to change my hairdresser.

2.   She always cuts my hair too short.

3.   And I always have to wait.

4.   This time she made my bangs uneven.

5.   I need to find someone else.

The client reads the script aloud one sentence at a time.

Self-cuing strategies are suggested by the clinician when the client evidences difficulty expressing the scripted information. Common self-cuing strategies include chunking utterances into shorter units and using gestures to communicate meaning.

The clinician videotapes the client reading the script to a familiar listener who is unaware of the script's contents. The listener is "coached" to glean the gist of the script, rather than trying to understand each word.

The three participants then evaluate the videotape to determine the success level of the scripted interaction, the aspects that the listener found most and least helpful, and alternative strategies that the client and listener might have used to improve the interaction.

The coaching and evaluation format is repeated with increasingly unfamiliar listeners, and new target behaviors are scripted into conversations.

USING THE CONTINUUM OF NATURALNESS

The degree of naturalness that we use in intervention must be determined by the nature and severity of a client's communication impairment and the client's responsiveness to different intervention strategies. Highly naturalistic activities are preferred only if they bring about improved communication abilities. Less naturalistic activities should be chosen if they are more effective in eliciting a target behavior. For example, children with language impairments may have difficulty inducing linguistic rules from natural interactions and may require more focused and explicit language input.

The approaches that form the continuum are not mutually exclusive. A combination of strategies may be appropriate for a particular client. For example, one communicative objective may be accomplished most efficiently using a highly structured CD strategy, whereas the client's needs for another objective may be met through naturally occurring activities. Often, programming for the same objective may make use of several activities that can range in naturalness from highly structured to highly natural. Fey (1986) reminded clinicians that only if two activities are *equally effective* in eliciting a particular linguistic structure or communicative intention is the naturalistic one preferred, because it will more likely promote the use of the newly acquired target behavior in everyday speaking situations.

Following are examples of intervention activities at various points along the continuum of naturalness for some of the children and adults we have been discussing.

DATA COLLECTION

The collection of data on client performance has three primary purposes.

1. It permits the clinician to track the client's progress from one session to another.

2. It provides documentation of the efficacy of a particular intervention strategy or set of strategies.

3. It maximizes clinician effectiveness.

For naturalistic intervention approaches, videotaping is the data collection procedure of choice because it permits a permanent audio and visual record. Frequently, repeated viewing of an interaction/session is necessary to fully

DARRELL, A PRESCHOOLER WITH UNINTELLIGIBLE SPEECH

Target behavior: Increase ability to produce three-syllable words correctly

Drill: Clinician names a set of picture cards with three-syllable words (tomato, banana, etc.). After each label, Darrell is cued to repeat the word. Each time all three syllables are produced, he receives a token. With 40 tokens, he can "buy" a turn throwing darts at a dart board.

Hybrid: Clinician and child play the game I Spy with a picture of fruits and vegetables that Darrell has practiced saying. Darrell chooses which one to name on his turn; the clinician points to the one he names.

Daily: Clinician and child make a Thanksgiving collage together. The cut-outs include many of the fruits and vegetables Darrell has been practicing naming. As they work, the clinician names some of these or asks Darrell to name them. She praises Darrell when he names them correctly, either in imitation, in response to her request to name, or spontaneously.

JONAH, A 7-YEAR-OLD WITH A HEARING IMPAIRMENT

Target behavior: Improve classroom listening skills using appropriate amplification

Drill: Jonah imitates clinician's instructions (drawn from those typically used by classroom teacher) and acts each one out as he imitates. Clinician reinforces correct actions.

Hybrid: Clinician and Jonah play "Army," taking turns being "Sarge." Sarge gives instructions (written on slips of paper, following teacher instructions, and drawn from an army hat). The partner must correctly follow the instruction.

Daily: Clinician works with Jonah in class during an instructional activity. Using prompts and cues, she encourages him to write down the instructions, asks questions about what he does not understand, adjusts his hearing aid if needed, and so forth.

ANNA, A SEVENTH-GRADE STUDENT WITH A LEARNING DISABILITY

Target behavior: Use of *because, if,* and *so* to produce cause/effect complex sentences

Drill:	The clinician explains the use of conjunctions, such as *because, if,* and *so,* to link ideas in sentences. The clinician presents simple sentences on cards, along with the conjunctions written on paper "hooks." Anna combines each pair with the given conjunction, following the clinician's model.
Hybrid:	The clinician reads Anna a cause/effect selection from a classroom textbook. The clinician provides several models of retelling the passage, using sentences with the conjunctions practiced. Then, Anna is asked a question that she can answer with a similar conjoined sentence.
Daily:	Clinician runs a "study group" with Anna and some other students who are struggling with a classroom textbook selection that discusses cause and effect. The students are encouraged to discuss the selection. The clinician occasionally models sentences using the target conjunctions within the context of the discussion.

MARLENE, AN ADULT WITH APHASIA

Target behavior: Improve client's use of the self-cuing strategy of sentence completion for retrieving verbal labels

Drill:	Clinician presents a list of incomplete sentences, such as "We use a broom to sweep the _____ ," for the client to imitate and complete.
Hybrid:	Clinician collects several identical pairs of cards depicting objects necessary to perform daily activities and demonstrates the sentence completion strategy for the client to imitate. After imitative practice of the strategy, the clinician shuffles the deck and gives each player five cards. The clinician explains that the goal of this activity is to make pairs for all of the cards in the player's hand by taking turns, asking one another, "Do you have a _____ ?"
Daily:	The client selects three daily activities (e.g., brushing teeth, making coffee, watering the plants). The clinician and client make a list of items necessary to perform each task. The client uses the sentence completion self-cuing strategy, "I need a _____ " to request each item.

RICHARD, WANTS ESOPHAGEAL SPEECH

Target behavior: Increase client's use of appropriate prosody

Drill:	Clinician writes pairs of sentences that contain the same subject, verb, and object. Each sentence is written on a separate card

with a different word underlined (e.g., I want coffee; I want <u>coffee</u>). The clinician points to one card at a time and produces each sentence for the client to imitate.

Hybrid: Using the same set of cards as above, the clinician places a pair of cards face up on the table and asks a question for the client to answer using the prosodically appropriate sentence with exaggerated stress (e.g., Q: <u>Who</u> wants coffee?; A: <u>I</u> want coffee; Q: <u>What</u> do you want? A: I want <u>coffee</u>).

Daily: Client chooses reading passages from magazines or newspapers. The clinician highlights the words that receive primary stress. The client reads aloud each passage concentrating on emphasizing the appropriate words.

THOMAS, HAS A FLUENCY DISORDER

Target behavior: Decrease client's stuttering moments and reduce anxiety associated with dysfluencies

Drill: Clinician reads passage and engages in voluntary stuttering on predetermined words. The client imitates each of the voluntary stutters.

Hybrid: Clinician introduces a board game such as Jeopardy! and explains that the client is the contestant. After reviewing the technique of pull-outs (Van Riper, 1973), the client is instructed to use one or more pseudo or real dysfluencies in response to game questions and to modify stuttering moments using pull-outs. (Pull-outs involve stopping a dysfluency in the middle of the stuttering moment, mentally rehearsing the intended word using an easier stuttering pattern, and then reproducing it.)

Daily: The client's task is to enter a situation that previously has been identified as mildly fearful and use the pull-out technique. Example situations include: calling a family member on the telephone, making an appointment for a haircut, and asking for directions.

describe and analyze the client's verbal and nonverbal communicative behaviors. Videotaping may not be possible at all times and in all settings, though. Alternative data collection methods include the development of checklists, rating scales, graphs, audiotapes, and use of multiple observers, each focusing on a different behavioral component. Data recording forms can be developed for group as well as individual sessions. The type of notation system used to chart data yields different kinds of information. A binary system records whether a behavior is correct/appropriate or incorrect/inappropriate. An interval rating scale gives more qualitative information because behaviors are rated on a continuum (e.g., degree of accuracy or appropriateness). It also is desirable to code whether the client's behavior is gestural, vocal, or verbal, or a combination thereof. In addition, data collection procedures should allow the clinician to distinguish between imitative, prompted, self-corrected, and spontaneous responses. Figures 6.2 and 6.3 present two examples of forms that can be used to track client behaviors. You may want to try coming up with your own to track the behaviors elicited in some of the examples we reviewed previously.

CONCLUSION

The aim of all intervention is to improve communicative behavior. This means that even though clinicians structure their therapy to achieve specific, measur-

Name:_____   Behavioral objective:_____

Clinician: _____   Reinforcement type/schedule: _____

Date: _____   Materials: _____

Trials

Task	1	2	3	4	5	6	7	8	9	10	% correct

Figure 6.2.   Example of a data log. (Key: + = correct; − = incorrect; A = approximation; S = self-correction; NR = no response.)

Clinician: _____   Date: _____

Client

				Objective						# Responses					# Correct responses					% Correct				
1	2	3	4	5	6	7	8	9	10	11	12	13	14	15	16	17	18	19	20	21	22	23	24	25
26	27	28	29	30	31	32	33	34	35	36	37	38	39	40	41	42	43	44	45	46	47	48	49	50

Client

				Objective						# Responses					# Correct responses					% Correct				
1	2	3	4	5	6	7	8	9	10	11	12	13	14	15	16	17	18	19	20	21	22	23	24	25
26	27	28	29	30	31	32	33	34	35	36	37	38	39	40	41	42	43	44	45	46	47	48	49	50

Client

				Objective						# Responses					# Correct responses					% Correct				
1	2	3	4	5	6	7	8	9	10	11	12	13	14	15	16	17	18	19	20	21	22	23	24	25
26	27	28	29	30	31	32	33	34	35	36	37	38	39	40	41	42	43	44	45	46	47	48	49	50

Client

				Objective						# Responses					# Correct responses					% Correct				
1	2	3	4	5	6	7	8	9	10	11	12	13	14	15	16	17	18	19	20	21	22	23	24	25
26	27	28	29	30	31	32	33	34	35	36	37	38	39	40	41	42	43	44	45	46	47	48	49	50

Figure 6.3.   Sample group therapy data sheet.

able goals, the true objective is to increase clients' overall ability to use communication in real, functional settings. When clinicians assess the effectiveness of intervention, it is this larger goal that needs to be kept in mind. In addition, we need to remember that our goal is to help clients communicate better, not to adopt a philosophy of therapy or join a "school" of intervention. We should, in other words, take advantage of ALL of the intervention approaches available to us and match each goal for each client to the most effective technique for that particular objective. Chances are, this will change over time. Although very structured CD intervention may work for some clients early in the course of intervention, they are likely to need more naturalistic approaches later. Other clients may require a naturalistic approach early on, during the "warming up and getting to know each other" period, and may be more willing to tolerate structured formats later. Whatever activities or sequences clinicians decide to employ, their obligations are always to maximize communicative effectiveness for the client. Part of the way that clinicians do this is by being aware of the range of therapeutic options available and choosing the most appropriate for each situation. Another part is by carefully monitoring the efficacy of their intervention by keeping data throughout the course of the intervention. Tracking client behaviors allows us to know when our intervention strategies have achieved their goals so that we can move on to others or even, if we are very fortunate, have clients "graduate" from intervention. Performance data also tell us when our strategies are not working and need to be changed to provide a better match to the client's needs. Communication intervention, then, involves continual and thoughtful monitoring. That is why it takes a clinician, not a technician, to do it.

REFERENCES

Crystal, D., Fletcher, P., & Garman, M. (1976). *The grammatical analysis of language disability: A procedure for assessment and remediation.* London: Edward Arnold.

Ewing, S. (1999). Group process, group dynamics, group techniques with neurogenic communication disorders. In R. Elman (Ed.), *Group treatment of neurogenic communication disorders* (pp. 9–17). Woburn, MA: Butterworth-Heineman.

Fey, M.E. (1986). *Language intervention with young children.* San Diego: College-Hill Press.

Fey, M.E., Cleave, P., Long, S., & Hughes, D. (1993). Two approaches to the facilitation of grammar in children with language impairment: An experimental evaluation. *Journal of Speech and Hearing Research, 36,* 141–157.

Hart, B., & Risley, T. (1975). In vivo language intervention: Unanticipated general effects. *Journal of Applied Behavioral Analysis, 13,* 411–420.

Holland, A. (1995). *Current realities of aphasia rehabilitation: Time constraints, documentation demands and functional outcomes.* Paper presented at Mid-America Rehabilitation Hospital, Overland Park, KS.

Hubbell, R. (1981). *Children's language disorders: An integrated approach.* Upper Saddle River, NJ: Prentice Hall.

Leonard, L. (1975). Modeling as a clinical procedure in language training. *Language, Speech, and Hearing Services in Schools, 6,* 72–85.

Nelson, K. (1985). *Making sense: The acquisition of shared meaning.* New York: Academic Press.

Olswang, L., & Bain, B. (1991). Intervention issues for toddlers with specific language impairments. *Topics in Language Disorders, 11,* 69–86.

Paul, R. (2001). *Language disorders from infancy through adolescence.* St Louis: Mosby.

Rogers-Warren, A., & Warren, S. (1980). Mands for verbalization: Facilitating the generalization of newly trained language in children. *Behavior Modification, 4,* 230–245.

Roth, F.P., & Worthington, C.K. (2001). *Intervention resource manual for speech-language pathology* (2nd ed.). San Diego: Thompson-Singular Press.

Scollon, R. (1976). *Conversations with a one-year-old.* Honolulu: University Press of Hawaii.

Shriberg, L., & Kwiatkowski, J. (1982). Phonological disorders III: A conceptual framework for management. *Journal of Speech and Hearing Disorders, 47,* 242–256.

Van Riper, C. (1973). *Speech correction: Principles and methods.* Upper Saddle River, NJ: Prentice Hall.

1. What are the three basic purposes of intervention?

2. What are the three components of a behavioral objective?

3. Discuss the sequence of steps used to do a task analysis.

4. Describe three points along the continuum of naturalness of intervention activities.

5. Describe a drill activity to teach correct /s/ production to a 5-year-old client.

6. Describe three types of language used in facilitative play.

7. Name six steps involved in incidental teaching.

8. Create an activity for a client with aphasia, using a conversational coaching approach.

9. Compare and contrast two means of clinical data collection.

10. What is meant by "hybrid" intervention techniques?

7

Interviewing, Counseling, and Clinical Communication

Kevin M. McNamara

As audiologists and speech-language pathologists (SLPs), we need to be effective in sharing information with clients across the entire continuum of clinical services: interviewing and counseling clients; documenting evaluation findings; developing treatment plans; recording outcomes; and educating family members, teachers, medical personnel, and caregivers regarding a client's communication needs. In each of these tasks, information must be conveyed clearly and understandably to clients, families, educators, other care providers, and administrators. To successfully accomplish this, we need to learn sensitive and efficient strategies for sharing information with the people that we serve. Our effectiveness in communicating information will contribute a good deal to the quality of the therapeutic relationships that we establish with our clients. It will impact our ability to advocate for appropriate services and equipment for those that we serve, as well as obtain adequate funding for those services. Poorly written clinical documentation can severely compromise a clinician's professional credibility (Roth & Worthington, 1996), and a poor oral communication style can negatively impact our ability to establish trusting relationships with clients and to relate vital clinical information to them. Part of our job as clinicians for people with communication disorders is to be skilled communicators ourselves.

BASIC PRINCIPLES OF ORAL AND WRITTEN CLINICAL COMMUNICATION

As clinicians, we rely on a set of principles governing effective communication in order to exchange information with those that we serve in a manner that is sensitive and appropriate to their needs. Information shared either orally or in writing should be presented in a manner that is concise, well organized, and related to a clearly stated topic. Sensitivity must be shown to issues such as a listener's or reader's language style, emotional needs, and level of familiarity with the topic being discussed. In the case of written reports, audiologists and SLPs may be writing for a mixed and sometimes unknown audience of readers, many of whom will differ from us in terms of educational backgrounds, language styles, and cultural perspectives. Unlike direct verbal exchanges, in which a listener has an opportunity to provide verbal and nonverbal feedback in order to clarify or expand the information being presented, there is not always an immediate opportunity for readers to ask for clarification or to confirm their understanding of written information. In order to increase our effectiveness in both oral and written communication, some general principles of effective clinical communication follow.

PRINCIPLES OF EFFECTIVE CLINICAL COMMUNICATION

In both oral and written presentations:

- Clearly introduce the topic about which you are writing or speaking.

- Organize all information in a logical, cohesive manner by subtopic.

- Avoid using technical language whenever possible. Use vocabulary and a language style easily understood by the people with whom you are communicating.

- Explain technical terms (when you cannot avoid using them) parenthetically or by stating examples.

- Use objective terms such as *observed, completed,* or *demonstrated;* avoid vague or judgmental terms such as *appears* or *seemed*.

- Avoid redundancy unless you are summarizing key concepts.

- Use people-first language (e.g., "a man with aphasia," "a person who stutters"), rather than referring to people as disabilities (e.g., "an aphasic," "a stutterer").

During direct verbal exchanges:

- Attend to the comfort of your listener.

- Explain the purpose of your discussion.

- Organize questions and informational statements in an orderly, sequential manner.

- Establish trust by being an active, empathetic, and nonjudgmental listener.

- Allow the person(s) with whom you are communicating to be an active participant in the conversation, ensuring opportunities for him or her to respond to questions, make comments, and ask questions.

- Remember that individuals comprehend information differently. Provide sufficient time for your listener to process and react to your statements.

- Be sensitive to and respectful of cultural differences and their impact on interpersonal communication. Avoid imposing your own cultural values, especially if they appear to conflict with those of your listener.

- Watch for both verbal and nonverbal cues from your listener to see if you are presenting your message in a way that is understandable and culturally acceptable. Rephrase, expand, or eliminate statements and questions based on these cues.

- Enlist the aid of interpreters to assist in situations in which you must verbally communicate with people who do not comprehend English or other languages in which you are proficient. Exercise extra caution in these situations to ensure that your message is being translated appropriately and that you accurately comprehend the information being conveyed to you via an interpreter.

The information that you convey to people during the course of their engagement with you can at times be difficult or even painful for them to hear. A family in the initial phase of identifying their child's hearing loss or communication impairment or an adult faced with a newly acquired communication disorder due to neurological damage or disease process must come to terms with a new and unfamiliar disability. This change in status may have a significant impact on a family's hope and expectations for their child or an individual's own perception of self-worth (Shames, 2000). As new clinicians, you may be tempted to avoid confronting your clients with "bad news" regarding their prognoses for improvement or limited achievements in therapy. In addition, you may at times be asked by clients or administrators to provide information that you do not have or be pressured to say or write things that you do not believe or cannot substantiate through research or clinical data. Above all else, clinicians are bound by ethical practice to be honest in all interactions with their clients, as well as with those people and agencies that support them. The Code of Ethics of the American Speech-Language-Hearing Association (ASHA) clearly stresses your responsibility for truthfulness in all aspects of your clinical practice. It states,

Individuals shall honor their responsibility to the public by promoting public understanding of the professions, by supporting development of services designed to fulfill the unmet needs of the public, and by providing accurate information in all communications involving any aspect of the professions. (ASHA, 1994, p. 2; see Chapter 2)

It is possible, however, to share difficult information with your clients in a manner that is supportive, sensitive, and truthful if you employ the basic principles of effective clinical communication.

OVERVIEW OF FORMATS USED TO GATHER AND CONVEY CLINICAL INFORMATION

The formats that you use to share information with your clients and those individuals and agencies that support them are influenced by a number of factors. The type of information being conveyed, as well as the audience with whom it is being shared, may in part determine whether you use a structured versus informal or a written versus oral format. Specific speech-language pathology or audiology programs or facilities may follow policies that dictate the use of particular formats for documenting evaluation results, intervention programs, and outcome data. For example, early intervention programs for children from birth to 3 years of age, school-based services for children 3–21 years of age, and geriatric speech pathology and audiology services funded by Medicare all have documentation requirements, formats, and time lines influenced by federal, state, and local policies.

Reviews of Existing Records

You have an obligation as a clinician to consider the needs of the people that you serve in the context of their home, school, work, family, and social interactions (Tomblin, 2000). A review of existing records can provide vital pieces to the puzzle revealing an individual's communication needs in those settings. Other audiologists or SLPs, as well as other medical, therapeutic, or educational service providers, may have already seen the clients who now seek your assistance. These previous contacts may yield medical reports, educational records, previous speech-language and audiological evaluations, and documents summarizing past intervention. You can gain knowledge of previous medical, cognitive, psychological, or psychiatric diagnoses, as well as previously documented information regarding an individual's social, adaptive, and educational functioning, from such reports. This will allow you to make more appropriate decisions regarding evaluation strategies, efficacy of intervention, and specific management goals, and avoid recommending intervention protocols that may be contraindicated by medical status or previously unsuccessful therapy. Remember that clients or their guardians ultimately control to whom information is released, and that "the confidentiality precept applies to both oral and written communication between clients and clinician and includes reports and other clinical records" (Silverman, 1999, p. 15; see Chapter 2).

CASE EXAMPLE 1

Mr. Rodrigues, a 78-year-old man, has just been transferred from an acute care unit in a local hospital to a short-term rehabilitation unit of a skilled nursing facility. He experienced a stroke approximately 2 weeks ago and received speech therapy in the hospital setting prior to his transfer. He has been admitted to the rehabilitation unit with doctor's orders for speech therapy evaluation and treatment of residual communication and swallowing problems secondary to his stroke.

If you were the SLP evaluating Mr. Rodrigues in the skilled nursing facility you could, theoretically, assess both his communication and swallowing status without looking first at the information available from his previous stay in the hospital acute care unit. By doing so, though, you would miss vital information essential to the safe and effective management of this client. For example, it would be essential for you to review information regarding his ability to swallow safely, as determined by a modified barium swallow (MBS) study performed in the hospital setting, prior to initiating dysphagia (swallowing) therapy. Implementing therapy procedures or diet modifications and feeding protocols based on insufficient information about the patient's functioning in this area may put him at risk for aspiration or other related and potentially life-threatening medical complications such as pneumonia. Specific information regarding the nature of the client's brain damage, as revealed through a CT scan, and more general medical information regarding the individual's overall health status will help you to determine a realistic prognosis for improvement of his communication and swallowing skills. Access to this information would allow you to understand the etiology of the client's impairment better and to make more appropriate treatment decisions that are consistent with his medical status and potential for improvement.

CASE EXAMPLE 2

Susan, a 7-year-old girl with a severe bilateral sensorineural hearing loss, has recently moved with her family to a new home in a different state. She currently wears two behind-the-ear hearing aids. She has been referred to a local audiologist's office for an audiological re-assessment and to explore the possibility of being fitted with an FM system to enhance her classroom listening skills.

In Susan's example, it is essential that as the new audiologist you have an opportunity to review previous findings regarding this young girl's hearing status in order to monitor for potential deterioration of hearing across time. A review of previous audiological evaluations, recommendations for hearing aids and other assistive listening devices, and follow-up documentation of audiological intervention will allow you to make better decisions regarding your own assessment and management of the child's audiological needs. In addition, reviewing related educational and speech-language pathology records will allow you to understand the functional, social, and academic communication needs of the child better and to offer recommendations for equipment and audiological management strategies that are appropriate for those needs and settings.

As you review existing records, you must remember that "information from other professionals can potentially lead to a biased view of your client's condition" (Shipley & McAfee, 1998, p. 5). It is essential to balance your own clinical observations and findings with the information reported from other sources when making diagnostic and intervention decisions.

Interviews

One of the most useful ways we can gain insight into the needs and backgrounds of our clients is by directly interviewing them and the people who care for them. An **interview** is an organic, fluid, and multifaceted process that is guided by the clinician and constructed by all participants (see Figure 7.1). It is a vehicle for gathering relevant information and educating people on issues related to communication disorders. It is also the first opportunity to begin to establish a trusting and cooperative relationship with clients and their families. It is a task that requires clinicians to employ active listening skills (Luteman, 1991; Shames, 2000); to be sensitive to individual personal, cultural, and linguistic styles (Battle, 1998); and to exercise flexibility in both their approach to questioning and responses to the information being shared. In addition to your clients and their families, you may interview doctors (general practitioners or specialists such as otolaryngologists, neurologists, or pediatricians), nurses, caregivers, classroom

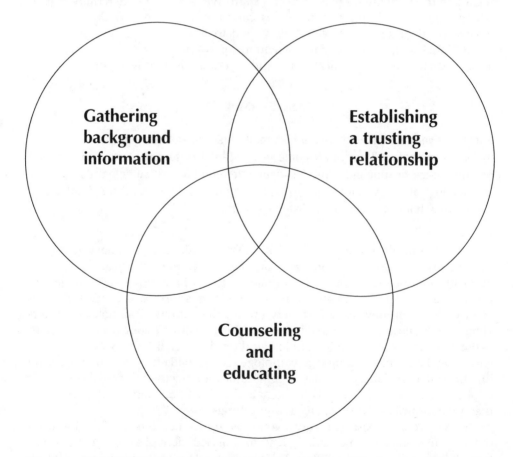

Figure 7.1.   The interrelationship of counseling, questioning, and trust building in a clinical interview.

teachers, special educators, social workers, vocational counselors, and clinicians from other disciplines including physical and occupational therapists and psychologists.

Establishing Trust

Shapiro (1999), in his discussion of interviewing parents of children who stutter, noted the importance of beginning a clinical interview in a positive and supportive manner. He stated that

Too often the communication problem becomes the immediate focus rather than the people with whom we are interacting. A social greeting enables clinicians and clients to begin the journey as co-equal participants in a shared process, and helps to establish a social and personal foundation. Before we can respect and respond to each other's roles and responsibility as clients or clinicians within the clinical process, we must first value each other as people. The importance of establishing positive rapport cannot be overstated. (p. 225)

Being sensitive to differences in cultural styles can help clinicians better establish respect and trust during an interview. For example, Latino clients and their families may view an initial period of informal talking as an appropriate prelude to more serious discussions, whereas an attempt to discuss such issues immediately may be considered rude (Anderson & Fenichel, 1989; Zungia, 1992). African Americans (and members of many other cultural groups), however, may find it disrespectful if too casual an approach is taken during an interview. Professionals are cautioned to address family members in a formal manner, using titles and surnames, unless specifically invited to do otherwise, or risk impeding the establishment of respect and trust (Willis, 1992).

Using Appropriate Question Formats to Elicit Information

Clinicians rely on a variety of question types to elicit information during an interview. **Open-ended questions** are typically used to initiate an interview, allowing the person being questioned to establish the direction of the interview by expressing issues that he or she hold as priorities. These questions encourage the client to be an active participant rather than a passive respondent in the interview process. Hall and Morris (2000) noted that by using open-ended questions, clinicians, while controlling the general background areas being explored, do not control the range of responses elicited from a client or how extensively the person responds. Questions or statements such as "How can I help you today?" or "Tell me about the trouble you're having hearing" allow you to relinquish some of the control held in an interview to the respondent, leading to increased trust and willingness to share information about sensitive and important issues.

After the client has had an opportunity to express priority concerns by responding to open-ended questions, you may find it necessary to use **closed questions** to elicit more specific information or narrow the range of response. There are a finite number of possible answers to questions such as "How much did your son weigh when he was born?" or "When was the date of your last hearing evaluation?" The use of such question forms allows the interviewer to regain more control of the interview and focus on more specific clinical issues. A particularly narrow form of closed questions are those requiring only a "yes" or "no" response. These types of questions require the respondent to confirm or deny statements made by the clinician and allow the client no control over the intent or direction of the question.

As with all interpersonal interactions, cultural values and styles may impact how a person responds to certain question forms. For African Americans, direct questions may at times be seen as harassing, and silence on the part of African American listeners may denote their refutation of what they perceive as an accusation rather than acceptance of that statement (Shipley & McAfee, 1998). Latino clients, out of respect for people in professional roles, may refrain from openly expressing disagreement with a clinician's statements, even though they may not agree with him or her (Langdon & Cheng, 1992). Members of some Asian cultures, to avoid offending a person, may say what they think the listener wants to hear, rather than what they themselves believe (Roseberry-McKibbin, 1995). Gender differences also play a part in how an interviewee may respond to questions, and this especially may be the case with some Middle Eastern cultures that place restrictions on the content and format of interactions between people of different genders. Even within our broader collective American culture, differences in communication styles often demonstrated by men and women may lead to miscommunication. This can be seen in a woman's affirmative head nod to indicate active listening and empathy with the speaker and a man's use of the same gesture to convey agreement (Maltz & Borker, 1982). A more comprehensive discussion of multicultural issues related to communication disorders can be found in Chapter 10.

Case History Questionnaires

A written **case history questionnaire** is a tool that is used to gather and organize information regarding the nature of speech, language, and hearing concerns; general developmental and health history; educational background; and history of related support services. By presenting both general and specific questions, it attempts to elicit a client's perception of the communication disorder and its impact on daily communication needs. Case history questionnaires may be broad in their scope of questions related to basic communication functions or may be customized to include questions related to specific issues such as hearing loss, central auditory processing disorder, fluency or voice disorders, and augmentative communication needs. Separate formats are typically used for adults and children (see Figure 7.2 for an adult format).

In some practice settings, clients or caregivers are asked to complete a case history questionnaire prior to arriving or a few minutes before the start of their initial diagnostic evaluation. You must be cautious, however, that you do not create barriers for people who are attempting to gain access to clinical services by making their first task the completion of a long, jargon-filled, and often confusing and intimidating questionnaire form. Alternatively, case history questionnaires may be more flexible in use as a guide for question topics during person-to-person diagnostic or intake interviews. As students, you may find the structure offered by such forms useful as you develop skills in the areas of interview and

Name: _____ Date: _____

1. How old were you when your hearing loss was first identified?

2. What have you done about your hearing loss?

3. What do you feel is the cause of your hearing problem?

4. Has a physician examined your ears?
   Who?   Date of last examination?

5. Have you experienced pain in either of your ears?   When?
   Describe.

6. Have you ever had ear infections (running ears)?
   Which ear?   When?

7. Have there been any changes in your hearing in the last 6 months?

   Last year?

   Last 2 years?

8. Do you have any allergies?
   Describe.

9. Do you ever feel dizzy?   How often?

10. Does your hearing seem better on some days than on others?

11. Have you ever worn a hearing aid?

Figure 7.2.   Sample questions found on an audiological case history form for adults.

evaluation. Try not to rely too much on the rigid format of written case history questionnaires during client interviews, though, as inflexible use of these forms may interfere with efforts to modify your interpersonal and language styles to better meet the needs of the people whom you are interviewing (Haynes & Pindzola, 1998; Shapiro, 1999).

Evaluation Reports

Written **diagnostic evaluation reports** are used to summarize information obtained in both audiological and speech and language evaluations. These reports serve as an official record of assessment findings, diagnoses, and recommendations (Meitus, 1983) and as a written description of the hearing and communication profiles of the individuals who are being evaluated. They are legal documents that, as is the case with all of our written documentation, may be called into legal proceedings to determine service provision and liability issues. The actual format for an evaluation report will vary across settings and sometimes by individual clinician or supervisor and may include specific outlines for individually written reports, or in some cases prewritten forms or checklists into which the details and interpretations from an individual client's evaluation are inserted. There are even software programs that, after the clinician inserts individual details, will generate a customized written summary report. Regardless of the format used, most evaluation reports contain specific sections presenting identifying and background information, a summary of test results and diagnostic observations, interpretations of findings, prognosis for improvement, and recommendations. A well-written diagnostic report is one that presents all information in an organized and sequential manner and efficiently integrates all diagnostic data, interpretations, and recommendations. We will examine the structure of a diagnostic report in greater detail later in this chapter.

Oral Reports/Conferences

Throughout our interactions with clients, we share information orally as well as in writing. You will continue to answer questions from your clients and their family members and caregivers regarding intervention procedures and outcomes. With their written permission, you may share information concerning your client's communication needs with teachers, program administrators, and insurers in order to advocate for the materials, resources, or funding necessary for adequate treatment of their communication disorders. The expanding role that SLPs and audiologists play in providing collaborative intervention rather than direct services has increased the frequency and importance of orally reporting information regarding our clients' communication needs to others collaborating to support these individuals (ASHA, 1991, 1993).

Case conferences are focused opportunities to present information to or about your clients. During these exchanges, you may follow a more outlined and systematic approach to sharing information than you do in more casual oral reports. The specific content may be dictated by the purpose of the conference, as well as by the needs of the participants. Examples of formal case conferences include individual meetings with clients and families to discuss evaluation and treatment outcomes and teacher conferences to discuss a student's communication needs in the classroom setting. Clinicians working in hospitals or rehabilitation centers may meet with other therapists, medical personnel, caregivers, and family members to discuss the client's progress in therapy and his or her multidisciplinary service needs. Regardless of the setting, audiologists and SLPs are responsible for presenting information in a succinct and organized manner that is easily understood by clients as well as those supporting them.

Treatment Plans

After an initial assessment of speech, language, and/or hearing needs has been completed, a determination is made regarding the need for intervention. This decision is based in part on evaluation findings, client and family priorities, program eligibility requirements, and other related factors. Once the decision for intervention is made, a formal **treatment plan** is developed. Formats for treatment plans may be determined by both federal and state regulations governing a particular type of service delivery program, as well as by the standards and protocols associated with individual practice settings. Examples of comprehensive treatment plans that outline a broad range of supports and outcomes within and outside the realm of communication include school-based **individualized education programs (IEPs), individualized family service plans (IFSPs)** for children from birth to 3 years old who are enrolled in early intervention programs, and **overall plans of service (OPS)** for adults with developmental disabilities.

In addition to these comprehensive plans, clinicians may develop treatment plans that outline individual sessions of speech, language, and audiology intervention in greater detail. These plans usually include long-term goals and short-term objectives related to speech, language, hearing, and other communication needs. Targeted communication behaviors are identified, as well as the conditions under which they are expected to occur, and measurable criteria for success are stated for each behavior. Intervention techniques, activities, and materials are listed as well. Such plans serve as a guide from which we organize and implement individual therapy sessions and are similar in purpose to the lesson plans developed by classroom teachers. During your clinical training, you will be asked to develop and implement treatment plans that offer a greater level of detail than experienced clinicians rely on in order to facilitate your understanding of intervention and documentation processes.

SOAP Notes

Therapeutic intervention is a dynamic process in which continual changes to therapy objectives and activities are made in response to a client's performance, as well as to new information revealed through ongoing assessment. The **SOAP note** *(Subjective, Objective, Assessment, Plan)* is a format often used in medical and other settings to record and analyze data specific to a client's ongoing performance in therapy (Golper, 1998). SOAP notes are documents summarizing the clinician's observations regarding a client's level of attention and participation in therapy, *(subjective)*, specific data regarding performance on therapy tasks *(objective)*, interpretation of those subjective observations and objective data *(assessment)*, and recommendations for future action based on that interpretation *(plan)*. SOAP notes may be quick handwritten entries in an individual's chart in a hospital or rehabilitation setting or may take the form of more extensive reports summarizing a person's progress in therapy. The SOAP note format may also be used for reporting more detailed diagnostic findings.

INDIVIDUAL TREATMENT PLAN FOR SPEECH-LANGUAGE THERAPY

Long-term goal(s):

1. José will increase his recognition and use of picture communication symbols in order to express needs and participate in classroom activities.

Short-term objective(s):

1. José will match 10 newly introduced picture symbols depicting classroom materials with the actual objects they represent with 80% accuracy.

2. José will point to the above-mentioned picture symbols presented on a picture symbol communication board when named by the clinician with 80% accuracy.

3. José will request a minimum of two items needed during a classroom activity by pointing to an appropriate picture symbol on a picture symbol board with no more than verbal prompting from the clinician.

Procedures:

Verbal instruction, object/picture matching, visual modeling of targeted behavior, physical cueing, verbal reinforcement

Activities:

1. Object/picture matching using the "Treasure Hunt" game

Objectives targeted during activity: 1

Materials needed: Picture symbol cards, corresponding objects

2. Arts and crafts project on curriculum-based reading theme

Objectives targeted during activity: 2, 3

Materials needed: Picture communication board, corresponding objects, craft material, storybook

A BRIEF PROGRESS NOTE IN A SOAP FORMAT

S: Mr. Smith was alert and oriented during today's session. Nursing reported an increase in his waking hours and general orientation to surroundings since yesterday evening. Mr. Smith's wife was present during the last half of therapy and reported that he was frustrated the night before at his inability to "find the right words."

O: Mr. Smith pointed to pictures of familiar household items with 75% accuracy (15 of 20) when named by the clinician, and with 80% accuracy (8 of 10) by function. He named 20% (2 of 10) of the same pictures with maximum cueing from the clinician. Severe dysarthria persisted, negatively impacting speech intelligibility. Imitation of lingual movements (tongue tip elevation, lateralization, and tongue retraction) was slow and labored.

A: Mr. Smith continues to demonstrate severe word finding problems, negatively impacting functional communication, as well as limited speech intelligibility secondary to oral motor weakness. An increase in word recognition and overall alertness and orientation to communication partners was noted since the last treatment session.

P: Continue speech therapy 30 minutes per day, targeting increased word finding and speech intelligibility. Provide picture board of common objects to facilitate word finding when conversing with wife and nurses. Counsel wife regarding strategies to facilitate word finding and repair communication breakdowns.

Progress Reports

At periodic intervals throughout the course of your clients' treatment, you will be required to summarize and document their cumulative progress toward achieving targeted intervention goals and to make recommendations regarding their need for continued therapy. These intervals are typically determined by the regulations governing the specific program in which the service is being provided, as well as by funding source requirements, and may vary from 1 month or less to 1 year or more. In these days of increasing demands on clinicians' time, and increasingly limited funding for our services, it has become critical for us to make carefully documented decisions regarding the continued need for intervention based on client outcome data. ASHA called for an "unbroken stream of activity seeking to provide the effectiveness of clinical procedures"(1995, p. 37). **Progress reports** are used as vehicles to summarize and review a client's cumulative achievement of intervention goals and objectives across a specific period of time and to outline the future direction of intervention. Typically, such reports contain brief background information, a summary of specific goals and objectives, a data-based analysis of the client's progress in those areas, an interpretation of those data and other related factors including prognosis for change, and recommenda-tions regarding the need for and direction of future intervention.

Discharge Summaries

Discharge from audiology and speech-language pathology services is based on a number of interrelated factors. These may include a client's progress (or lack of progress) toward targeted objectives, achievement of functional communication status, successful fitting and use of hearing aids or other assistive listening devices, funding limitations, and a client's changing priorities regarding commu-nication intervention. A **discharge summary** is a written report of a client's cumulative progress from the initiation of therapy to his or her discharge. As in the case of a progress report, a summary and interpretation of an individual's accomplishments and continued needs are made based on a review of cumulative client performance data, on our judgment regarding the person's prognosis for further change, and on other related variables. Recommendations for necessary posttreatment supports or services are typically offered.

Professional Correspondence

SLPs and audiologists often exchange information regarding clients with other professionals serving those same individuals. A variety of written correspondence formats are used to share client information, including **referral letters** to other service providers, **follow-up letters** to those referring clients for audiology and speech-language pathology services, and requests for the release of information from other service providers. At times we write **letters of justification** to advo-cate for diagnostic or therapy services, hearing aids, FM systems, communication devices, and other supports for our clients. In all cases, written permission must be obtained from a client before any information can be released between prac-titioners or agencies, and clients have the final decision about what information, if any, may be released.

REPORTING DIAGNOSTIC FINDINGS

It is essential for SLPs and audiologists to share diagnostic assessment findings in a manner that is efficient, well organized, and clearly understood by all who need access to this information. This process begins with a verbal review of findings shared with your client and his or her family or caregivers immediately after the completion of the evaluation and continues with a written summary of findings that becomes a permanent record of this information.

Evaluation Feedback

It is a general expectation of anyone seeking the help of professionals to have at least some feedback regarding findings immediately following an evaluation. Think about your last trip to your general physician for a comprehensive physi-cal examination. Although you know that your doctor will not have the results of blood tests, throat cultures, biopsies, or other lab tests immediately following your examination, you would expect him or her to take a few minutes to summarize the general findings of his or her evaluation and implications regarding your overall health status. Failure to do so would certainly leave you in a state of uncertainty and anxiety, potentially reducing your confidence in the physician's ability to effectively evaluate and manage your health needs. Individuals who seek our help in diagnosing hearing loss, swallowing, speech, language, and other communication disorders have a similar need for immediate feedback from us, and they experience many of the same concerns if we neglect to provide a summary of our findings at the conclusion of our evaluation.

How can you immediately summarize your evaluation findings before you have had time to score tests, transcribe language samples, or carefully analyze the relationship between all of the diagnostic data collected during the course of an evaluation? First, clearly state that all comments made during follow-up counseling sessions are only your first impressions of diagnostic findings and will be subject to possible revision after you have had time to carefully analyze the information that you have collected. Review the purpose of the assessment activities that your client has just completed and your initial impression of the outcomes of each of those activities in order to help the client begin to better understand both the reasons for those activities and their implications concerning his or her communication status. Such a review provides you with a systematic and sequential structure through which to begin to relay your findings and helps you to convey information in smaller segments more easily processed by your client.

In addition to providing a mechanism to summarize evaluation results, engaging in postevaluation feedback presents an opportunity for audiologists and SLPs to continue the process of educating clients about communication disorders that began during the preassessment interview—this is the next step in developing a partnership between client and clinician. As is the case during an initial interview, the style in which you present information when counseling a client after an evaluation is as important as the content. Haynes and Pindzola (1998) cautioned to "refrain from being didactic; do not lecture your clients. Focus on sharing options rather than giving advice"(p. 49). You should begin your discussion with a summary of strengths demonstrated by the client and transition to areas of weakness in measured increments based on your perceptions of his or her ability to accept and process that information. Incorporate information abut normal processes of hearing and communication, and relate this information to the profile of communication strengths and needs that you have identified for your client. Again, as in all clinical interactions, use language that is readily understood by clients, their family, and their caregivers. You must be alert to both verbal and nonverbal signals from your listeners regarding their level of understanding and you should paraphrase or modify the style and content of your statements accordingly. Remember that the counseling following a diagnostic assessment often takes place immediately after a long and sometimes arduous evaluation session that may leave the participants fatigued and emotionally drained. Too much technical information, information that is presented in a rapid and confusing manner, or information that is presented in a style inconsistent with the culture of the individual or family may be difficult to understand. Because some individual and cultural interaction styles may preclude a listener from letting you know that he or she does not understand what you are saying, you must not assume that a client has comprehended your message simply because he or she or the family members are nodding their heads or verbally agreeing. You should allow opportunities for asking follow-up questions, and you should listen carefully to the content of those questions to judge the person's comprehension of concepts or information that you have presented.

By maintaining a flexible style in which you encourage ongoing comments and questions from your clients as you present diagnostic findings, you will create a two-way flow of communication rich with opportunities for further clarification of information and the establishment of a trusting therapeutic relationship. Remember that counseling remains an ongoing dynamic process woven into the continuum of an audiologist or SLP's clinical activities and does not end with the reporting of diagnostic findings. You must be prepared to develop and maintain an appropriate counseling role throughout the entire course of intervention.

Maintaining Appropriate Professional Boundaries

As we establish trusting and empathetic relationships with our clients through effective interview and counseling strategies, we may set the stage for those individuals to engage in the process of *transference*. From a psychodynamic standpoint, this concept refers to the process by which "the counselor becomes the object for, target of, and the symbol of the client's emotional expressions" (Shames, 2000, p. 79). Shames noted that this transference is a natural result of establishing a trusting relationship between client and clinician. These emotional expressions from a client can take many forms, from personal questions to romantic inclinations, and Shames cautioned clinicians to try to understand the function of these expressions and to not view them as necessarily a personal threat. Clinicians, however, may share their own personal feelings only if the expression of those feelings will facilitate the therapeutic process. Stone and Olswang (1989), however, noted the importance of establishing limitations on the content, focus, and style of the counseling efforts of SLPs and audiologists. They suggested that expression of attitudes and questions relating to the presenting communication disorder is within an appropriate content boundary for audiologists and SLPs; however, other topics not related to communication disorders are out of bounds and may necessitate referral to other sources of support.

Diagnostic Evaluation Reports

A diagnostic evaluation report serves as a tool for organizing, integrating, and interpreting information regarding a person's hearing and communication skills. A thorough report summarizes background information pertaining to an individual's presenting concern, gives results of evaluation measures and observations, and allows for a discussion of the implication of those findings as related to the person's communication needs and potentials. Like all clinical records, diagnostic reports are legal documents that serve as documentation of assessment activities and findings long after the diagnostic event has passed. Both audiology and speech-language pathology reports are divided into subsections to more clearly organize information. The exact formats and section headings of reports may vary from setting to setting but typically include sections for background information, test results and other diagnostic data and observations, a summary section, and a final section with recommendations based on the findings of the evaluation. In some settings, these sections follow the SOAP format discussed previously but employ the same basic organizational strategy. Figure 7.3 shows an outlined format for a typical speech and language diagnostic report from a university speech and hearing clinic.

Identifying Information All reports begin with a section identifying the individual who was evaluated, as well as other pertinent information regarding the type, setting, and date(s) of evaluation. The name(s) of the clinicians who conducted the evaluation, as well as their credentials, must be clearly listed. Other identifying information, including the client's address and telephone number, primary languages, parents or guardians if appropriate, and referral source, is typically included. It is extremely important to list complete and accurate identifying information to facilitate record keeping and assure confidentiality.

Background History Most diagnostic evaluations are at best a snapshot in time, reflecting the test data and observations collected during a limited time frame and often under conditions that do not represent the functional communication environments of the person being tested. One way that you can attempt to compensate for this partial view of your client's communicative competency is to summarize background information collected through written case histories, record reviews, and personal interviews with the client, his or her family, educators, or other caregivers. This summary should be a succinct overview of medical and developmental diagnoses related to the presenting communication concerns; findings of previous speech, language, and audiological evaluations; as well as evaluations from other disciplines and reviews of any past or current speech, language, or audiological intervention. In the case of children, background summaries typically include birth and developmental history appropriate for the age of the client, as well as information regarding educational placement and other related support services. For adults, educational and vocational history is usually summarized. The individual's primary and any secondary languages should be identified, as well as any other considerations unique to the person that may impact on the interpretation of evaluation findings.

Results In the *results* section of a diagnostic report, all standardized tests and nonstandardized assessment procedures are listed, along with a brief explanation of what each test or procedure attempted to accomplish. Normative test scores, data from nonstandardized evaluation tasks, and behavioral observations are listed in a brief narrative or table format. In speech and language evaluation reports, this section may contain a summary of communication strengths and weaknesses, whereas in audiological evaluation reports the results of a client's response to trial fittings of hearing aids, FM systems, and other assistive listening devices may be summarized. A description of the testing conditions, duration of testing, adaptations to standardized test administration protocols, and the level of

Initial Communication Evaluation

Name: _____

Date of birth: _____ Chronological age: _____

Address: _____

Telephone (home): _____ (work): _____

Parent/guardian/spouse: _____ Relationship to client: _____

Referral source: _____ Date of evaluation: _____

Supervisor: _____ Clinician: _____

Background

- State referral information/reason for evaluation.

- Summarize birth/developmental history as appropriate.

- Identify primary language(s).

- Comment on findings of previous communication evaluations and other related evaluations.

- List medical/developmental diagnoses that relate to presenting communication disorder.

- Identify educational placement/modifications (children).

- Summarize history of past and current speech-language intervention; contacts made with other service providers.

Evaluation conditions

- Describe testing conditions (location, length of time, use of interpreter, augmentative communication, etc.).

- Describe client behavior during evaluation (attentiveness, cooperation, etc.).

- State your level of confidence in your findings, based on the above factors.

Figure 7.3.   Initial communication evaluation.

Results

- List standardized tests used, describe their purpose, and list scores obtained.

- List observed and derived data from nonstandardized evaluation tasks (MLU, frequency of stuttering, summary of language strengths and weaknesses, etc.).

Interpretation

- Describe findings related to presenting communication concerns (receptive language, expressive language, oral motor skills, speech production, voice, fluency, hearing, etc.).

- Synthesize data listed in the *Results* section.

- Answer diagnostic questions you posed when planning the evaluation.

- Conclude with a short statement summarizing findings, diagnosis, and contributing factors.

- State prognosis for improvement.

Recommendations

- State all recommendations as options to consider, not mandates to follow.

- Present menus of options to achieve same result, if possible.

- Include suggestions for additional evaluations and related services, when appropriate.

- Provide suggestions for therapy goals and objectives, as well as frequency and duration of therapy, when appropriate.

_____   _____
John Doe, B.A.   Jane Smith, M.A., CCC/SLP
Graduate Student Clinician   Supervising Speech-Language Pathologist

cooperation and attention demonstrated by the individual being assessed is typically included to assist in appropriately interpreting evaluation results. Detailed analysis of evaluation findings, however, is usually reserved for the *interpretation* section of the report.

Interpretation   Once you have successfully summarized all of the data that you have collected during the course of the audiological or speech and language evaluation, you must then interpret those data to draw conclusions regarding the communication status of the individual. Similar to research projects, all communication evaluations begin with the evaluator framing a series of questions regarding the client's communication and hearing status (Tomblin, 2000). These questions guide the evaluator in the choice of tests and assessment protocols to be administered and provide the foundation for interpreting all evaluation results. In the *interpretation* section of an evaluation report, the author compares and interprets the data collected in relation to these questions or hypotheses. Because the data collected during an evaluation do not always point to the same conclusions, you must consider these data in relation to client behavior, evaluation conditions, pertinent background information, and other related factors if you hope to make a thoughtful interpretation of their meaning and draw conclusions relevant to your initial questions. You will not always be able to definitively answer the questions that you initially set out to explore during the evaluation. Based on careful interpretation of diagnostic data, however, you should be able to integrate and summarize the knowledge related to those questions that you have gained through the evaluation process in this section of the diagnostic report and identify what diagnostic questions remain fully or partially unanswered. Based on this summary, you must also include a statement of **prognosis,** estimating the likelihood that the individual can improve (or maintain) communication or hearing skills.

> Example: Prognosis for improvement of Johnny's speech intelligibility through the elimination of developmentally atypical phonological processes appears fair to good given the delayed emergence of more typical phonological patterns noted in today's evaluation, his stimulability for more accurate sound productions, and his strong family and educational support systems.

Recommendations   The *recommendations* section of a diagnostic report is often the first, and sometimes the only, section to be read by the numerous individuals who will review this document. In this section, recommendations regarding the need for follow-up intervention are stated based on the data collected during the evaluation and the conclusions outlined in the preceding *interpretation* section. The recommendations section reflects the culmination of the diagnostic process and serves as an important tool for determining an individual's need and eligibility for service. You may make recommendations for additional testing, either within the domain of the current evaluation or by professionals in other disciplines, and/or suggestions for related services. Equipment needs, including hearing aids and other assistive listening devices, augmentative communication devices, or educational materials can be stated. Suggestions for modifications to home, educational, and vocational routines and environments are sometimes included to better enhance communication skills in those settings. Potential therapy goals and objectives and suggestions regarding the frequency, duration, and model of intervention may be outlined in this section. Realistic recommendations should be offered based on the individual client's needs and the priorities and values held by the person, his or her family, and their community. Other factors include the individual's health status and the availability of time, money, and other resources necessary to implement those recommendations. Recommendation statements usually take the form of numbered or bulleted statements but may at times include more narrative descriptions of recommended intervention strategies, adaptive equipment, or environmental or educational modifications.

EXAMPLES OF RECOMMENDATION STATEMENTS

1. Anita will benefit from speech and language intervention targeting the development of age-appropriate language and phonological skills necessary for her successful participation in academic tasks and social routines. Specific focus should be placed on:

   - Increasing speech intelligibility through the elimination of the phonological patterns of fronting and final consonant deletion

   - Increased use of age-appropriate syntax, including auxiliary verb forms, prepositions, and the possessive marker /s/

   - Increased comprehension of vocabulary related to curricular and social demands

2. Anita should continue to be monitored regularly for signs of middle ear infection and receive medical intervention as needed to minimize the risk of transient hearing loss due to middle ear infection.

3. The SLP should collaborate with the classroom teacher to develop intervention activities that can be supported in the context of classroom-based activities.

CONTRIBUTING TO COMPREHENSIVE SERVICE PLANS

SLPs and audiologists often serve as contributing members of interdisciplinary service teams. In this capacity, you will be called on to assist in the development of comprehensive service plans outlining the educational or rehabilitative supports offered to your clients. The formats of these plans will vary based on the age of the client and the service delivery setting. Regardless of their format, all comprehensive service plans serve as a legal mechanism for detailing the supports to be offered to an individual, the time lines for delivery of these services, the people responsible for providing these supports, and the mechanisms for evaluating outcomes.

Individualized Education Programs

The Education for All Handicapped Children Act (PL 94-142) was passed in 1975, ensuring a free and appropriate public education and related services for all children regardless of their disability. This act has been amended and re-authorized several times over the ensuing years and is currently encompassed in the Individuals with Disabilities Education Act (IDEA) Amendments of 1997 (PL 105-17). The law specifies, among other things, that educators develop an annual IEP for children ages 3–21 who are determined eligible for special education services. An *IEP* is a comprehensive written document identifying the specialized resources needed to maximize the academic success of students who have met eligibility requirements due to academic-based learning impairments, including speech, language, and hearing disorders. The process leading to the development of an IEP begins with the informal identification of students with special needs by classroom teachers; parents; family members; or specialists such as SLPs, psychologists, or social workers. A prereferral screening process is used to estimate the nature and extent of the student's problems and their potential impact on academic success. If, after an initial period in which trial strategies and modifications to academic tasks and classroom routines are implemented, the child continues to exhibit problems that are likely to have a negative impact on academic success, a more formalized evaluation process is initiated. In this phase, the SLP serving the school may be asked to complete and document a more comprehensive speech and language evaluation if communication problems appear to contribute to the child's academic difficulties. This evaluation may include both standardized testing and nonstandardized assessment and observation of the student communicating in classroom or other social settings. An interdisciplinary **planning and placement team (PPT)** reviews the results of this evaluation, along with the results from evaluations by educators and professionals in other disciplines who may have been called into the process, to determine the appropriateness of special education services based on state and federal eligibility criteria. If eligible, an IEP is developed at a PPT meeting to outline specific educational services and modifications designed to meet the student's individualized learning needs. The IEP document is typically handwritten on a prepared fill-in-the-blank form and is completed by the conclusion of the PPT meeting.

The components of an IEP are clearly specified in the public law. The IEP document begins with a cover sheet with identifying information regarding the student, his or her family, participating team members, and the reason for the PPT meeting. Subsequent sections summarize the student's present level of educational performance in the areas of health and development (including vision and hearing); academic, cognitive, and social/emotional/behavioral skills; motor and communication abilities; activities of daily living; and vocational domains. These summaries are generated from observations of classroom performance, parent reports, and direct assessment results. Not all domains may be reviewed, given the age and presenting concerns of the student. The SLP participating on the planning and placement team may be called on to contribute both formalized evaluation findings and more incidental observations of the student's communication skills as part of this discussion and should employ the principles of effective oral and written communication discussed previously in order to clearly present findings. Based on this cumulative information, the team ultimately decides if the student's disability affects his or her involvement and progress in the general academic or preschool curriculum and makes a determination regarding eligibility for service.

Once eligibility has been determined, the team proceeds to formulate and record annual goals and short-term objectives based on the student's needs. Broad-based goals, including those in the communication domain, are written in functional terms that directly relate to the student's success in an academic environment and are followed by measurable short-term objectives or benchmarks that support those goals. Methods of evaluating progress and a schedule and place for reviewing and recording student outcomes are also included in this section (see Figure 7.4).

The team then documents the specific education resources allocated to the student. These include services such as speech-language therapy, physical therapy or other supports, the hours per week those services will be delivered, beginning and ending dates, and the parties responsible for implementing the service (see Figure 7.5). The instructional site (e.g., regular classroom, resource room, related services office) for each service is identified, as well as the need for assistive technology (including communication devices, FM systems, and other communication aids). Any modifications to the school schedule are also listed, as are accommodations for students with hearing and vision impairments, behavior challenges, or limited English proficiency.

A placement summary outlines the rationale for the type and location of educational placement chosen, as well as exit criteria from special education. IDEA '97 mandates that school systems provide education for all students in the *least restrictive environment*. Modifications and adaptations in general education settings are indicated, including specialized instructional strategies; organizational supports; behavior management support; testing procedures; and adaptations to materials, books, and equipment (see Figure 7.6).

An SLP's role in the IEP process continues after the development of the initial plan and involves subsequent implementation and review of the components of the IEP related to communication. Audiologists, although not always physically present during planning and placement team meetings, also contribute to the development and implementation of IEPs for students with hearing impairments or central auditory processing disorders, through consulting with the team, writing diagnostic reports, and communicating to the team via the school-based SLP.

Individualized Family Service Plans

When the Education for All Handicapped Children Act of 1975 was re-authorized as the Education of the Handicapped Act Amendments of 1986 (PL 99-457) it

MEASURABLE ANNUAL GOAL AND SHORT TERM OBJECTIVES*

☐ Academic/Cognitive ☐ Social/Behavioral **X Communication** ☐ Gross/Fine Motor ☐ Employment/Post Secondary Education**

☐ Self Help ☐ Community Partic.*** ☐ Independent Living**** ☐ Health ☐ Other: (specify) _____

☐ **Check here if the student is 13 or older.**(Note: Page 4-A, Transition Summary, must be completed if this box is checked)

Measurable Annual Goal*: # 1 _Eric will demonstrate improved receptive language skills allowing him to better participate in grade level curricular activities_

Eval. Procedure: _10_

Perf. Criteria: _____

(%, Trials, etc:) _____

Short Term Objectives/Benchmarks

Obj # 1 _Eric will demonstrate understanding of 2 step directions related to academic routines by listening to each complete direction, restating the direction, and correctly following the instruction._

Eval. Procedure: _1,3_

Perf. Criteria: _A_

(%, Trials, etc;) _75%_

Obj. # 2 _Eric will demonstrate comprehension of later developing "wh" questions "when", "why", and "How" by:_

a) _correctly pointing to picture cards representing correct responses to targeted question forms_

Eval. Procedure: _1,3_

Perf. Criteria: _A_

(%, Trials, etc;) _75%_

b) _producing correct verbal responses to targeted question forms in the context of curriculum based activities._

Perf. Criteria: _____

(%, Trials, etc;) _____

Indicate Dates For Reporting

Progress in Boxes Below

9/30	10/31	11/28	1/5
2/2	3/3	4/30	6/1

Report Progress Below (Use Reporting Key)

S	S
S	

Report Progress Below (Use Reporting Key)

S	S
A	M

Report Progress Below (Use Reporting Key)

S	S

206

Obj # 3 _Eric will demonstrate comprehension of prepositional concepts "under", "behind", "in front of",_
and "next to" by pointing to appropriate picture stimuli or manipulating objects during structured therapy
activities _____

Perf. Criteria: A _____

_____ **(%, Trials, etc:) 90%**

NS	S	S

Evaluation Procedures		Performance Criteria	
1. Criterion-Referenced/Curriculum Based Assessment	7. Behavior/Performance Rating Scale	A. Percent of Change	F. Duration
2. Pre & Post Standardized Assessment	8. CMT/CAPT	B. Months Growth	G. Successful Completion of Task/Activity
3. Pre & Post Base Line Data	9. Work Samples, Job Performance or Products	C. Standard Score Increase	H. Mastery
4. Quizzes/Tests	10. Achievement of Objectives (Note: use with goal only)	D. Passing Grades/Score	I. Other: (specify) _____
5. Student Self-assessment/Rubric	11. Other: (specify) _____	E. Frequency/Trials	J. Other: (specify) _____
6. Project/Experiment/Portfolio	12. Other: (specify) _____		

Progress Reporting Key: (indicating extent to which progress is sufficient to achieve goal by the end of the year)   **M** = Mastered   **S** = Satisfactory Progress - Likely to achieve goal   **U** = Unsatisfactory Progress - Unlikely to achieve goal   **N** = No Progress - Will not achieve goal   **NI** = Not Introduced   **O** = Other: (specify)

Figure 7.4.   Example of goal and object documentation on an IEP. (Courtesy of the Connecticut State Department of Education, © 2000.)

SUMMARY: SPECIAL EDUCATION, RELATED SERVICES, AND REGULAR EDUCATION

Special Education	Goal #	Hours/wk	Staff Responsible	Start Date	End Date	Site
Reading instruction	5,6	5	Special education teacher	9/1/00	6/5/00	2
Related Services						
Speech-language pathology	1,2,3	2	Speech-language pathologist Speech Asst.	9/1/00	6/5/00	1,4
Occupational therapy	4		Occupational therapist	9/1/00	6/5/00	1

Instructional Site (Indicate all that apply)
1. Regular Classroom   2. Resource Room   3. Self-contained Classroom   4. Related Service Office/Classroom
5. Community-based   6. Other (specify): _____

Figure 7.5.   Identifying educational support services on an IEP. (Courtesy of the Connecticut State Department of Education, © 2000.)

introduced Part H in order to create a federally supported mechanism for the provision of early intervention services for children from birth to 3 years of age who demonstrated substantial and measurable delays in key developmental areas. More recently, IDEA '97 has re-authorized that legislation and changed Part H to Part C. Early intervention services include adaptive/self-help skills (e.g., bathing, feeding, dressing), cognitive skills, physical development (e.g., gross and fine motor skills, hearing, vision), social and emotional development, and receptive and expressive communication skills. Services provided through this program are based on the concept of *family-centered practice* (see Chapter 12), with the child's family serving as key determiners of the type and focus of intervention services. Assessment and intervention are implemented in the child's natural environment, and a major focus is placed not only on the specific developmental needs of the child but also on the needs of the child's family. Service is provided through a **transdisciplinary service delivery** team in which family members are key players. They are supported by other team members, such as early intervention educators, SLPs and audiologists, occupational and physical therapists, nurses, and social workers, any of whom may serve as an overall case manager for the family.

Upon referral, a child undergoes a transdisciplinary developmental evaluation by two or more members of the birth-to-3 team. If the child meets eligibility requirements, team members will meet with the family to develop an IFSP. Throughout this process, the child's family is encouraged to identify their child's likes and dislikes, as well as his or her strengths and areas of need. A written IFSP document is developed to capture this information and will ultimately serve as the comprehensive guide to the family's individualized support (see Figure 7.7).

More global family needs, such as access to health care or adequate shelter or the needs of other siblings, are also discussed, in recognition of the impact that such considerations have on the child's development. Early intervention specialists assist the family in identifying their priorities for support and then aid in developing a plan to meet those needs, helping the family to access needed services both within and outside of the birth-to-3 program. At times, the priorities stated by families may differ with the priorities set by other team members, including SLPs and audiologists, but family-generated priorities always take precedence. This information is documented in the written IFSP document (see Figure 7.8). Once the child's strengths and needs and the family's priorities are identified, a plan of services and supports is developed. As is the case in an IEP, the type of supports, the service providers responsible, and the location and schedule of services are outlined (see Figure 7.9).

The completed IFSP document becomes the working guide to the child and family's participation in the birth-to-3 program. It will be reviewed by the early intervention team periodically throughout the period the child is enrolled in the program and revised as needed to better serve the child and family. As is the case with all of the clinical intervention and documentation formats we have discussed so far, you must rely on a style of presenting information that is clear, supportive, and respectful to the needs of the families with whom you are working.

Individualized Transition Plans

Students from ages 14 to 21 who are in continued need of specialized educational services are, under the provisions of IDEA '97, afforded additional planned assistance to facilitate their transition from an educational environment to an appropriate vocational or supported adult service setting. An **individualized transition plan (ITP)** is developed as an integrated component of these students' IEPs, and is designed to identify the specific skills and supports that the students will need to make a successful transition. The focus of goals and objectives may shift somewhat at this point from academic to independent living, community participation, and prevocational skills. An effort is made to involve members from the student's current educational team and representatives from adult support agencies in this transitional planning process. The transition plan is recorded as part of the overall IEP document (see Figure 7.10).

Overall Plans of Service

Many individuals with mental retardation and other developmental disabilities are supported in habilitative settings with 24-hour supervision. At one time, these were mostly institutional facilities housing large numbers of people with disabilities. Due to the nationwide movement to support people with disabilities in least restrictive settings, there has been a major reduction in the numbers of such people residing in large institutions. This has resulted in a substantial increase in the number of people with all types and severity of developmental disabilities who reside in smaller community-based homes. Many of these residential programs receive funding under a federal program for **intermediate care facilities for persons with mental retardation (ICFs/MR).** ICFs/MR regulations require that a formalized written plan of habilitative treatment, known as an *OPS*, be developed based on an interdisciplinary team's evaluation of a person's developmental needs and potentials. Both SLPs and audiologists may play a direct or consultative role on this team, depending on the needs of the individual. The

COLLABORATION/SUPPORTS FOR SCHOOL PERSONNEL

Modifications/Adaptations in Regular Education - Including Nonacademic and Extracurricular Activities	Sites/Activities Where Required and Duration	Required Supports for Personnel and Frequency and Duration of Supports
Materials/Books/Equipment: □ Alternative Text □ Consumable Workbook □ Modified Worksheets □ Manipulatives X Access to Computer □ Tape Recorder X Supplementary Visuals □ Large Print Text □ Spell Check □ Calculator X Assistive Technology: (specify) *FM Auditory Trainer* □ Other: (specify) _____	*Regular Classroom, resource room*	*Speech-language pathologist to train classroom teachers and aid in use of FM during first 2 weeks of school year*
Tests/Quizzes/Time: X Preview Test Procedures X Test Study Guide X Simplify Test □ Prior Notice of Tests □ Oral Testing Wording □ Limited Multiple Choice □ Student Write on Test □ Shortened Tasks □ Hands-on Projects □ Reduced Reading X Alternative Tests □ Objective Tests □ Extra Credit Options □ Extra Time–Written Work X Extra Time–Tests X Extra Time–Projects X Extra Response Time X Modified Tests □ Pace Long Term Projects X Rephrase Test Questions/Directions □ Other: (specify)	*Regular Classroom, resource room*	*Special education teacher and speech-language pathologist to consult with regular classroom teacher regarding multi-modality teaching strategies.*
Grading: □ No Spelling Penalty □ No Handwriting Penalty X Grade Effort + Work □ Grade Improvement □ Course Credit □ Base Grade on IEP □ Base Grade on Ability □ Modified Grades □ Pass/Fail □ Audit Course □ Other: (specify)	*Regular Classroom, resource room*	
Organization: X Provide Study Outlines X Desktop List of Tasks **B** List Sequential Steps X Post Routines X Post Assignments X Give One Paper at a Time X Folders to Hold Work □ Pencil Box for Tools □ Pocket Folder for Work □ Assignment Pad X Daily Assignment List X Daily Homework List □ Worksheet Formats □ Extra Space for Work Assign Partner □ Other: (specify)	*Regular Classroom, resource room*	

			Regular Classroom
Environment:			
X Preferential Seating	❑ Clear Work Area	❑ Study Carrel	❑ Other: (specify) _____	*All settings*
Behavior Management/Support:			
X Daily Feedback to Student Sign Homework	X Chart Progress	❑ Behavior Contracts ❑ Parent/Guardian	
X Positive Reinforcement Sign Behavioral Chart	❑ Collect Baseline Data	❑ Set/Post Class Rules ❑ Parent/Guardian	
❑ Cue Expected Behavior Positive Reinforcement	X Structure Transitions	❑ Break Between Tasks ❑ Time Out from	
❑ Proximity/Touch Control		❑ Contingency Plan ❑ Other: (specify) _____	
Instructional Strategies:			*Regular Classroom, resource room*
X Check Work in Progress	❑ Immediate Feedback	X Pre-teach Content X Have Student Restate Information	
X Extra Drill/Practice	X Review Sessions	X Review Directions X Provide Lecture Notes/Outline to Student	
X Use Manipulatives Assisted Instruction	❑ Modified Content	X Assign Study Partner ❑ Computer	
X Monitor Assignments	X Provide Models	X Repeat Instructions X Support Auditory Presentations with Visuals	
X Multi-Sensory Approach	X Highlight Key Words	❑ Oral Reminders X Display Key Vocabulary	
X Visual Reinforcement Bank	❑ Pictures/Charts	X Visual Reminders X Provide Student With Vocabulary Word	
❑ Mimed Clues/Gestures	X Concrete Examples	❑ Use Mnemonics ❑ Personalized Examples	
❑ Number Line	❑ Other: (specify) _____		

Figure 7.6.   Educational modifications as outlined on an IEP. (Courtesy of the Connecticut State Department of Education, © 2000.)

211

OPS is then implemented on a 24-hour basis by the professional, paraprofessional, and direct care staff who support the individual with developmental disabilities in order to provide consistent active treatment. The OPS is reviewed by team members quarterly and revised annually. As is the case with the development and implementation of school-based IEPs, our role in the development and implementation of an OPS is varied. It may include initial evaluation and annual

---

Name: _Tonya Williams_   Date: _2/19/01_

1. Indicate the dates and types of evaluations or assessment reports that were used to develop this plan.

Eligibility evaluation of 2/14/01 & 2/16/01, parent interview, and family assessment of 2/16/01

2. Summarize additional observations by family and other team members of the child's abilities, strengths, and needs in day-to-day routines. Areas to include:

• Your child's likes and dislikes

• Your child's frustrations

• Daily routine/activities

• Bathing, feeding, dressing, and toileting (adaptive self-help skills)

• Thinking, reasoning, and learning (cognitive skills)

• Moving, hearing, vision, and health (physical development)

• Feelings, coping, and getting along with others (socioemotional development)

• Understanding, communicating with others, and expressing self with others (communication skills)

Tonya spends most of the day at home with her mother and grandmother, where she often plays in her room alone. In addition, she spends 3 hours each morning in a home-based child care center where she reportedly separates herself from the other children. She enjoys playing with stuffed animals. She likes to line them up in neat rows, move them, and line them up again. Tonya also spends time repeatedly stacking plastic rings on a post. She becomes quickly frustrated when someone tries to move her stuffed animals or other toys out of the order in which she placed them. At these times she will vocalize loudly and quickly restore her toys to their original order. Tonya becomes agitated when her mother and grandmother cannot figure out what she wants. She does not, however, appear to change strategies in order to make her needs known. Tonya is beginning to feed herself soft foods with a spoon and prefers cold foods to hot foods. She has not yet shown a readiness for toilet training.

See background information contained in eligibility report for more detailed developmental information.

Figure 7.7.   Summary of a child's present abilities, strengths, and needs. (Courtesy of the Connecticut Birth to Three System, December 1999.)

Family information for the individualized family service plan

Tonya lives with her mom and grandmother. The family enjoys watching television and visiting Tonya's aunt at her home across town. They are very involved in church activities and turn to their church for emotional support. Both mother and grandmother state that they "have not slept well since Tonya was born" and constantly worry over her well being.

What would be helpful for you or your family in the months and year ahead? (Family outcome)

*   Help in learning how to teach Tonya to "play like other kids"

*   Assistance in finding safe, affordable housing

*   Medical resources when family members are sick

What assistance or information will you need to achieve this outcome?

*   Help in applying for financial assistance for housing and health care

*   Someone to show the family how to play with Tonya

*   Toys and books

Figure 7.8.   Summary of a family's concerns, priorities, and resources as they relate to enhancing their child's development. (Courtesy of the Connecticut Birth to Three System, December 1999.)

Name: _Tonya Williams_   Date of birth: _2/3/98_   Date: _2/19/01_

What is going to happen	Delivered by (discipline responsible)	Location	How often	How long	Start date
Instructional home visit	Early intervention specialist (teacher)	Family's home	Once per week	1 hour	3/5/01
Speech therapy consultation	Speech-language pathologist	Family's home	Once per month	1 hour	4/2/01
Nursing consultation	Nurse	Family's home	Twice per month	1 hour	3/12/01

Figure 7.9.   Early intervention services and supports. (Courtesy of the Connecticut Birth to Three System, December 1999.)

TRANSITION PLANNING SUMMARY

1. Statement of Transition Service Needs for students age 14 and older: (Must be completed at each Annual Review following a student's 13th birthday) *Mary will benefit from coordination of educational, pre-vocational, and community participation supports to prepare her to function at her optimum capacity in a supported vocational or community experience program.*

2. Student Preferences/Interests - document the following: (Sections 2, 3, and 4 must be completed at each Annual Review following a student's 15th birthday)

a) Was the student invited to attend her/his Planning and Placement Team meeting?   **X** Yes   ☐ No

b) Did the student attend?   **X** Yes   ☐ No

c) How were the student's Preferences/Interests, as they relate to planning for Transition Services, determined?   **X** Personal Interviews   ☐ Informal/Formal Testing

X Vocational Assessments   ☐ Comments at Meeting   **X** Other: (specify) *Interview of student's family*

d) Summarize student preferences/Interests as they relate to planning for Transition Services: *Mary has demonstrated an interest in pre-vocational activities and community experiences that involve consistent routines, physical activity, and opportunities to socialize with others. Activities that Mary has experienced and responded favorable to include volunteer activities ("Meals on wheels"), landscape work and gardening, and building maintenance. She demonstrated a distinct dislike of sedentary assembly work, unpredictable schedules, and work routines with long periods of inactivity, as evidenced by her verbal and behavioral responses to such experiences.*

3. Agency participation:

a) Were any outside agencies invited to attend the PPT meeting?   **X** Yes   ☐ No (If no, specify reason) _____

b) If yes, did the agency's representative attend?   **X** Yes   ☐ No

c) Has any participating agency agreed to provide or pay for services/linkages?   ☐ No   **X** Yes (specify) *4 hours/week pre-vocational training & community experience.*

4. Justification Statements for Transition Services not being addressed:

a) If an annual goal and related objectives were not developed for Independent Living or Community Participation, provide a justification statement.

NA (Goals developed)

b) If Activities/Training are not provided in both the <u>Community</u> and the <u>Classroom</u>, provide a justification statement:

NA - Activities/Training are provided in <u>both</u> locations

5. At least one year prior to reaching age 18, the student must be informed of her/his rights under IDEA, if any, which will transfer to her/him at age

NA   (Student will not be 17 within 1 Year)

Figure 7.10.   ITP summary incorporated into an IEP. (Courtesy of the Connecticut State Department of Education, © 2000.)

re-assessment of communication skills; implementation, documentation, and review of direct and consultative therapy services; and written and verbal updates on client progress for family, support staff, and professional team members.

CONCLUSION

As you have seen in the previous discussions, the act of obtaining, relaying, and documenting clinical information is a multifaceted task that requires you to integrate writing abilities, interpersonal skills, cultural sensitivity, and clinical knowledge in order to serve clients, their families, and their caregivers effectively. It is a process in which form does not follow function but rather blends with it to create an effective format for information sharing. It is a process that you will refine throughout the entire course of your clinical education and subsequent professional practice as audiologists and SLPs. We will serve our clients most effectively if we remember that in addition to increasing their communication skills, we have an obligation to continually refine our own.

REFERENCES

American Speech-Language-Hearing Association. (1991). A model for collaborative service delivery for students with language-learning disorders in the public schools. *ASHA, 33*(Suppl. 5), 44–50.

American Speech-Language-Hearing Association. (1993). Guidelines for caseload size and speech-language service delivery in the schools. *ASHA, 35*(Suppl. 10), 33–39.

American Speech-Language-Hearing Association. (1994). Code of ethics. *ASHA, 36*(Suppl. 13), 1–2.

American Speech-Language-Hearing Association. (1995). Collecting outcome data. *ASHA, 37*(11/12), 36–38.

Anderson, P.P., & Fenichel, E.S. (1989). *Serving culturally diverse families of infants and toddlers with disabilities.* Washington, DC: National Center for Clinical Infant Programs.

Battle, D.E. (1998). *Communication disorders in multicultural populations* (2nd ed.). Boston: Butterworth-Heinemann.

Education for All Handicapped Children Act of 1975, PL 94-142, 20 U.S.C. §§ 1400 *et seq.*

Education of the Handicapped Act Amendments of 1986, PL 99-457, 20 U.S.C. §§ 1400 *et seq.*

Golper, L.G. (1998). *Sourcebook for medical speech pathology* (2nd ed.). San Diego: Singular Publishing Group.

Hall, P.H., & Morris, H.L. (2000). The clinical history. In J.B. Toblin, H.L. Morris, & D.C. Spriestersbach (Eds.), *Diagnosis in speech-language pathology* (2nd ed., pp. 65–82). San Diego: Singular Publishing Group.

Haynes, W.O., & Pindzola, R.H. (1998). *Diagnosis and evaluation in speech pathology* (5th ed.). Needham Heights, MA: Allyn & Bacon.

Individuals with Disabilities Education Act Amendments of 1997, PL 105-17, 20 U.S.C. §§ 1400 *et seq.*

Langdon, H.W., & Cheng, L.L. (1992). *Hispanic children and adults with communication disorders: Assessment and intervention.* Gaithersburg, MD: Aspen Publishers.

Luteman, D.M. (1991). *Counseling the communicatively disordered and their families* (2nd ed.). Austin, TX: PRO-ED.

Maltz, D., & Borker, R. (1982). A cultural approach to male-female miscommunication. In J.J. Gumperz (Ed.), *Language and social identity: Studies in international sociolinguistics* (pp. 146–216). Cambridge, MA: Cambridge University Press.

Meitus, I.J. (1983). Clinical report and letter writing. In I.J. Meitus & B. Weinberg (Eds.), *Diagnosis in speech-language pathology* (pp. 287–301). Needham Heights, MA: Allyn & Bacon.

Roseberry-McKibbin, C. (1995). *Multicultural students with special language needs: Practical strategies for assessment and intervention.* Oceanside, CA: Academic Communication Associates.

Roth, F.P., & Worthington, C.K. (1996). *Treatment resource manual for speech-language pathology.* San Diego: Singular Publishing Group.

Shames, G.H. (2000). *Counseling the communicatively disabled and their families: A manual for clinicians.* Needham Heights, MA: Allyn & Bacon.

Shapiro, D.A. (1999). *Stuttering intervention: A collaborative journey to fluency freedom.* Austin, TX: PRO-ED.

Shipley, K.G., & McAfee, J.G. (1998). *Diagnosis in speech-language pathology: A resource manual.* San Diego: Singular Publishing Group.

Silverman, F.H. (1999). *Professional issues in speech-language pathology and audiology.* Needham Heights, MA: Allyn & Bacon.

Stone, J.R., & Olswang, L.B. (1989). The hidden challenge in counseling. *ASHA, 31,* 27–31.

Tomblin, J.B. (2000). Perspectives on diagnosis. In J.B. Toblin, H.L. Morris, & D.C. Spriestersbach (Eds.), *Diagnosis in speech-language pathology* (2nd ed., pp. 3–33). San Diego: Singular Publishing Group.

Willis, W. (1992). Families with African American roots. In E.W. Lynch & M.J. Hanson (Eds.), *Developing cross-cultural competence: A guide for working with young children and their families* (pp. 121–150). Baltimore: Paul H. Brookes Publishing Co.

Zungia, M.E. (1992). Families with Latino roots. In E.W. Lynch & M.J. Hanson (Eds.), *Developing cross-cultural competence: A guide to working with young children and their families* (pp. 151–179). Baltimore: Paul H. Brookes Publishing Co.

1. Describe at least four principles of effective oral and written communication.

2. Discuss the advantage of using an in-person interview rather than a written case history questionnaire to gain background information from your clients.

3. Name three cultural factors that may influence a person's responses to interview questions.

4. Explain the importance of follow-up counseling as a component of diagnostic assessment.

5. What criteria are used to determine if a particular topic is appropriate for an audiologist or SLP to address during a clinical counseling session?

6. Describe the components of an individual treatment plan for speech-language therapy.

7. Compare and contrast the purpose of the following documents: individual treatment plan, SOAP note, progress report, and discharge summary.

8. Contrast the structure and purpose of at least two comprehensive service plan formats.

Public Policies
Affecting Clinical Practice

Nickola Wolf Nelson
Yvette D. Hyter

Public policies influence all aspects of clinical service provision at all age levels, from early infancy through late adulthood. They play a significant role in determining how clinical decisions are made, as well as where and when clinical services will be provided and how (and if) they will be reimbursed. Public policies vary with and are related to the broader systems in which clients are assessed and treated—home, educational, employment, or health care settings. Moreover, they are constantly changing.

That is both the good news and the bad news. The good news is that ineffective policies can be modified, which can be especially reassuring when a policy has clear negative effects. It is also the case, however, that policies with positive effects can be changed in negative ways. Therefore, vigilance must be maintained, and professionals should always be ready to assume advocacy roles on behalf of individuals with communication disorders and the services that they need.

This chapter provides overviews for several key pieces of public legislation that have implications for clinical service provision. We also discuss the role of advocacy with regard to polices that have an impact on practice in speech-language pathology and audiology. We start by defining important terms used in **public policy** discussions.

DEFINING PUBLIC POLICY

Public policy can be defined as any action (or lack thereof) taken by local, state, or federal officials to address a given problem (Dye, 1998). Public policies are established at the federal, state, and local levels and they can occur in many forms, such as laws, rules, and court decisions. They may apply to the development of programs, the distribution of money or benefits, or the extraction of taxes (Dye, 1975, 1998; Lieurance, 1993).

Essential to understanding public policies and how they can be changed is to become aware of the level at which they are established and whether they are laws, regulations, or guidelines. **Laws** begin as bills that move through legislative committees, are passed by legislative bodies, and are signed into law by executive officials, who then become responsible for implementing them. **Regulations** for a particular law are designed to govern interpretation of the law and its implementation. They are generally more detailed than the law and may be generated by the executive agencies charged with implementation. Before final passage, proposed regulations are generally open for a period of public comment. Before they can be changed, both laws and regulations require action by the regulatory and legislative bodies that originated them. In addition, **case law** may influence how policies are implemented when disputes taken to court result in decisions that have implications broader than the single case.

Guidelines may be established by entities such as communities, school districts, health care agencies, hospitals, or professional associations. Guidelines suggest ways to implement and monitor public policies established at state and federal levels. Although guidelines may be treated as "policies," they do not have the weight of law. Overinterpretation of guidelines as law is sometimes responsible for excessive layers of complexity or paperwork that were not intended by the developers of the original policy—but they also are often easier to change.

We turn now to a discussion of some specific pieces of legislation; specifically Section 504 of the Rehabilitation Act of 1973 (PL 93-112), the Americans with Disabilities Act (ADA) of 1990 (PL 101-336), the Individuals with Disabilities Education Act (IDEA) Amendments of 1997 (PL 105-17), **Medicare,** and **Medicaid.** All of these have important implications for practice in speech-language pathology and audiology. As part of this discussion, we touch on influences on the implementation of these laws by another piece of legislation, the Balanced Budget Act (BBA) of 1997 (PL 105-33).

SECTION 504 OF THE REHABILITATION ACT OF 1973

Section 504 of the Rehabilitation Act of 1973 is civil rights legislation. It specifies that no otherwise qualified individual with a disability shall be excluded from participation in, be denied the benefits of, or be subjected to discrimination under any program or activity receiving financial assistance from the federal government—including public elementary, secondary, and postsecondary schools. To qualify for accommodations under Section 504, individuals must be identified as having a physical or mental impairment that substantially limits one or more of their major life activities. Section 504 covers conditions that currently do not qualify as disabilities under IDEA, including attention-deficit/hyperactivity disorder. Section 504, however, carries no funds to pay for its provision, whereas IDEA does.

Protection from discrimination in education agencies means that schools must make reasonable accommodations, such as structural alterations and modifications of classroom materials and procedures. Educational agencies must ensure that their students have access to nonacademic services as well. At the postsecondary level this might include access to housing comparable to that provided for students without disabilities. Other modifications in academic programs might include extra time to complete assignments, adjustments in length of assignments, use of peer tutors, provision of visual aids, audiotaping of lectures, or use of specialized curricular materials. Modification of tests might include giving tests orally or on audiotape, allowing more time to complete tests, allowing students opportunities to dictate answers, altering the test format, or using enlarged type. Provision of auxiliary aids and devices might include interpreters, FM amplification systems, and other forms of assistive technology. In requiring schools to be accessible, Section 504 does not require that every part of a school be accessible to students with disabilities, as long as its programs as a whole are accessible. Evaluations under Section 504 must be conducted with procedures that are 1) validated for the specific purpose for which they are used, 2) administered by trained personnel, 3) tailored to assess specific areas of educational need, and 4) selected to ensure that, when a test is administered to a student with impaired sensory, manual, or speaking skills, the test results reflect the student's aptitude or achievement rather than reflecting the student's impairment.

Parents of school-age children with disabilities have a right to be notified of their **due process** rights under this civil rights legislation, as well as how to file a grievance with the school district. Parental rights also include a right to be notified when eligibility is determined, when an evaluation is planned that might result in a significant change in the student's status, and when re-evaluation or other actions are proposed that might affect the student's program of accommodations. Parents should be aware that their child's evaluation must use information from multiple sources, that they have a right to examine all relevant records and request changes, and that they have a right to receive information in their native language or primary mode of communication.

AMERICANS WITH DISABILITIES ACT

The ADA's three basic purposes ensure that people with disabilities will enjoy equal opportunity to 1) participate fully in society, 2) live independently, and 3) enjoy economic self-sufficiency through removal of barriers. The legislation is divided into five areas, or "titles," addressing employment, public services, public accommodations operated by a private entity, telecommunications, and miscellaneous other issues.

Title I applies to *employment.* It requires employers with 15 or more employees, employment agencies, labor agencies, and labor-management committees to make accommodations for qualified employees. Such individuals are defined as those who have a disability but can perform the essential functions of an employment position with or without reasonable accommodation.

Title I prohibits discrimination in job application procedures; the hiring, advancement, or discharge of employees; employee compensation; job training; and other terms, conditions, or privileges of employment. Reasonable accommodations include job restructuring, modification of work schedules, acquisition or modification of equipment or assistive devices, adjustment or modification of examination materials or training materials or policies, provision of qualified readers or interpreters, and so forth. Procedures for determining reasonable accommodations include 1) analyzing the requirements of the job, 2) identifying potential accommodations in consultation with the person with the disability, and 3) considering the preferences of the individual when deciding which options to pursue.

Title II applies to *public services* provided in public entities such as schools and colleges. It ensures that policies are in place to protect the educational opportunities of individuals with disabilities and to guard against discrimination.

Title III applies to *public accommodations operated by a private entity.* It protects the rights of individuals with disabilities to gain access to places of lodging, bars and restaurants, places of exhibition or entertainment, places of recreation, places of education, places where social services are offered, and stores and shopping centers. For example, architectural accessibility modifications must be made to remove architectural and structural barriers in existing facilities when "readily achievable." If not readily achievable, the entity must provide alternative methods for gaining access to the public accommodations. New buildings are required to comply fully with ADA accessibility requirements. Some strategies for removing architectural barriers include 1) installing ramps, 2) repositioning shelves, 3) adding raised markings on elevator control buttons and lowering the panels, 4) creating designated parking spaces, 5) installing accessible door hardware, 6) widening doors and doorways, and 7) installing grab bars in toilet stalls.

Title IV applies to *telecommunication services.* It requires the provision of technical support for people with hearing and speech impairments. This area is responsible for telephone systems with TTY (teletypewriter) devices to be made available to the public in such facilities as airports and restaurants.

Title V applies to *due process* provisions. It includes notice that courts may award attorney's fees to prevailing parties, that retaliation and coercion against people with disabilities seeking enforcement are prohibited, and that the law does not invalidate any federal, state, or local laws. Although the ADA is enforced through court actions, parties are encouraged to resolve disputes through methods other than litigation when appropriate.

INDIVIDUALS WITH DISABILITIES EDUCATION ACT

IDEA was amended in 1997 with PL 105-17. It was the latest revision of legislation passed originally in 1975 as PL 94-142, the Education for All Handicapped Children Act. The purpose of IDEA is to ensure that all children with disabilities have access to a *free appropriate public education* (FAPE) in the *least restrictive environment (LRE)*. IDEA has four major parts. *Part A* includes definitions and general provisions; *Part B* specifies how services are to be provided to preschool and school-age students; *Part C* specifies requirements for service provision to infants and toddlers and their families; and *Part D* includes provisions for supporting research, personnel preparation, technical assistance, and dissemination of information for improving the education of children with disabilities.

Part B, which regulates the provision of services for children with disabilities from ages 6 to 21 years, also includes *Section 619*, which regulates provision of services for preschool-age children (3–5 years) in most states. The LRE requirements of Part B specify that, whenever appropriate, children with disabilities must be educated with children without disabilities. Children with disabilities have **individualized education programs (IEPs),** which include statements of 1) the child's present levels of educational performance; 2) measurable annual goals, including benchmarks or short-term objectives; 3) special education and related services to be provided, including supplementary aids and services; 4) the extent, if any, to which the child will not participate with children without disabilities in the regular class; 5) any modifications in administration of state or districtwide assessments of student achievement; 6) the projected date for the beginning of the services and the anticipated frequency, location, and duration of those services; 7) a description of transition services needed (at least by age 14), and 8) methods for measuring and reporting the child's progress toward annual goals on a schedule at least as frequent as general education reports of progress are made. IEPs must be revised at least annually and they must be designed in such a way as "to enable the child to be involved in and progress in the general curriculum" (Section 614 [a] [1] [A] [ii] [I]).

In developing each child's IEP, the *IEP team* considers the strengths of the child, the concerns of the child's parents and teachers, and the results of the initial evaluation or most recent evaluation of the child. The IEP team consists of 1) the parents of the child with a disability; 2) at least one general education teacher of such child (if the child is, or may be, participating in the general education environment); 3) at least one special education teacher, or where appropriate, at least one special education provider of such child; 4) a representative of the local education agency; 5) at the discretion of the parent or the agency, other individuals who have knowledge or special expertise regarding the child, including related services personnel; and 6) whenever appropriate, the child with a disability. A sample IEP appears in Figure 8.1.

Part C describes provisions for services to meet the needs of *infants and toddlers with disabilities.* Children served under Part C have **individualized family service plans (IFSPs)** rather than IEPs. (Children between 3 and 5 years may have either an IEP under Section 619 of Part B or an IFSP under Part C, depending on their own state's organizational system.) IFSPs define the service unit as the family rather than the child. Development of IFSPs requires decisions to be made about a family's service needs and mandates family representation in the decision-making process. The content of IFSPs includes statements of 1) the infant's or toddler's present levels of development; 2) the family's resources, priorities, and concerns; 3) major outcomes expected; 4) specific early intervention services; 5) natural environments in which services shall occur; 6) projected dates of initiation of services and length; 7) identification of the service coordinator, and 8) steps to be taken to support the transition to preschool or other educational levels. IFSPs must be revised at least every 6 months. Figure 8.2 contains a sample of an IFSP.

MEDICARE, MEDICAID, AND THE BALANCED BUDGET AMENDMENTS

Prior to 1961, public policies aimed at assisting older adults consisted primarily of retirement supplements and benefits for the poor. In 1961, President John F. Kennedy sponsored a "Conference on Aging" to build national awareness of issues important to older adults. The outcome of this conference was identification of problems ("want-get gaps") that were distressing to older adults, such as

INDIVIDUALIZED EDUCATION PROGRAM MEASURABLE ANNUAL GOAL AND SHORT-TERM OBJECTIVES

Student: _____ DOB: _____ PPT DATE: _____

☐ Academic/Cognitive ☐ Social/Behavioral ☐ Communication ☐ Gross/Fine Motor ☐ Health ☐ Self Help ☐ Other: (specify) _____

☐ Employment/Post Secondary Education*** ☐ Community Participation** ☐ Independent Living** ☐ **Check here if the student is 13 or older.** If checked, **IEP/28-R99,** Transition Planning Summary must be completed. ***Required if Goals are written. **If this area is **NOT** addressed, there must be a Justification Statement on **IEP/28-R99,** Transition Planning Summary

Measurable Annual Goal # _____ :	Method of Evaluation	Performance Criteria	Report of Progress*			
			Nov.	Jan.	April	June
Short Term Objectives/Benchmarks						
Obj#:						
Obj#:						
Obj#:						

Evaluation Procedures	Performance Criteria	Report of Progress Key*
1=Criterion-Referenced/Curriculum Based Assessment	**A**=100%	**M**=Mastered
2=Pre & Post Standardized Assessment	**B**=90%	**S**=Satisfactory Progress (likely to achieve)
3=Pre & Post Base Line Data	**C**=80%	**U**=Unsatisfactory Progress (unlikely to achieve)
4=Quizzes/Tests	**D**=70%	**NP 1**=No Progress (will **Not** achieve) lack of prerequisite skills
5=Student Self-Assessment/Rubic	**E**=Standard Score Increase: ___	**NP 2**=No Progress (will **Not** achieve) need more time
6=Observation	**F**=Months Growth Increase: ___	**NP 3**=No Progress (will **Not** achieve) inadequate assessment
7=Work samples/Project/Experiment/Portfolio	**G**=Passing Grades/Score: ___	**NP 4**=No Progress (will **Not** achieve) excessive absences/tardiness
8=Job Performance or Products	**H**=Frequency/Trials: (e.g., 9/10) ___	**NI**=Not Introduced
9=Behavior/Performance Rating Scale	**I**=Duration: (e.g., 15 min, 1 per) ___	**O**=Other: (specify) ___
10=CMT/CAPT	**J**=Successful Completion of Task/Activity	
11=Achievement of Objectives *(Note: Use with goal Only)*	**K**=Other: (specify) ___	*Indicating extent to which progress is sufficient to achieve goal by the end of the year
12=Other: (specify) ___	**L**=Other: (specify) ___	

Figure 8.1.   Sample individualized education program form.

SAMPLE INDIVIDUALIZED EDUCATION PROGRAM (CON'T.)
MODIFICATIONS/ADAPTATIONS IN REGULAR EDUCATION-INLCING NONACADEMIC AND EXTRACURRICULAR ACTIVITIES AND COLLABORATION/SUPPORTS FOR SCHOOL PERSONNEL

Student: _____ DOB: _____ PPT Date: _____

Modifications/Adaptations in Regular Education-Including Nonacademic and Extracurricular Activities	Sites/Activities Where Required and Duration	Required Supports for Personnel and Frequency and Duration of Supports**
Materials/Books/Equipment:		
☐ Alternative Text ☐ Consumable Workbook ☐ Modified Worksheets ☐ Manipulatives ☐ Access to Computer		
☐ Tape Recorder ☐ Supplementary Visuals ☐ Large Print Text ☐ Spell Check ☐ Calculator		
☐ Assistive Technology: (specify) ☐ Other: (specify)		
Tests/Quizzes/Time:		
☐ Prior Notice of Tests ☐ Preview Test Procedures ☐ Test Study Guide ☐ Simplify Test Wording ☐ Oral Testing		
☐ Limited Multiple Choice ☐ Student Writes on Test ☐ Shortened Tasks ☐ Hands-on Projects ☐ Reduced Reading		
☐ Alternative Tests ☐ Objective Tests ☐ Extra Credit Options ☐ Extra Time-Written Work		
☐ Extra Time-Tests ☐ Extra Time-Projects ☐ Extra Response Time ☐ Modified Tests		
☐ Pace Long Term Projects ☐ Rephrase Test Questions/Directions ☐ Other: (specify)		
Grading:		
☐ No Spelling Penalty ☐ No Handwriting Penalty ☐ Grade Effort+Work ☐ Grade Improvement ☐ Course Credit		
☐ Base Grade on IEP ☐ Base Grade on Ability ☐ Modified Grades ☐ Pass/Fail ☐ Audit Course		
☐ Other: (specify)		
Organization:		
☐ Provide Study Outlines ☐ Desktop List of Tasks ☐ List Sequential Steps ☐ Post Routines ☐ Post Assignments		
☐ Give One Paper at a time ☐ Folders to Hold Work ☐ Pencil Box for Tools ☐ Pocket Folder for Work ☐ Assignment Pad		
☐ Daily Assignment List ☐ Daily Homework List ☐ Worksheet Formats ☐ Extra Space for Work ☐ Assign Partner		
☐ Other: (specify)		
Environment:		
☐ Preferential Seating ☐ Clear Work Area ☐ Study Carrel ☐ Other: (specify)		
Behavioral Management:		
☐ Daily Feedback to Student ☐ Chart Progress ☐ Behavior Contracts ☐ Parent/Guardian Sign Homework		
☐ Positive Reinforcement ☐ Collect Baseline Data ☐ Set/Post Class Rules ☐ Parent/Guardian Sign Behavioral Chart		
☐ Cue Expected Behavior ☐ Structure Transitions ☐ Break Between Tasks ☐ Time Out From Positive Reinforcement		
☐ Proximity/Touch Control ☐ Contingency Plan ☐ Other: (specify)		
Teaching Strategies:		
☐ Check Work in Progress ☐ Immediate Feedback ☐ Pre-teach Content ☐ Have Student Restate Information		
☐ Extra Drill/Practice ☐ Review Sessions ☐ Review Directions ☐ Provide Lecture Notes/Outline to Student		
☐ Use Manipulatives ☐ Modified Content ☐ Assign Study Partner ☐ Computer Assisted Instruction		
☐ Monitor Assignments ☐ Provide Models ☐ Repeat Instructions ☐ Support Auditory Presentation with Visuals		
☐ Multi-Sensory Approach ☐ Highlight Key Words ☐ Oral Reminders ☐ Display Key Vocabulary		
☐ Visual Reinforcement ☐ Pictures/Charts ☐ Visual Reminders ☐ Provide Student with Vocabulary Word Bank		
☐ Mimed Clues/Gestures ☐ Concrete Examples ☐ Use Mnemonics ☐ Personalized Examples		
☐ Number Line ☐ Other: (specify)		

Figure 8.1. *(continued)*

Figure 8.1. *(continued)*

OBJ WL1

WRITTEN LANGUAGE: EARLY AND MIDDLE STAGES

CHILD: _____ AGE: _____ SCHOOL: _____ GRADE/LEVEL: _____ Date: _____

SPEECH-LANGUAGE PATHOLOGIST: _____ OTHERS IMPLEMENTING OBJECTIVES: _____

GOAL: The child will demonstrate skill for decoding and comprehending written words, sentences, paragraphs, and texts, and for writing short paragraphs that make sense.

PRESENT LEVELS OF PERFORMANCE:

PART A. PHONOLOGICAL AWARENESS

SHORT-TERM OBJECTIVES: THE CHILD WILL:	INDIVIDUAL THERAPY		MINICLASSROOM		CLASSROOM		COMMENTS/ TECHNIQUES/ EVALUATION
	Date In.	Date Accom.	Date In.	Date Accom.	Date In.	Date Accom.	
A. demonstrate phonological awareness skills for associating sounds and symbols by performing activities such as those listed below (80% success level in each of the contexts selected for at least 2 sessions):							
1. segment words into their constituent phonemes in order to:							
a. "stretch" particular sounds in words (i.e., extend continuants or repeat stops), as requested by an adult ("cat, stretch the /k/ sound" → /k-k-kaet/; "sock, stretch the first sound" → /sssok/);							
b. delete a sound in the position specified in a word which has been pronounced by an adult ("If I say rope, you say ope; If I say sock, you say ock; If I say shoe, you say ____");							
c. tell what sound a word starts with;							
d. tell what sound a word ends with;							
e. identify the vowel sounds in single syllable words;							
f. pronounce words with separated phonemes after they have been pronounced as whole words by an adult ("cat" → /k/-/ae/-/t/);							
2. synthesize sounds and syllables spoken individually by an adult, and say them so that they can be recognized as nonsense words (i.e., nonwords that conform to the orthographic and phonological structure of English) or real words, retaining the number and sequence of sounds from the separated model;							
3. analyze sound patterns of words with sufficient skill to be able to:							
a. tell whether or not two words are the same;							

The portion on written language is from Nelson, N.W. [1988]. *Planning individualized speech and language intervention programs* (pp. 345–346). Austin, TX:PRO-ED.

OBJ WL1

WRITTEN LANGUAGE: EARLY AND MIDDLE STAGES

Date: _____

CHILD: _____

SHORT-TERM OBJECTIVES: THE CHILD WILL:	INDIVIDUAL THERAPY		MINICLASSROOM		CLASSROOM		COMMENTS/ TECHNIQUES/ EVALUATION
	Date In.	Date Accom.	Date In.	Date Accom.	Date In.	Date Accom.	
b. tell whether or not two words rhyme;							
c. tell how many syllables are in a word;							
d. tell which syllable in a word is accented;							
4. associate sounds and symbols with sufficient skill to be able to:							
a. pick the following letter symbols from an array to match their associated spoken phonemes:							
b. write the following letter symbols to match their associated spoken phonemes:							
c. say the sound usually indicated by the following letter symbols:							
d. name the letter indicated by the following symbols:							
e. show differential knowledge of such metalinguistic terms as "letter," "sound," "word," and "syllable," by responding appropriately to such mixed directions as "Tell me what letter this is," and "Tell me what sound this is";							
f. select written syllables and nonsense words to match spoken sound patterns, using previously learned phoneme/letter correspondences;							
g. read nonsense words;							

Referral Date _2-11-01_

Person Referring _D. Smith_

Today's Date _2-12-01_

Agency Initiating IFSP _Public School_

Child Information

Social Security # _1-11-11-1111_

Child's Legal Name _Janna Johnson_		Nickname _Janna_	Date of Birth _11-1-99_	Sex: M/F
Address _123 Main Street, Any town, USA_		Phone (home) _555-5555_		Phone (daycare) _555-5554_
Address		Medical Insurance # 123456789		
School District of Residence _Any town Schools_	County _Any town_	Ethnic Heritage _African Am._		Native Language _English_

Name	Relationship to Child	Birth date (Optional)	Address	Phone (home)	Phone (work)
Mike Johnson	_Father_	_3-15-71_	_Same as above_	_Same_	_555-1212_
Sharika Johnson	_Mother_	_8-29-71_	_Same as above_	_Same_	_555-1234_
Issac Johnson	_Brother_	_7-13-97_	_Same_	_Same_	_----_

If parent/guardian needs an interpreter, give language:

Agencies and Persons Working with the Family (Fill in anytime)

Start Date	Agency	Contact Person (s)	Phone	Type of Service or Title	End Date	Send Copy of IFSP?
_11-5-99_	_Health Services Hosp._	_Isabel Jones_	_222-2222_	_Audiologist_		_X_
_1-5-00_	_Any town Public School_	_Diane Smith_	_333-3333_	_Speech Language Pathologist_		

Child's Strengths and Needs

Child's Name _Janna Johnson_		Birth Weight _7.2_	Birth date _11-1-99_	Number of Wks premature _NA_

Area	Present Level of Development		Date	Name/Type of Evaluation	Person Doing Evaluation	Agency
	Parent Input	Professional Input				
General	_Very expressive, and "laid back". A good baby_	_Speech therapy, Continued hearing impaired services after a cochlear implant_	_1-15-01_	_Cognitive screening_	_Developmental Psychologist_	_Anytown Schools_
Hearing	_Doesn't respond to sound but does to gestures_	_Profound bilateral hearing imp._	_11-5-99_ _12-15-99_	_Neonatal screening ABR_	_Audiologist_	_Health Services Hospital_
Communication	_Follows eyes, coos and makes sounds_	_Age appropriate so far_		_Rossetti Infant-Toddler Scale_	_SLP_	_Anytown Schools_

Child Eligibility

Part C of IDEA	_X_ Yes	☐ No	☐ Unknown	(Based on: Established Condition _deafness_	Developmental Delay _____

Service Plan

Service Coordinator _D. Smith_ Services Coordinator Phone # _333-0300_				
Interim	_X_ Initial	Review	Annual	Transition (90 days before entry into new program or third birthday – whichever comes first.)

OUTCOMES	WHO & WHAT	WHERE, WHEN & HOW	DATE SERVICE		PAYOR	REVIEW *
What would we like to have happen, by when, and how will we know when it happens.	What service or activity is needed and Who will do it.	When will the services occur, How often, How long each time, Individual or Group	Begins	Ends	Who will pay for it	Date/ Rating/ Comments
1) _Cochlear implant (3-5-01)_	1) _Univ. Hospital_	1) _Implant programming_	_3-5-01_	_When complete_	_Private insurance + Medicaid_	
2) _Understand and say words by age 2 (at least 50)_	2) _Speech/ Lang Pathologist, Speech language therapy_	2) _Parent-toddler group 60 min. 2x/week; 20-30 min. Individual Tx with family_	_2-17-01_		_Public School_	
3) _Take part in family discussions by age 3 (make comments and ask Qs)_	3) _Hearing Impaired Teacher Consultant_	3) _Home Visit 1x/month: 45 min Individual Tx_	_1-18-00_		_Public School_	
4) _Play normally with other children by age 4_	4) _Early Intervention Coordinator_	4) _Weekly home or clinic consultation by H.I Consultant_	_11-1-99_	_ongoing_	_Public School_	

Figure 8.2.   Sample individualized family service plan.

228

health and income maintenance; retiring with dignity; and issues pertaining to housing, transportation, and social isolation (Brown, 1996). This conference set the stage for the development of several key pieces of legislation, including the Older American's Act of 1965 (reauthorized in 2000 as the Older American Act Amendments [PL 106-501]), Medicare, and Medicaid (Brown, 1996). The purpose of the Older American's Act was to help older people by providing funds to states for programs and services such as education about nutrition, hot meals, transportation, legal assistance, and materials to train service providers in the area of gerontology (Gelfand, 1999).

Medicare

The Social Security Act of 1935 (PL 74-271), which had been passed under the leadership of President Franklin D. Roosevelt, was originally designed to alleviate conditions of poverty. Medicare was established in 1965 as Title 18 to the Social Security Act. It was an initial attempt by the government to assist individuals to meet the costs of adequate health care. Medicare assistance is administered by the *Health Care Financing Administration* and is available to individuals older than 65 who are eligible for benefits based on their employment before retirement. It is also available to individuals younger than age 65 who have renal disease or a disability (Gelfand, 1999). Medicare has two parts: *Part A* provides prepaid hospital insurance and *Part B* offers optional additional medical insurance.

Part A finances hospital insurance through a payroll tax. Consequently, those who are eligible for Medicare do not pay additional premiums for the hospital insurance, which covers inpatient care in hospitals, **skilled nursing facilities (SNFs),** and hospice for a limited number of days in any benefit period. A **benefit period** includes the time from when one first enters the hospital up to and including the day of discharge from the hospital. The longer the stay in the hospital, the more out-of-pocket costs are charged to the patient and the less costs are covered by Medicare. For example, the first 60 days are covered by Medicare after the patient has paid a deductible, which is typically equivalent to one day's stay in the hospital (Dye, 1998). For days 61–90, the patient pays a co-payment for each day of hospital stay (New York State Bar Association [NYSBA], 1996).

Part A benefits also cover limited days in a SNF. SNFs (previously known as *nursing homes*) are identified as such because they include a percentage of residents who require services from skilled professionals such as nurses and rehabilitation specialists. For the first 20 days in a SNF, Medicare pays 100% of the costs. For days 21–100, there is a co-payment (e.g., Medicare pays 80%, patient and family pay 20% of costs). After 100 days, the patient must have a pay source other than Medicare. Pay sources may include private pay, Medicaid, or other supplemental insurance plans (Patricia A. Walker, personal communication, January 23, 2000). Part B of Medicare consists of medical insurance, which is financed through a monthly premium paid by the patient. In the year 2000, eligible people paid approximately $45.50 per month for this insurance, but the rate was scheduled to increase. After an annual deductible of $100 is met, Medicare Part B pays 80% of "reasonable and necessary charges" for covered services.

Most services covered under Part B are limited to long-term, rehabilitative care. There is little emphasis on preventative care because routine checkups, glasses, dental care, and prescriptions are not covered under Part B services (Brown, 1996). Part B, however, will cover such services as home health services, physician medical and surgical services, supplies (including drugs that cannot be self-administered), diagnostic services, physical therapy, home dialysis, X-rays, surgical dressings, casts, orthopedic devices, oxygen tanks, wheelchairs, ambulance services, prosthetic devices (but not dentures), and immunizations (NYSBA, 1996). In 2001, Part B does not cover hearing aids, but as of January 2001, coverage of augmentative and alternative communication devices (referred to by Medicare as "speech generating devices or SGD") was added for people eligible for Medicare for whom need can be justified (http://www.aac-rerc.com).

Some programs have been established to fill the gaps in Medicare services to older adults of low socioeconomic status and to those with disabilities. One program is **Medigap,** consisting of supplemental insurance to cover what Medicare does not. Although there are 10 Medigap policies (Gelfand, 1999), each of which offers a different benefit package, there are services that are common to each Medigap package. These core services include co-insurance for Medicare Part A, 365 days of hospital coverage after Medicare benefits end, 20% of doctors fees not covered by Medicare, and the first 3 pints of blood needed each year (Gelfand, 1999).

Managed care organizations (MCOs) provide additional forms of supplemental insurance to Medicare recipients. MCOs manage or control health care expenditures by closely monitoring how service providers (e.g., hospitals, physicians) treat their patients and by evaluating the necessity, appropriateness, and payment efficiency of health services. The oldest types of MCOs are **health maintenance organizations (HMOs).** HMOs provide a range of care on a prepayment basis; individuals continue to pay Medicare Part B premiums and the HMO receives payment from the federal government for each HMO member equivalent to 95% of the average Medicare costs. HMOs cover many costs that are not covered by Medicare, such as prescription drugs and eyeglasses; however, some speech-language pathologists (SLPs) have experienced problems with HMOs when attempting to get approval for necessary SLP services.

HMOs contract with or employ service providers and pay for a *minimum* of 2 months or 60 visits (whichever is more) per condition for a combination of SLP, occupational therapy (OT), and physical therapy (PT) services. Some HMOs, unfortunately, interpret these visits as the *maximum* rather than the minimum, resulting in inadequately provided SLP services. Consider the following two cases.

CASE EXAMPLE 1

Mrs. Robinson, an outpatient at Cedar Rehabilitation Services, was referred by an ear, nose, and throat specialist to Ms. Downs, an SLP, for voice therapy following medical treatment for vocal nodules. For each of the next 6 months after receipt of the referral, the HMO refused to approve treatment. When treatment was approved, it was approved for three visits only. Ms. Downs felt that three visits simply were insufficient to serve this client adequately. She continued to advocate with the HMO to justify additional sessions and wrote to her legislators about problems in the health care financing system that were affecting their constituents' access to adequate health care.

CASE EXAMPLE 2

Mr. Rivers resided in a SNF for 2 years prior to having a stroke. Following the stroke, he was evaluated by Ms. Jackson, the SLP on staff, who found that Mr. Rivers required dysphagia treatment. The SLP recommended treatment for 5 days per week for 3 weeks. Mr. Rivers' HMO, however, approved 5 days per week for 1 week. The SLP provided dysphagia treatment for 1 week, during which time she trained the nursing staff to feed and support Mr. Rivers during meal times. Ms. Jackson reported that the limited time approved for therapy did not allow the opportunity to establish and monitor a routine with the nursing staff charged with managing the care of Mr. Rivers. Consequently, the staff often forgot to use the food and liquid thickener and frequently did not assist Mr. Rivers during mealtime. He suffered several episodes of aspiration and eventually reverted to his original swallowing problem. Like Ms. Downs, Ms. Jackson continued to advocate with the HMO to justify more treatment sessions and communicated with Mr. Rivers' legislators about the dangers inherent in the current system, some of which were life threatening.

Medicaid

Congress established Medicaid in 1965 under Title 19 of the Social Security Act. Funding for Medicaid comes from state, federal, and city taxes. Hence, it is a *federal/state matching program* because both the state and federal governments must contribute to it. Also, it is run by the state with guidelines from the federal government, resulting in variability in eligibility benefits from one state to the next.

Medicaid is an **entitlement program** that was created to pay medical bills for people of low socioeconomic status who have no other financial means to pay for medical care. An entitlement program refers to expected government benefits for groups for which Congress has set eligibility criteria, such as age, income, retirement, disability, or unemployment. If one meets the criteria established by the government, then he or she is entitled to the benefits offered through the program (Dye, 1998). Most Medicaid spending goes to older adults and to younger adults with disabilities. In addition, anyone receiving public assistance (*Supplemental Security Income [SSI]*, or *Temporary Assistance for Needy Families [TANF]*) is automatically eligible for Medicaid.

Medicaid covers such services as payment to hospitals, coverage of prenatal and delivery services for those with no other insurance, and services to families of low socioeconomic status who do not receive cash assistance. Moreover, it also covers long-term nursing home care but only after beneficiaries have exhausted all of their other income and forms of payment. Most benefits are limited to long-term rehabilitative care with little emphasis on preventive care.

Legislation was passed in 1996 to restructure Medicaid funding and to fill in some of the gaps previously not covered by Medicaid. The Personal Responsibility and Work Opportunity Reconciliation Act of 1996 (PL 104-93) created mandatory categories of eligibility with assistance to pregnant women and children younger than 6 years with a family income below 133% of the poverty level; children 6–12 years in families with income below 100% of the poverty level and with optional coverage for children ages 13–18; children receiving foster care and adoption assistance; and individuals with disabilities who meet income and resource standards as determined by states (NYSBA, 1996). This act eliminated the **fee-for-service finance structure** and introduced a **capitated finance structure.** In a fee-for-service finance structure, service providers are compensated by paying the fee for each service provided. Typically, the providers agree to discount their fees by a certain percentage in exchange for referrals from the paying source (e.g., an HMO). Alternatively, in a capitated finance structure system, the HMO pays the service provider a set amount of money per enrollee per month for a defined set of medical services. For example, the provider may receive $.40 per enrollee per month to provide audiological services or $.04 per enrollee per month to provide speech-language pathology services.

BALANCED BUDGET AMENDMENTS

On August 1, 1997, former president William J. Clinton signed into law the Balanced Budget Amendment (BBA), which was designed to balance the national budget. The BBA included provisions to reduce overall spending on Medicaid and to slow the growth of Medicare spending over 5 years. It also included funds for preventative benefits not previously provided, such as mammograms, diabetes self-management, and prostate and colorectal cancer screenings. Caps were placed on spending under the BBA that would result in some programs receiving more funds and other programs receiving less funds, causing agencies and providers to compete for funding. As often occurs, those most affected by budget cuts are those most vulnerable—individuals who are older, are of low socioeconomic status, or have disabilities.

One result of the caps on spending was the $1,500 cap on Medicare outpatient rehabilitation services, which affected SLP, OT, and PT services. Specifically, this cap required SLPs and PTs to share a maximum of $1,500 for Part B Medicare services for each patient. Several problems rose from this cap, but two primary concerns were that 1) the shared cap forced patients to choose between two vital services and 2) patients in SNFs or rehabilitation agencies who had used up their $1,500 limit would have to leave their current placements to seek help in hospital outpatient facilities that were less accessible.

The Balanced Budget Refinement Act (BBRA) of 1999 (PL 106-113) was signed into law on November 29, 1999, by former president Clinton, resulting in a 2-year moratorium on the $1,500 cap on Medicare Part B services for outpatient SLP, OT, and PT services beginning January 2000 until December 2001. Through this "refined" act, speech-language pathology service was reinstated as an independent service no longer linked with PT; this made it possible for SLPs and PTs to be reimbursed separately. The BBRA was brought about through the actions of Senator Charles Grassley [R-IA] and Representative Richard Burr [R-NC] who introduced the legislation with the help of other elected representatives and through the advocacy of special interest groups such as ASHA, the American Occupational Therapy Association, and the American Physical Therapy Association.

ADVOCACY

It is difficult to imagine how one could be an effective, ethical practitioner and not be actively involved in understanding, implementing, and influencing public policy. Thinking of oneself in the **advocacy** role may conjure up intimidating images of visits to Capitol Hill in Washington, D.C. This is one important avenue and not nearly as scary as it may seem at first, but active advocacy roles may also be assumed at the level of the individual client.

As we have discussed, policies are in place to govern who is eligible for service and who will pay for it, as well as how services are delivered. SLPs and audiologists are responsible for seeing that individuals receive services according to the policies written to address their needs. This means that professionals must know how to conduct assessments and write reports that will maximize their ability to deliver high-quality services. For example, this includes responsibility to advocate for clients who at first may appear not to qualify for services because of someone else's overly strict interpretation of eligibility guidelines. It also refers to advocacy efforts in calling and writing to third party payers on behalf of individual clients who have been denied funding for needed services.

CASE EXAMPLE 3

Mr. Watson is an SLP who works in a school district with a long-standing policy that students with language delays are not eligible for services unless formal tests show a discrepancy between cognitive I.Q. scores and language quotient scores. Brian is a child with a history of preschool language problems involving phonology and syntax. In first grade, Brian is struggling with phonemic awareness, reading decoding, and spoken and written language comprehension but with cognitive skills in the "low normal range" that are not significantly above his language test scores. Mr. Watson has been reading the literature and can find no support for the cognitive referencing "policy." He advocates for Brian's eligibility for service on the principle that consideration of Brian's individualized needs for specialized instruction under federal policy supercedes a local policy that reduces individualized decision making. Brian is placed on Mr. Watson's caseload and receives services. At the same time, Mr. Watson initiates a study group to reconsider the wisdom of the local guidelines.

Advocacy at the individual client level also may include working with others to make policy implementation effective. For example, one of the provisions of IDEA is that children with disabilities are expected "to be involved and progress in the general curriculum...and to participate in extracurricular and other nonacademic activities; and to be educated and participate with other children with disabilities and non-disabled children" (Part B, Section 614 [d] [1] [A] [iii] [II-III]). Implementation of this policy may require some personal advocacy efforts by SLPs and audiologists with school district and building staffs to increase opportunities for individual clients to participate with their peers and be active in the general education curriculum.

CASE EXAMPLE 4

Ms. Ramirez has been working as an SLP for a year in an elementary school in which the students with special needs have traditionally been served in separate class-rooms or pulled out for speech-language therapy. She is concerned that this approach is not meeting the students' needs and begins to work with the early and later elementary special education teachers to bring more aspects of the general education curriculum into the special education classroom. She also explores more ways for the students with disabilities to participate actively with their peers in the general education classrooms.

Advocacy at the individual client level also includes responsibility to instruct clients and their families about how to advocate for themselves. This includes informing clients about relevant public policies, helping them acquire strategies for communicating their needs to others consistent with those policies, and providing consultation about due process for remedying problems if they arise. Consultation may also be provided to individuals and families who want to know how to play an active role in advocating for policy changes themselves.

In addition to being an advocate for individuals, it is important to consider extending advocacy efforts to broader issues of practice. Local, state, and federal policies govern areas such as professional certification and licensure, as well as access to care for people with disabilities and other aspects of clinical decision making. When policies (or lack thereof) have negative effects on how professional services are provided, it is the responsibility of professionals to advocate for changes in those policies.

Advocacy Strategies

Grass roots advocacy involves efforts of individuals. This type of advocacy is particularly effective because it is individuals who are eligible to vote for policy makers. Professional associations often guide the process, however, making it less daunting. Associations serve as a resource for clarifying the issues, for keeping individuals informed, and for setting up opportunities for members to communicate with key policy makers.

Understanding Current Policy and How to Change It   The first step for individuals who wish to influence existing policy is to obtain a copy of the actual wording of the current policy. This involves a series of steps to find out 1) where the policy is printed (this usually can be done through the Internet), 2) which government body or agency made the policy or rule, 3) whether the policy might have flexibility that was previously not noticed, and 4) whether one's immediate employer or reimbursement agency might have room to negotiate a variation that will overcome the particular problem or concern. If current policy still clearly presents a problem, professionals have three choices (Nelson, 1998):

1. *Study the rationale for the policy and decide to accept it.* In some cases, investigating the rationale for a policy may lead to greater understanding about why the policy was established, and the professional may decide that there is no need to influence change.

2. *Seek approval for a policy exception.* If a policy includes any room for negotiation or for exceptions, the professional may pursue such options. Obtaining permission for an exception to the rule may make it possible to gather additional data, which can then be used to make a case for widespread change if it still seems desirable.

3. *Work to change the official policy.* If a policy clearly needs changing, professionals have an obligation to work within official systems to advocate for change.

Communicating Directly with Policy Makers   The framing of a new bill requires direct involvement with legislators, particularly those on the committee where the bill will first be considered. Professional associations sometimes employ lobbyists who are familiar with this complicated process and know best how to influence it. If the change needed is at the level of regulation rather than legislation, it may be more appropriate to start by communicating with the agency of the executive branch of government that is responsible for implementing the policy. One important question in such cases is whether the agency expects the regulations to be open for change any time soon.

When communicating directly with policy makers, it is important to note that most employers do not allow their employees to write letters with political implications on agency stationery. Political advocacy messages should be conveyed as personal communications by individuals. This makes it clear that a constituent's views do not necessarily represent the official positions of the individual's employers. In fact, personal communications coming from constituent's home addresses to legislative representatives and senators (state or national) gen-

Table 8.1.   Checklist for advocacy letters

Short: Is my letter one page or less in length?

Direct: Is my letter to the point?

Client-based rationale: Does my letter show how the proposed policy or change will influence the lives of the constituents of the person to whom I am addressing the letter?

Data rather than emotions: Does my letter provide information that will help the policy maker decide (rather than making an emotional plea)?

Ask for a specific action: Does my letter make it clear what action I am requesting from the policy maker?

Responsive: Does my letter indicate who I am and how I may be contacted for further information? (This also implies that I will follow up with the policy maker to express appreciation for considering my input, and if appropriate, to thank the policy maker for action consistent with my request.)

Personal: Is my letter on my personal stationery unless I have obtained specific permission to use the stationery of the agency where I am employed?

erally have the most meaning for policy makers. Table 8.1 summarizes considerations for writing advocacy letters or e-mail messages.

Working within Professional Associations   Some of the most effective efforts to influence change are guided by members of professional associations working together. ASHA, for example, keeps its members informed of policies and their implications, both through its web page (http://www.professional.asha.org) and its publications, particularly *The ASHA Leader*. ASHA's Government Relations and Public Policy Board is responsible for developing an annual public policy agenda to prioritize the advocacy activities of the association. The goal is to address issues that are of major concern to speech-language-hearing scientists, SLPs, audiologists, and those that they serve. Two examples of the effectiveness of this agenda setting strategy (Moore, 2000) were observed in 1999 when 1) a campaign of letters, telephone calls, e-mails, and visits to Capitol Hill by consumers and ASHA members led to the suspension of the $1,500 cap (introduced in the BBA) on funding for rehabilitation outpatient services (SLP, OT, and PT) that could be covered by Medicare Part B; 2) a similar campaign, fortified by an ASHA-led coalition of 20 organizations, resulted in the passage of the "Newborn and Infant Hearing Screening and Intervention Act" (Boswell, 2000).

At a minimum, professionals who pay their dues to professional associations help to maintain the organizations so that they can monitor public policy and communicate with their members, the public, and policy makers. At a level of slightly greater involvement, professionals can make voluntary contributions to groups that are in a position to lobby directly for change, using strategies that include financial contributions to political campaigns of candidates. At the most active level, professionals can become personally involved by writing letters, sending e-mail messages, and making telephone calls or personal visits to policy makers. Individual SLPs and audiologists have played important roles in the development and modifications that have been made over the years in many of the key pieces of legislation discussed in this chapter.

CONCLUSION

Public policies guide many aspects of clinical decision making. It is the responsibility of professional practitioners to understand how public policies are generated, legislated, and regulated. Although professionals are expected to implement public policies, they also can question the wisdom of some policies, and when problems are evident, it is professionals' responsibility to advocate for change. Effective advocacy involves gathering and presenting data in a way that communicates a need clearly to policy makers. Among the United States of America's policies that are important for the practice of speech-language pathology and audiology are Section 504 of the Rehabilitation Act, the ADA, IDEA, Medicare, Medicaid, and the BBA.

REFERENCES

Americans with Disabilities Act (ADA) of 1990, PL 101-336, 42 U.S.C. §§ 12101 *et seq.*
Boswell, S. (2000). Congress funds newborn hearing screening. *The ASHA Leader, 5*(1), 1.

Brown, D.K. (1996). *Introduction to public policy: An aging perspective.* Lanham, MD: University Press of America.

Dye, T.R. (1975). *Understanding public policy* (2nd ed.). Upper Saddle River, NJ: Prentice Hall.

Dye, T.R. (1998). *Understanding public policy* (9th ed.). Upper Saddle River, NJ: Prentice Hall.

Education for All Handicapped Children Act of 1975, PL 94-142, 20 U.S.C. §§ 1400 *et seq.*

Gelfand, D.E. (1999). *The aging network: Programs and services* (5th ed.). New York: Springer Publishing.

Individuals with Disabilities Education Act (IDEA) of 1990, PL 101-476, 20 U.S.C. §§ 1400 *et seq.*

Individuals with Disabilities Education Act Amendments (IDEA) of 1997, PL 105-17, 20 U.S.C. §§ 1400 *et seq.*

Lieurance, E. (1993, October). *Speak up! Get involved in public policy.* (Available on-line at http://www.muextension.missouri.edu/xplor/hesguide/famecon/gh3970.htm)

Moore, M. (2000). '99 victories in Congress spur 2000 strategies. *The ASHA Leader,* 5(2), 1.

Nelson, N.W. (1998). *Childhood language disorders in context: Infancy through adolescence.* Needham Heights, MA: Allyn & Bacon.

New York State Bar Association Young Lawyers Section. (1996). *Senior citizens handbook.* (Available on-line at http://www.nysba.org/public/sencitizens/schandtoc.html)

Rehabilitation Act of 1973, PL 93-112, 29 U.S.C. §§ 701 *et seq.*

Social Security Act of 1935, PL 74-271, 42 U.S.C. §§ 301 *et seq.*

1. Differentiate among the forms (e.g., laws, regulations, guidelines, court decisions) that public policies may take, agencies that may generate them, and problems that they might address.

2. Describe two ways in which Section 504 differs from IDEA with regard to school-age children.

3. Describe some modifications that might be covered under Section 504 for post-secondary students.

4. What are the three basic purposes of the ADA; what is covered under each of its five titles; and how is the law enforced?

5. What are the two major purposes of IDEA, and what is covered under each of its four main parts? Within Part B, what age group does Section 619 cover?

6. Compare and contrast IEPs and IFSPs.

7. When was Medicare first passed and as part of what law? What does HCFA do? Who is eligible for Medicare coverage? What are the differences between Part A and Part B of Medicare coverage?

8. Who is covered under Medicaid and how does it differ from Medicare?

9. What were some of the problems associated with the BBA of 1997? How did the BBRA resolve them, and what lobbying efforts led up to it?

10. What strategies could you use in dealing with policies that you think should be changed?

Clinical Service Delivery

Paul W. Cascella
Mary H. Purdy
James J. Dempsey

Speech-language pathologists (SLPs) and audiologists provide a broad range of professional services aimed at assessing, treating, and preventing speech, language, voice, hearing, swallowing, and related communication disabilities. Estimates have identified that there are about 3 million Americans with speech-language impairments and roughly 21–28 million Americans with hearing impairments (American Speech-Language-Hearing Association [ASHA], 1994b). As professionals, we strive to create service delivery models that can accommodate the range of communication disabilities, while at the same time, matching the particular needs of each individual. **Service delivery models** are the systems that we use to organize speech-language and hearing programs within our employment settings. These models define our roles in the rehabilitation of people with communication disorders.

This chapter introduces contemporary service delivery models and work settings within the field of communication disorders. In discussing service delivery, we talk about the formats by which services are rendered, including where, when, and with whom services are provided. To illustrate service delivery, this chapter highlights specific work settings, some of which you will be assigned to during your educational program, and others that are more unique and less often included in professional preparation.

SERVICE DELIVERY FEATURES

To open this chapter, it is important that you become familiar with the core vocabulary that distinguishes one service delivery model from another. In service provision, particular features characterize each approach.

Direct and Indirect Services

Direct services occur when you work in a hands-on format with an individual client or a group of clients. In medical speech-language pathology, an example of a direct service is when the client comes to your office for treatment at a rehabilitation facility or when you practice swallowing with patients in their hospital room. **Indirect services** occur when you do not have hands-on contact with the client; instead, you consult with family members, teachers, and/or medical personnel about the client's communication needs. An example of this occurs when a classroom teacher follows your suggestion and deliberately emphasizes the way that particular sounds are pronounced during a "letter of the week" activity in a kindergarten class.

Clinical and Consultative Services

The terms *clinical* (or "pull-out") and *consultative* (or "push-in") are examples of direct services often utilized with school children ages 3–21. In a **clinical service delivery model,** the SLP typically takes children out of their general classroom, providing intensive one-to-one or small-group instruction in a separate location. A clinical model is advantageous when trying to initially teach children particular speech-language skills and when standardized testing needs to be completed. A clinical model can also be utilized when the child needs a less distracting environment and when the treatment protocol warrants privacy. This is necessary, for example, among students who stutter and need a safe place in which to talk about their feelings. The clinical model is also utilized within medical speech-language pathology.

Consultative services occur when the classroom teacher and the SLP structure small groups within the classroom, and the clinician specifically works with the one or two groups who have children with speech-language goals. An advantage of this approach is that the children can generalize and practice speech-language skills within the context of general classroom activities. In addition, this approach enables the teacher to directly observe the clinical strategies used by the SLP. Another format for the consultative approach has the SLP providing guidance to family members and professional colleagues (i.e., general and special education teachers, nursing home workers, group home personnel, **nurses,** early intervention teachers, **psychologists**) who work more directly with the client. This can occur, for example, when we teach parents how to provide home-based language models. Also, following our own diagnostic evaluation, we might make recommendations to a nursing home staff about how to keep a client with Alzheimer's disease less confused during daily situations.

In both clinical and consultative situations, there needs to be considerable scheduling coordination that does not interfere with classroom learning activities for school children. For example, in a clinical model, classroom teachers may become concerned about the amount of time and instruction that the child misses when taken from class. In consultative services, classroom curricula and activities must be flexible enough to accommodate the incorporation of speech-language goals. Consultation partnerships require professionals from different disciplines to work together in an effort to integrate client goals, objectives, and intervention strategies. In these partnerships, participants bring their own expertise to their professional colleagues when they design instruction, problem solve, and share teaching responsibilities.

Individual and Group Services

Individual services are intense and one-to-one in nature, whereas **group services** include two or more members, most of whom are working on similar speech-language skills. Individual services are usually direct and strive to make therapy more meaningful and relevant so that the client can generalize skills beyond the isolated treatment context. In contrast, group services more naturally foster social communication and the generalization of skills. An example of this can be found in many university clinics that conduct individual and group intervention for adults with **aphasia.** Individual services might focus on skill practice and strategies, whereas group sessions enable clients to receive natural feedback from their peers. Another example of group services occurs in a **self-contained classroom** when the SLP is the primary educator providing both academic instruction and intensive speech-language remediation. An example of this occurs when clinicians run their own class for preschoolers who need a focused speech-language program.

Multi-, Inter-, and Transdisciplinary Models

SLPs are often asked to work with their professional colleagues from education, medicine, and allied health (i.e., physical therapy, occupational therapy) so as to conjointly develop intervention plans that are unified and coordinated by content, objectives, and strategies (see Table 9.1). There are currently three models that identify the relationships shared by team members in the facilitation of client progress. The first two—interdisciplinary and multidisciplinary—are often interchanged depending on the work setting, and both are popular in medical settings and schools. In a **multidisciplinary** model, each individual discipline conducts its own assessment and develops discipline-specific goals with minimal integration of these goals across disciplines. Each discipline has its own plan for the client, with goals reflecting only their own field of expertise.

In an **interdisciplinary** model, each discipline conducts its own particular assessment; however, there is ongoing communication among professionals about the results of these assessments. This discussion fosters complimentary goal development so that as each discipline creates its plan for the client, professionals incorporate elements of the goals and objectives of related fields. For example, when working with individuals with traumatic brain injury, language sequencing may be one objective for the SLP. As part of the program, you might have the client write the steps associated with daily tasks. When doing so, the client can be given instructions about pen holding and eye–hand coordination, strategies that were suggested by the **occupational therapist (OT).** Likewise, during occupational therapy, the OT will include sequencing as part of therapeutic activities.

Table 9.1. Service delivery professionals

	Birth-to-3	School settings	Medical settings
Physiatrist			✓
Neurologist			✓
Nurse	✓	✓	✓
Nurse's aide			✓
Occupational therapist	✓	✓	✓
Physical therapist	✓	✓	✓
Speech-language pathologist	✓	✓	✓
Social worker	✓	✓	✓
Rehabilitation aides and paraprofessionals	✓	✓	✓
Recreational therapist			✓
Psychologist	✓	✓	✓
Neuropsychologist			✓
Child care worker	✓		
Special education teacher	✓	✓	
Pediatric developmental specialist	✓	✓	✓
Dietician			✓
Chaplain			✓
School counselor		✓	
General education teacher	✓	✓	

In a **transdisciplinary** model, team members have an ongoing dialogue in which they share information, knowledge, and skills in order to develop and implement a single integrated client services plan. In this model, a single assessment of the client is completed in unison by professionals from several disciplines. Together, they review assessment data and weave together objectives reflective of all the disciplines. Then, the team typically authorizes one person who, along with the family, becomes responsible for carrying out the client's treatment plan. In a transdisciplinary model, the family and the client are respected as key decision makers, with support coming from the primary interventionist and other team members as it is needed. The transdisciplinary model is often used in birth-to-3 service provision and among children and adults with severe developmental disabilities.

PROFESSIONAL GUIDELINES FOR SERVICE DELIVERY

In both speech-language pathology and audiology, there are guidelines from ASHA and the American Academy of Audiology (AAA) that provide direction about clinical activities within service delivery and work settings. These guidelines establish professional practice parameters for everyday clinical activities (see Table 9.2).

CONTEMPORARY ISSUES IN SERVICE DELIVERY

Historically, speech-language service delivery has concentrated on the one-to-one or small-group treatment approach in which client skills are strengthened

Table 9.2.   Service delivery guidelines from ASHA and the AAA

Organization	Guideline
ASHA and AAA Codes of Ethics	Provides an ethical code governing clinician behaviors and actions
ASHA and AAA scope of practice guidelines	Describes the broad range of services and supports offered by these professions
ASHA preferred practice guidelines	Outlines acceptable client care, clinical processes, and anticipated outcomes
ASHA practice guidelines	Recommends clinical practice parameters
ASHA position statements	Describes policies in matters of professional practice

through a hierarchy of task demands and prompts. Service delivery has seen vast changes since the 1970s, and service delivery models in 2001 reflect evolving government agencies, health care management, educational philosophy, and human services principles. As service providers, we need to be aware of these issues and recognize how they impact service delivery, regardless of the work setting in which we are employed (see Table 9.3).

EDUCATIONAL WORK SETTINGS

SLPs work in a variety of educational settings for children from birth to age 21. Here, we introduce you to some of the programs that you are likely to participate in as part of your graduate clinical practica.

Early Intervention Programs

Chapter 8 discusses the public policies that affect clinical practice, including public laws that govern early intervention services. Early intervention applies to children from birth to kindergarten, and two systems of early intervention exist, one for children from birth to 3 years, and the second for preschoolers (age 3 until kindergarten).

Birth-to-3 services emphasize that the family of the child with a disability is the recipient of the services. This means that we must understand family-guided practice that is both culturally sensitive and specific to each family's circumstance. In this model, family members are integral to the design, implementation, and evaluation of services, and they are considered partners with education and rehabilitation professionals in their child's developmental growth (Rini & Whitney, 1999). Birth-to-3 service provision most often operates using a transdisciplinary model by designing a single integrated **individualized family service plan (IFSP).** When speech-language objectives are recommended for the child, these are designed to coincide with objectives being addressed across other areas of development. The primary interventionist represents every discipline, and, for example, when we assume that role, we would facilitate not only communication skills but also any other goals on the child's IFSP (i.e., fine and gross motor skills, **cognition,** socialization, adaptive behavior, transition). In this model, service provision occurs in a variety of settings (i.e., the child's home, child care center, a clinic, segregated and inclusive playgroups, and/or library storytime) and our roles may be direct or indirect, individual or group, and consultative.

Table 9.3.   Contemporary issues that impact service delivery

Issue	SLPs are being challenged to:
Functional communication	Develop protocols that relate to classroom curricula, independent living and vocational skills, and the natural situations in which our clients communicate.
Assistive and instrumental technology	Increase their technical competence with augmentative and alternative communication (AAC), assistive technology, and medical technology (e.g., ventilators, tracheostomies, nasendoscopy, videofluoroscopy).
Managed care	Prioritize the measurement of clinical outcomes and treatment efficacy, with an emphasis on accountability.
Inclusion	Ensure that communication supports assist children with special needs as they gain access to the regular education curriculum.
Multicultural issues	Provide services that are culturally sensitive and culturally applicable.
Transition services	Help our clients make life transition decisions (e.g., high school to work, reintegration to employment after adult onset disorders).
Regulations and accreditation	Stay familiar with the regulatory and accreditation guidelines governing service delivery.
Self-advocacy, family involvement, client rights	Respect clients and family members as integral participants in designing, implementing, and evaluating the effectiveness of treatment programs.
Eligibility and exit criteria	Balance the opinions of clients, families, and regulatory bodies who may have different opinions about when services are warranted and/or when services are no longer needed.
Speech-language pathology assistants and paraprofessionals	Use support personnel.

A primary goal of many birth-to-3 programs is to mainstream young children with disabilities so as to provide rich peer language models and promote social development. In doing so, the interventionist becomes responsible for creating educational activities that adapt everyday routines by training child care providers and promoting social skills with peers.

Preschool and School-Based Services

Data from the 1995 ASHA omnibus survey indicated that 24% of school-based SLPs work in preschool settings, 45% serve children in the early elementary years (ages 6–11), and 25% serve children ages 12–17. The average caseload for school clinicians is 46 children, slightly higher than the ASHA recommendation of 40, and children are most often served in group sessions (44%). Table 9.4 identifies the distribution of communication disorders within schools.

Among school SLPs, particular service delivery models seem to occur for particular communication disorders. A traditional clinical model is prevalent for children with disorders of articulation/phonology, fluency, voice, and language. Classroom-based models are often utilized for children with augmentative communication needs, as well as children with language disorders, cognitive-communication needs, and central auditory processing disorders. Collaborative/

Table 9.4.   Percentage of communication
disorders served by school-based clinicians

Language	42%
Articulation/phonology	28%
Cognitive-communication	13%
Central auditory processing	5%
Augmentative communication	4%
Fluency	3%
Voice	2%
Dysphagia	1%
Aural rehabilitation	1%
Orofacial myofunctional	1%
Communication instruction	<1%

consultation models occur most frequently for children with language concerns and cognitive communication needs.

As Chapter 8 notes, children are eligible for speech-language services through the Individuals with Disabilities Education Act (IDEA) of 1990 (PL 101-476), the planning and placement team process, and the individualized education program. IDEA is the most often used mechanism for providing special services to students with disabilities; however, other legislative acts also serve that purpose (see Table 9.5). IDEA supports about 5.5 million school-age children (ages 3–21), and is the largest support mechanism for students with special needs served through federal legislation.

School-based speech-language services require the child to be labeled "speech or language impaired" or to have a primary diagnosis that includes speech-language concerns (i.e., specific learning disability, autism spectrum disorder, mental retardation, hearing impairment, attention-deficit/hyperactivity disorder). About 25% of students in special education have "speech or hearing impaired" as their primary diagnosis, making it the second largest special education disability classification. Of this group, nearly 80% are primarily educated in the general education environment. To qualify for speech-language services, the child's communication disability must negatively influence classroom learning. For example, children with a mild articulation problem may not qualify for speech services, as that problem is not likely to interfere with academic performance. Table 9.6 outlines IDEA-mandated school speech-language pathology services.

Within school-based services, clinicians are likely to be assigned nonclinical tasks shared by the entire teaching staff. This might include performing lunch and bus duty, assisting with kindergarten registration, creating hallway bulletin boards, and helping with school plays and concerts. These additional duties may seem unfairly time burdensome, given our large caseloads, travel between schools, and lack of planning time. Yet, these duties provide opportunities to interact cooperatively with the other faculty and enable the clinician to observe and stimulate children out of the typical classroom and therapy context.

Table 9.5. Examples of legislative efforts that impact service delivery to schools

Individuals with Disabilities Education Act (IDEA) Amendments of 1997 (PL 105-17)	This act stresses that students with special needs be given educational supports to succeed in the general education classroom. These supports can include modifications to the classroom teaching format, differentiated instruction, content enhancement (i.e., preteaching), cooperative learning, and/or assistive technology.
Section 504 of the Rehabilitation Act of 1973 (PL 93-112) and Title II of the Americans with Disabilities Act (ADA) of 1990 (PL 101-336)	These laws prohibit discrimination against people with disabilities by guaranteeing public access and accommodations. Section 504 may apply to children who do not qualify as educationally disabled based on IDEA '97, but for whom speech-language services accommodate the child in the general education setting.
Head Start Act of 1964	This act provides comprehensive health, education, dental, and social services to young children (birth through preschool) who meet certain economic guidelines, and allows for the placement of up to 10% of preschoolers with disabilities.
Goals 2000: Educate America Act of 1994 (PL 103-227)	Goals 2000 is part of the educational reform movement that encourages the nation's public schools to help all students reach rigorous academic and occupational standards.
School-to-Work Opportunities Act of 1994 (PL 103-239)	This act is aimed to create transition services that integrate academic and occupational learning so that graduating high school students can find productive roles in the American workforce.

246

Table 9.6.   IDEA '90 requirements for school-based speech-language services

Identification	Students must be screened to determine whether they have speech-language concerns in need of further assessment.
Assessment	Students who are potentially eligible for speech-language services must participate in nonbiased assessment of their strengths, weaknesses, disorders, and/or delays.
Treatment	Students deemed eligible for services are entitled to receive free and appropriate speech-language intervention services in the least restrictive environment.
Consultation/Counseling	Family members and educators who are primarily responsible for the child with disabilities are entitled to ongoing discussion about the child's problem and its remediation plan.
Referral	Children with communication disorders are entitled to the professional advice of related education and rehabilitation disciplines.

MEDICAL WORK SETTINGS

There are a wide variety of medical facilities in which we may work (see Table 9.7). Typically, the children and adults who are patients in these facilities sustained an injury or suffer from an illness that resulted in a communication and/or swallowing disorder (see Table 9.8). In each of these settings, our role typically includes assessment, development of a treatment plan, and patient–family education, although the proportion of these duties may vary depending on the setting. Individuals typically transition from one setting to another as the course of recovery and goals of rehabilitation change. This progression through various settings is referred to as the **continuum of care (COC).** As part of the treatment team, we often participate in the decision to transition people. See information on pages 250–251 for an example of how patients may progress through the COC.

The specific way in which services may be delivered vary among settings. Service delivery in medical settings is often influenced by various regulatory bodies. One of the major issues related to service delivery in medical settings is the concept of **managed care.** This is the collective term for approaches to the delivery of health care that attempt to control quality while containing costs. Third party payers that cover the costs of rehabilitation (e.g. Medicare, private insurance) now have a great influence in determining the number of sessions an individual may receive and may even influence how he or she progresses through the COC.

Table 9.7.   Medical settings in which a speech-language pathologist (SLP) may be employed

Acute care hospital
Rehabilitation units and hospitals
Outpatient rehabilitation centers
Transitional living centers
Residential care facilities
Home health care

Table 9.8.   Medical conditions that may result in communication and/or swallowing disorders

Medical conditions	Communication and swallowing disorders
Stroke	Aphasia
Traumatic brain injury	Dysarthria
Progressive disease	Apraxia
Spinal cord injury	Cognitive-linguistic disorder
Head and neck tumors	Dysphonia
Brain tumors	Aphonia
Dementia	Speech-language delay/disorder
Vocal fold abnormalities	Dysphagia
Acquired immunodeficiency syndrome	
Respiratory disorders	
Congenital and genetic disorders	
Premature birth	

Other regulatory bodies that may influence service delivery are the accreditation commissions. The **Joint Commission on the Accreditation of Health Care Organizations** and the **Commission on the Accreditation of Rehabilitation Facilities** both have regulations that must be met regarding documentation, amount of therapy provided, communication among team members, goal setting, and inclusion of the patient in the plan for his or her treatment. In these work settings, we must adhere to the guidelines imposed by both the insurance companies and the accrediting bodies.

Acute Care Hospital   A person is admitted to the acute care hospital due to a need for rapid medical management. As a result, these individuals are often medically unstable and cannot tolerate long assessment or treatment sessions. In addition, the length of time they remain in the hospital has been reduced due to changes in insurance coverage and alternative medical management techniques. Therefore, the clinician's role is typically that of a consultant. You are responsible for evaluating the person in order to determine the presence, type, and severity of the communication or swallowing disorder, and educating him or her, the family, and the staff regarding the findings and recommendations of the evaluation. For example, you may receive a referral from a **neurologist** to evaluate a patient who was admitted with the diagnosis of a **stroke** who now has difficulty speaking and swallowing. You evaluate the person and determine that his speech is difficult to understand due to severe **dysarthria.** He also has a severe **dysphagia** and cannot eat or drink safely. Following the evaluation, you recommend speech therapy to develop an **augmentative and alternative communication (AAC)** system and we train him, the family, and the staff in use of the system. We also recommend an alternative method of feeding, such as a **nasogastric tube.** Although the patient receives feeding through the tube, we can concurrently begin work on exercises to improve both his speech and swallowing.

You also collaborate with medical and rehabilitation staff such as the **physical therapist (PT)** and the OT regarding the continued needs of the person and the most appropriate discharge destination. In the case mentioned previously, no other physical impairments were identified by the PT or OT, thus he was able to be discharged home and receive speech therapy through a home health care service.

Within many birthing acute care hospitals, premature infants or other infants with severe medical problems immediately after birth may be hospitalized in the **neonatal intensive care unit (NICU).** Many of these infants have feeding and swallowing problems that you may be asked to address. For example, you may receive a referral for a infant delivered at 32 weeks' gestation. She has numerous respiratory problems and an uncoordinated suck/swallow. You may observe and evaluate the infant during feedings and provide suggestions to the mother and staff.

Rehabilitation Units and Hospitals   Some acute care hospitals have a dedicated rehabilitation unit within the hospital. Other intensive rehabilitation programs are housed in specialized rehabilitation hospitals. Patients admitted to these inpatient programs are generally medically stable and are able to participate in several hours of therapy each day (combination of speech, occupational, physical, recreational, and/or psychosocial). Often, these are people who suffered a stroke or other brain injury. Our role is to assess the person and develop an appropriate treatment plan given the specific diagnosis and needs of the client. We also function as a member of a team. Depending on the philosophy of the rehabilitation program, the type of team may vary (multi-, inter-, transdisciplinary). In this setting, we will likely provide a combination of individual and group therapy. In addition, we may co-treat with another discipline. For example, if a patient has *cognitive impairments* that interfere with sequencing behaviors, we might do a treatment session with the OT in the kitchen. We would focus on assisting the person with organization and sequencing skills required to prepare a meal while the OT would address the person's hand and arm control and would train him or her in the use of adaptive equipment. The primary goals of therapy are to enhance communicative and cognitive functioning and to prepare the individual for discharge home.

Outpatient Rehabilitation Centers   Outpatient rehabilitation centers may be affiliated with an acute care or rehabilitation hospital or may be an independent center. People participating in these programs are transported from their homes to the center. Similar to inpatient programs, we will do an evaluation and set up an individualized treatment plan. The patient and his or her family are likely to have significant input into the goals of treatment. The individual may state, "I want to talk better so I can be understood on the telephone and get back to work." Goals typically are geared toward maximizing communicative functioning in the home and in the community as well as those communication skills necessary for returning to work or school. Again, we function as a member of the treatment team, which may vary, depending on the philosophy of the rehabilitation program. The intensity of treatment may vary from daily to once a week. Individual and group treatments are typically provided and co-treatments may occur. Some treatment may even occur in the community. For example, we may take a person to McDonald's to practice his or her verbal skills or use of an AAC system in ordering a meal.

Transitional Living Centers   **Transitional living centers** are geared toward those individuals who need to return to an independent lifestyle. Most residents in this type of program are young and have sustained a traumatic or other acquired brain injury as a result of something such as a motor vehicle accident. In this setting, you will work very closely with other rehabilitation staff, providing direct treatment toward self-management and community re-entry skills. For example, you may help the nurse develop a plan to teach the patient his or her medication schedule and compensate for memory problems, or you may address managing the individual's finances. Therapy is often provided in a group setting led only by SLPs or with other team members, depending on the focus of the group.

Residential Care Facilities   Individuals are admitted to a **residential care facility,** also referred to as a **skilled nursing facility,** if they need ongoing nursing and medical care and cannot be managed by family members in the home. These individuals may have the diagnosis of **Alzheimer's disease** or may have a progressive neurological disease such as **Parkinson's disease.** Your role and the goals of treatment will vary depending on the medical diagnosis, communication diagnosis, and whether the resident will ultimately be discharged home or if he or she will remain in the facility indefinitely. For example, you may see a person with swallowing problems due to Parkinson's disease who will remain in the facility for the rest of his or her life. His or her **prognosis** for improvement is not good. Therefore, your goal for intervention may be to train the staff to use some strategies to make swallowing easier and to recognize any sign of difficulty. Medicare regulations have greatly impacted the provision of speech therapy and other rehabilitation services within these facilities. Strict guidelines must be followed regarding the amount and type of therapy provided.

Home Health Care   People may be eligible to receive therapy in the home if they are considered "homebound"; that is, they are unable to leave their home. They may be transported by family members or by wheelchair van to their doctor appointments but do not leave their home for any other purpose. These individuals often require the services of a registered nurse and a home health aid. We might be seeing an **oncology** patient who had a portion of her tongue removed due to cancer. She is still very weak and cannot drive. She has had difficulty maintaining her weight due to swallowing difficulty and needs supplemental tube feeds, and her speech is slurred. The nurse may help with management of the tube feeds and a home health aid may assist her with bathing, dressing, and household chores. Your role is to help her with her speech and swallowing and to educate her and her caregivers regarding techniques that help her to be understood and that improve the safety of her swallow.

CASE EXAMPLE 1

How a patient may transition through the COC
<u>Stroke patient with right leg and arm paralysis and aphasia</u>
Bob is a 58-year-old man admitted to the *acute care hospital* with the diagnosis of a stroke. The SLP completes an evaluation and diagnoses a moderate aphasia. A PT and

an OT determine that he has a paralysis of his right side and is unable to complete basic activities of daily living (ADLs; e.g., dressing, bathing, cooking). Given his age, motivation, and potential for good progress, the rehabilitation team recommended he be discharged to an inpatient rehabilitation program.

At the *inpatient rehabilitation program*, the SLP begins intensive treatment. Bob is scheduled for 1 hour of individual speech therapy per day. He begins to make progress in his ability to understand directions and questions, expresses some basic thoughts and ideas, and reads sentences. Progress is also made in physical therapy and occupational therapy, although Bob continues to need moderate assistance to complete his ADLs. After 3 weeks, the rehabilitation team determines that his wife can manage Bob at home. After some family education and training, Bob was discharged home.

Once at home, Bob receives occupational therapy, physical therapy, and speech therapy through *home care services*. Rapid progress is made with his mobility and ability to perform his ADLs. The SLP continues to work on his language skills. After 4 weeks, Bob makes significant progress in all language areas. Physically, he can now get around the house and in and out of the car, so the PT discharges him. A referral to outpatient therapy is recommended.

Bob begins therapy at an *outpatient rehabilitation facility*. The focus of his speech and language program is now geared toward returning to work. He participates in individual and group therapy, as well as some activities in the community. After 4 weeks, Bob is ready to return to work on a part-time basis.

Private Practice

If you choose to work in a private practice, you have a lot of flexibility in choosing the setting in which you work. You may see individuals in a private office; you may contract with various facilities such as hospitals, rehabilitation agencies, schools, or group homes; or you may act primarily as a consultant. You can specify the types of communication disorders that you treat and accept only those referrals. Depending on the setting and type of client seen in private practice, you may work completely independently or be part of a team. For example, one SLP may specialize in management of communication disorders in children with autism spectrum disorders. She may contract with several school systems and be called on to evaluate a child, provide specific treatment recommendations, and train the teachers in management of the child. The SLP may also be hired by parents of children with communication disorders and provide therapy outside of school. Another SLP may have contracts with several nursing homes or hospitals. The facilities would contact her when needed and she would evaluate the client and set up a treatment plan. She may also be hired privately by a family to provide therapy when insurance runs out.

College and University

You may function as professors or clinical supervisors in a college or university setting. You may provide direct services to the clients, but your main role is to provide undergraduate and graduate education and supervise graduate student clinicians who are training to become SLPs. Services may be provided at a university-based clinic or in a variety of educational or medical settings with whom the university has a contract. If you function as a clinical supervisor, your role is to provide a foundation in the principles of diagnosis and treatment and expose the student to a wide variety of communication disorders often encountered in children and adults. You are also ultimately responsible for the treatment provided to the client. In this capacity, you may act as a consultant and provide a second opinion to school- or hospital-based SLPs or you may function independently.

SPECIALIZED SERVICE DELIVERY SETTINGS

Clinical practice sometimes finds SLPs working in particular settings that are less often a part of graduate practica experience. Here are a few examples.

Rural Service Delivery

Service provision to rural communities is influenced by the inherent shortage and isolation of rehabilitation personnel, the lack of teaching materials and equipment, and the possibility of a low socioeconomic environment, homes without telephones, and families without health insurance (Coleman, Thompson-Smith, Pruitt, & Richards, 1999). For effective service delivery, clinicians should understand the community's local flavor and its unwritten codes of social behavior.

Psychiatric Centers

If you decide to work in a psychiatric facility, you will likely meet individuals who have severe behavioral disabilities secondary to psychiatric illness, mental health concerns, social-emotional maladjustment, and/or mental retardation. For this population, you will need to develop an understanding of behavior management and the potential communicative function of aberrant behavior. In psychiatric centers, you will work with **psychiatrists, behavior modification specialists,** and psychiatric **social workers.**

Supported Employment

Supported employment occurs when people with physical and mental disabilities are provided with job support to achieve competitive employment through task accommodations, social skills training, and job coaching. Within this model, SLPs may be asked to consult on social skills instruction, problem solving, and non-verbal communication strategies (i.e., communication books) while working with the client's employer (Storey, Ezell, & Lengyel, 1995).

Prison Services

At the core of prison services is the political issue—should prisons punish or rehabilitate—and the clinical issue of whether speech-language services really impact a prisoner's current and future behavior. When services are available, you will likely find some prisoners highly motivated, whereas others are apathetic to their communication disorder. For security reasons, access to prisoners is often interrupted due to lockdowns, loss of privileges, and unpredictable scheduling changes (Crowe, Byrne, & Henry, 1999).

Group Home Settings

Small, local community group homes have gradually replaced large state institutions for people with developmental disabilities. Service provision to adults with developmental disabilities is often consultative in nature, and assessment includes both the person with developmental disabilities and the communication styles and group home patterns that facilitate or inhibit communication. Intervention less often focuses on developmental skills and, instead, considers how functional communication can be supported within everyday routines and community recreational events.

WORK SETTINGS FOR AUDIOLOGISTS

Audiologists practice their profession in a variety of settings. The majority of audiologists practice in some type of health care setting. A smaller number of audiologists practice in school systems, universities, and industrial environments.

Scope of Practice

In defining the scope of practice for the field of audiology, it is important to realize that audiologists are autonomous professionals. This means that they have earned the right to function independently. Individuals who seek the services of an audiologist can do so directly, without the referral of a physician. In order to maintain this autonomy, it is important that the audiologist provide services that fall under the true mission of the profession. .

The audiologist is involved in activities that identify, assess, diagnose, manage in a nonmedical fashion, and interpret test results related to disorders of human hearing, balance, and other neural systems. This would include traditional **behavioral audiologic tests** of hearing sensitivity (i.e., air and bone conduction thresholds) as well as **electrophysiological** tests (i.e., auditory brain stem response). The audiologist is uniquely qualified to assess the hearing sensitivity of children and adults. In addition to assessing peripheral hearing sensitivity, audiologists are also involved in evaluation and management of children and adults with **central auditory processing disorders.**

The audiologist often serves in a consultative capacity. When dealing with school-age children, the audiologist may be called on to consult with an educational team regarding educational implications of a hearing loss, educational programming, classroom acoustics, and classroom, as well as large-area, amplification systems for children with hearing impairments. Audiologists may also serve as consultants with regard to compliance with the **Americans with Disabilities Act (ADA)** of 1990 (PL 101-336). In this capacity, the audiologist may be called on to determine accessibility for people with hearing loss in public and private buildings and facilities. Many audiologists serve as expert witnesses for legal interpretations of audiological findings and general effects of hearing loss. Consulting with industry regarding prevention of noise-induced hearing loss and implementing **hearing conservation program** techniques has been a staple of the audiological profession for many years. Since the 1980s, many audiologists have gotten involved in consultation and provision of rehabilitation to people with balance disorders through habituation, exercise therapy, and balance retraining.

The scope of practice for the audiologist has been rapidly expanding since 1990. One area in which audiologists have become involved is in the use of **oto-scopic** examination and external ear canal management for removal of **cerumen.** In the past, cerumen management was a function performed exclusively by physicians or nurses. An ear canal that is clear of excessive cerumen is critical to obtaining an accurate audiological evaluation and impression of the external ear. In an attempt to expedite the diagnostic evaluation process, many audiologists have become involved in cerumen management.

Technological advances have led to additional activities becoming part of the audiological scope of practice. Many audiologists who are familiar with electrophysiological equipment now find themselves working in the operating room side by side with surgeons. In these instances, the audiologist is providing neurophysiologic **intraoperative monitoring** and cranial nerve assessment. The purpose of intraoperative monitoring is to try to alert the surgeon to possible nerve damage during surgery in an attempt to maintain complete nerve function.

Another technological advancement that has broadened the scope of practice of the audiologist is the **cochlear implant.** Audiologists are involved in determining candidacy for cochlear implants as well as fitting, programming, or mapping the device. Audiologists also provide rehabilitative services to optimize the benefits derived from the cochlear implant.

Although audiologists have been involved in newborn hearing screening programs for many years, legislation passed in many states during the 1990s has increased the need for involvement in this area. Many states now have mandated universal hearing screening for all individuals born in that state. The development of the **oto-acoustic emission (OAE)** test battery has provided one tool by which these universal screening programs can be carried out. The **auditory brainstem response (ABR)** also continues to be used for this purpose.

Audiologists are also involved in **tinnitus** assessment and management. New developments in nonmedical management of tinnitus using biofeedback, masking, hearing aids, education, and counseling have led to an increase in this area by many audiologists.

The reduction of communication disorders is a primary theme that runs through the activities of the audiologist. Audiologists screen for obvious speech-language disorders, are involved in the use of sign language, and provide rehabilitative services including speechreading and communication management strategies.

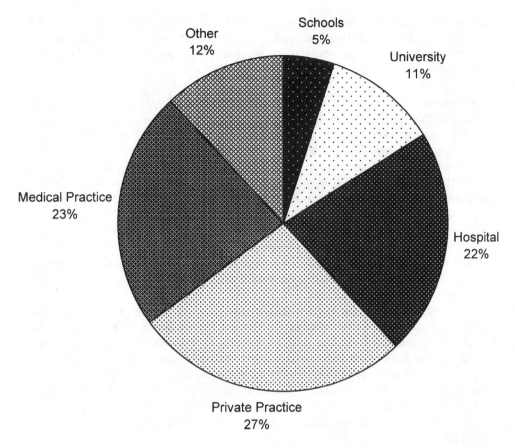

Figure 9.1.   Primary settings in which audiologists practice. (From Stach, B. [1998]. *Clinical audiology: An introduction* [p. 11]. San Diego: Singular Publishing Group; reprinted by permission.)

Practice Settings for Audiologists

Audiologists work in a wide variety of settings, and Figure 9.1 contains a breakdown of the primary settings in which they practice.

Schools   Those individuals who work in the school system are referred to as educational audiologists. Their role will be mainly rehabilitative in nature. The educational audiologist will work in a collaborative fashion with educators as a member of an interdisciplinary team. The educational audiologist will provide input about amplification issues as well as communication management, educational implications of hearing loss, educational programming, and classroom acoustics.

An example of a common scenario faced by an educational audiologist would be the case of a 10-year-old girl with a moderate to severe hearing loss who has recently moved into a town. As the educational audiologist in this setting, you will be called on to provide input to the child's educational team regarding use of an **FM amplification system** in the classroom. You will also provide information regarding the expected impact of the hearing loss on educational performance for this young girl.

Hospital   Approximately 20% of audiologists work in a hospital or medical center. In this setting, the audiologist is almost always an employee of the hospital. The hospital setting provides a broad array of duties for the audiologist. Diagnostic procedures will include in-depth electrophysiological and behavioral assessments of inpatients and outpatients of all ages. If the hospital is a birthing hospital, you will likely be involved in a universal neonatal hearing screening program. You may also be involved in hearing screenings and diagnostic evaluations of babies who spend time in the NICU. In many hospital settings, the audiologist will have the opportunity to be involved in intraoperative monitoring in order to measure the integrity of various nerves during surgical procedures. Audiologists are most likely to be involved in working with cochlear implants or be called on to assess the possible **ototoxic** effects of various types of drug therapies in a hospital environment.

One example of a clinical scenario in the hospital setting would be the case of the 20-year-old male who has cystic fibrosis. This patient's team of doctors has prescribed Amikin to help him with his breathing. This particular drug is known to have possible ototoxic side effects. The physicians have asked the audiologist to perform repeated serial audiograms in order to monitor the patient's hearing sensitivity very closely. Ototoxic effects are usually first evident as shifts in hearing sensitivity in the very high frequencies. Under these circumstances, we may choose to perform a combination of repeated high frequency audiograms as well as repeated OAE's.

Medical Practice   Approximately 23% of audiologists work in a medical practice. In this setting, the audiologist is most often an employee of the corporation that is usually managed by a physician or a group of physicians. The medical specialty of the physician who hires the audiologist is almost always **otolaryngology.**

In this setting, the duties of the audiologist will usually have a diagnostic emphasis. In addition to routine behavioral diagnostic measures of hearing sensitivity, the audiologist will often be called on to perform electrophysiological tests such as the ABR and **electronystagmography (ENG)** to assist the physician in making diagnoses regarding hearing and balance disorders.

An example of a common clinical scenario in a medical private practice could be seen in the case of a 62-year-old male who has been seen by the otolaryngologist with a complaint of episodes of dizziness. The physician has referred the patient to the audiologist for an audiological evaluation to measure hearing sensitivity and an ENG to evaluate the vestibular (balance) system. As audiologists working in this type of setting, we will be responsible for performing the requested tests and providing the results to the physician. Our role in this case is primarily diagnostic in nature and interpretation of test results will usually be left up to the otolaryngologist.

Private Practice   The practice setting that has grown most dramatically since the 1990s, and is most likely to continue to grow, is independent private practice. In 2001, almost 30% of audiologists work in this setting. One obvious reason for the growth in this area is related to a change in the official scope of practice guidelines for the profession. In the 1970s, dispensing hearing aids was not considered to be in the audiologist's scope of practice. Today, dispensing hearing aids is an integral part of the audiologist's duties and has provided the main source of income for many who are maintaining an independent private practice. Although diagnostic evaluations are an important part of most private practices, the emphasis is usually on the rehabilitative services of dispensing and fitting hearing aids.

Running an independent private practice is similar to running other small businesses. The challenges and risks, both financial and emotional, of such an endeavor are greater than in other professional settings. The rewards of a successful private practice, however, are equally great. Most private practitioners state that they experience a tremendous feeling of satisfaction in running their own businesses. In addition, the potential for financial benefit is great as well. Median earnings for a successful independent private practice are estimated to be between 33% and 100% higher than the salary of other audiologists (Stach, 1998).

An example of a common clinical scenario in an independent private practice would be illustrated by the case of a 72-year-old female who has noticed a decrease in hearing sensitivity. This individual has sought the advice of her family physician regarding her increase in communication difficulties. The physician has provided medical clearance for amplification to the individual and has referred her to the private practice. As audiologists in private practice, we will be responsible for assessment of the person's hearing sensitivity as well as selection and fitting of appropriate hearing aids. In addition to the formal test protocols that may be used, a good deal of our efforts will be rehabilitative in nature. We will spend significant time counseling the person regarding proper use of the instruments and establishing realistic expectations concerning aided performance.

Industry   Audiologists who work in industry are referred to as *industrial audiologists* or as *environmental audiologists.* Industrial audiologists are involved in the prevention of hearing loss to a greater extent than audiologists in other professional settings. A primary role of the industrial audiologist is to be a manager of an effective hearing conservation program.

An industrial hearing conservation program includes assessing the levels of noise exposure experienced by workers and performing baseline and annual audiometric evaluations, as well as providing recommendations for utilizing hearing protection devices. An important part of an effective hearing conservation program is providing education to workers and supervisory personnel regarding noise-induced hearing loss. In addition, many industrial audiologists will be called on to make suggestions for engineering and administrative controls that will reduce the levels of noise exposure to employees.

Universities   Some audiologists work at universities as professors or clinical supervisors. Although these professionals may be involved in clinical activities, their main role is to provide graduate-level education and training to audiology students. It is common for audiologists in these settings to divide their time between lecturing to graduate students regarding diagnostic and rehabilitative procedures and providing actual services to a clinical population.

Hearing Aid Manufacturers Companies that manufacture hearing aids employ some audiologists. In this setting, the audiologist will be responsible for bringing ideas to the company regarding design of instruments and communicative needs of individuals with hearing impairments. Audiologists working for hearing aid companies will often serve as in-house consultants to practicing audiologists regarding specific instruments produced by their company. These audiologists are available to provide hearing aid fitting suggestions over the telephone to other audiologists. On occasion, the audiologist working in this capacity will travel to various facilities as a product representative for their particular company.

CONCLUSION

SLPs and audiologists have a myriad of opportunities to match their personal interests and styles to a work setting. All settings in which we practice make high levels of demand in terms of productivity, accountability, and technical competence. But all provide the personal satisfaction that is unique to our profession, knowing that we are helping clients to engage in one of the most important human functions—communication.

REFERENCES

American Academy of Audiology. (1996). *Audiology: Scope of practice.* McLean, VA: Author.
American Speech-Language-Hearing Association (ASHA). (1994a). Code of ethics. *Asha, 36* (Suppl. 13), 1–2.
American Speech-Language-Hearing Association (ASHA). (1994b). *Communication fact sheet.* Rockville, MD: Author.
American Speech-Language-Hearing Association (ASHA). (1997). *Preferred practice patterns for the profession of audiology.* Rockville, MD: Author
American Speech-Language-Hearing Association (ASHA). (1998). *Survey of speech-language pathology services in school-based settings: National study, final report.* Rockville, MD: Author.
Americans with Disabilities Act (ADA) of 1990, PL 101-336, 42 U.S.C. §§ 12101 *et seq.*
Coleman, T.J., Thompson-Smith, T., Pruitt, G.D., & Richards, L.N. (1999). Rural service delivery: Unique challenges, creative solutions. *ASHA, 41*(1), 40–45.
Crowe, T.A., Byrne, M.E., & Henry, A.N. (1999). Prison services: The Parchman project. *ASHA, 41*(6), 50–54.
Goals 2000: Educate America Act of 1994, PL 103-227, 20 U.S.C. §§ 5801 et seq.
Individuals with Disabilities Education Act (IDEA) of 1990, PL 101-476, 20 U.S.C. §§ 1400 *et seq.*
Individuals with Disabilities Education Act Amendments of 1997, PL 105-17. 20 U.S.C. §§ 1400 *et seq.*
Rehabilitation Act of 1973, PL 93-112, 29 U.S.C. §§ 701 *et seq.*
Rini, D.L., & Whitney, G.C. (1999). Family centered practice for children with communication disorders. *Child and Adolescent Psychiatric Clinics of North America, 8*(1), 153–174.
School-to-Work Opportunities Act of 1994, PL 103-239, 20 U.S.C. §§ 6101 *et seq.*
Stach, B. (1998). *Clinical audiology: An introduction.* San Diego: Singular Publishing Group.
Storey, K., Ezell, H., & Lengyel, L. (1995). Communication strategies for increasing the integration of persons in supported employment: A review. *American Journal of Speech-Language Pathology, 4*(2), 45–54.

1. Describe some of the different service delivery features that influence the role of the SLP.

2. Contrast multi-, inter-, and transdisciplinary service provision.

3. Describe some of the contemporary factors affecting speech-language service provision in birth-to-3, public schools, and medical settings.

4. How is the work setting of the SLP in birth-to-3 services uniquely different than that of the school-based clinician?

5. Describe the parameters that contribute to a patient's progression through the COC.

6. Describe three different settings in which audiologists may practice.

7. How have recent technological developments broadened the scope of practice of the audiologist?

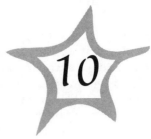

Issues of Cultural
and Linguistic Diversity

Brian Goldstein
Aquiles Iglesias

A personal story from the first author: As a speech-language pathologist (SLP) at Massachusetts General Hospital in Boston, I was asked to evaluate a 4-year-old Vietnamese-speaking child suspected of a speech-language delay. At the time, I was perplexed about how I, as a speaker of English and Spanish, would assess the speech and language skills of a child who did not speak the languages that I did. Moreover, I knew little about the cultural characteristics of the Vietnamese people. To prepare for this evaluation, I read material on Vietnam and the Vietnamese people, culture, and language. I also consulted with an individual from the Vietnamese Community Center about the culture, language, and dialect of the region from which this child emigrated. That individual, after some training, served as my interpreter during this assessment. The knowledge that I obtained from the individual at the community center and my training in a bilingual-bicultural emphasis graduate program allowed me to provide this child with an appropriate assessment.

Not every SLP will have access to individuals who can provide cultural and linguistic information about the client or will have been enrolled in a training program with a major focus on providing appropriate clinical management to individuals from culturally and linguistically diverse populations (although academic and clinical education that prepares students to practice in a multicultural society is mandated for accredited programs by the American Speech-Language-Hearing Association [ASHA, 1996a]). This chapter provides a road map to the linguistic and cultural differences found in the United States of America and shows how they impact the field of speech-language pathology so that if you are confronted with the challenge of providing clinical services to an individual who does not share your cultural and linguistic experiences, you might be better prepared for the process.

DEFINING CULTURALLY AND LINGUISTICALLY DIVERSE

Who is considered *culturally and linguistically diverse?* For the most part, normative information that we have about speech and language development and disorders has come from Caucasian, middle-class individuals. That is, we have tended to base our diagnostic and intervention approaches on one group. So, in a sense, everyone except that group would fall into the category of *culturally and linguistically diverse.* For our purposes, we are concerning ourselves with those groups designated by the U.S. Census Bureau as African Americans, Asian Americans, Hispanics/Latinos, and Native Americans.

DEMOGRAPHICS

Historically, the United States of America has been called a *melting pot* because immigrants from diverse countries came representing diverse races, ethnic groups, religions, languages, and so forth and then were thought to assimilate into mainstream (however *mainstream* is defined) American culture. The obvious disadvantage to assimilation was the loss of cultural and linguistic identities. A "mosaic" is the image more commonly used now to represent the way in which individuals new to the United States of America fit into the fabric of the country. That is, individuals retain some or all of their historical identities while, at the same time, create a new and different picture of the United States of America. In the future, that picture will continue to change. Table 10.1 shows U.S. population statistics from 1995 and projected for the year 2050 (U.S. Bureau of the Census, 1995).

By the year 2050, the percentage of African Americans/Blacks[1] in the United States of America's population will increase 2%. The percentage of individuals of Asian descent will almost triple. The percentage of individuals of Hispanic descent will almost double. The percentage of Native Americans will increase 1%. The percentage of Caucasians will decrease to slightly more than half of the population.

There is a misperception that individuals from culturally and linguistically diverse populations exist mainly in large, urban areas such as Chicago, New York, Philadelphia, and Los Angeles. That is clearly not the case. For example, there are large Spanish-speaking communities in Arkansas, Nebraska, and Oregon. There are Native Americans in North Carolina and Minnesota. There are sizeable Hmong (Cambodian) communities in Massachusetts and California. This linguistic diversity extends to speakers of English dialects as well. For example, Washington and Craig (1994) indicated that the number of children speaking African American English (AAE) is increasing and will continue to do so in the foreseeable future. Thus, children from culturally and linguistically diverse populations are well represented in our nation's school systems. In 1997, approximately 50 million children age 5–17 years were enrolled in the United States of America's school system, 10.5 million (21%) of whom were from culturally and linguistically diverse populations (U.S. Department of Education, 1998).

---

[1]Terms are those used by the U.S. Department of Commerce, Bureau of the Census.

Table 10.1. United States population statistics: 1995 and 2050

Group	1995		2050
African American/ Black	32 million	12.0%	14.4%
Asian American	9.2 million	3.4%	9.7%
Hispanic	27 million	10.1%	22.5%
Native American	2.0 million	0.75%	1.0%
Caucasian	195 million	73.5%	52.5%
Total	265.2 million		

From U.S. Department of Commerce.

Roseberry-McKibbin and Eicholtz (1994) surveyed school-based SLPs on a number of issues concerning students from culturally and linguistically diverse backgrounds, particularly those who spoke English as a second language. Based on the 1,145 surveys that were returned, Roseberry-McKibbin and Eicholtz found that 78% of SLPs had 0–3 students with limited English proficiency on their caseloads; 11% had 4–7 students; 4% had 7–10 students; and 6% had more than 10 students with limited English proficiency on their caseloads. The majority of SLPs were working with children of Hispanic descent, although they were also working with children of Chinese, Filipino, Hmong, Korean, Middle Eastern, Mixed European, Portuguese, and Vietnamese descent. Peters-Johnson (1998) surveyed school-based SLPs and found that 35% of 1,718 indicated that a percentage of students on their caseload spoke a language other than English, although only 10% of 1,718 respondents were proficient in languages other than English. So, if you are an SLP working almost anywhere in the United States of America, you are almost certain to encounter individuals from culturally and linguistically diverse backgrounds.

COMMUNICATION AND CULTURE

The way in which we communicate reflects, among many things, the culture in which we were raised. Parents socialize their children to be "good" communicators within their own community. Given the diversity that exists in the United States of America, SLPs may find that the ways in which parents interact with their children vary greatly. That variation may be reflected in the responses to tasks that we ask families to perform during the clinical management process. For example, during an evaluation of a child of Latino descent, a student clinician asked the parent of a 4-year-old boy to go into the diagnostic room and "play with your child as you do at home." The parent and the child entered the room that was full of toys and games appropriate for his age. After entering the room, the child promptly went to the kitchen area and began playing with the pots and pans. The mother sat nearby and observed the child play. Every once in a while, the mother would ask the child in Spanish to bring her something to drink or eat. He complied with all of her requests that were repeated more than twice. The child's verbal utterances were limited in quantity and quality. The graduate students in the observation room were dismayed because they felt that the interaction was stilted and the language sample was not very rich. They wondered why the parent did not ask questions, make comments or statements, or engage in play with her child. The students began to wonder whether the child's low verbal output, and possible delay, was due in part to the mother's interaction style.

The supervisor then asked one of the student clinicians to go into the room with a puzzle that was rather complex. The student was to ask the mother to explain to the child how to put the puzzle together. After being given the instructions, the mother asked her son to sit in a chair next to her. She began asking the child questions and making commands using a high number of nonspecific words (Where do you put this one? Put that one next to that thing.). The child's expressive language was more complex. Receptively, he appeared to understand all of his mother's utterances. The language output, however, was still less than one would expect of a 4-year-old child, and the student clinicians were almost positive that he had a language delay. Finally, the child's 6-year-old sister was brought into the room and allowed to play with her younger brother. The older child informed the younger child that they were going to play school, pulled out a book, and proceeded to play the role of the teacher reading the storybook *Goldilocks and the Three Bears* (What is the girl's name? What happened when she sat in papa bear's chair? What happened next?). The verbal output of the younger child amazed all who were participating in the evaluation. The 4-year-old used language for a variety of purposes, his sentences were complex, and his vocabulary was diverse.

The student clinicians were not prepared for the fact that different cultures interact with their children in different ways depending on the context and that there are cross-cultural differences in parent–child interaction and communication (Iglesias & Quinn, 1997). For example, adults do not necessarily engage in cooperative play with their children. Parents may see their role as more of a caregiver, and in a situation in which language is contextualized, parents may use a high degree of nonspecific vocabulary.

Providing appropriate services to individuals who come from cultures other than your own or speak languages other than your own necessitates that you gather cultural and linguistic information. You might read and study about various cultural groups, talk to and work with individuals from a variety of cultures, participate in the life of someone from another culture, and/or learn another language (Lynch, 1992). There are a number of specific *sociolinguistic* factors (both verbal and nonverbal) that might impact your interaction with a client and his or her family (Damico & Hamayan, 1992; Kayser, 1993; Lynch, 1992; Roseberry-McKibbin, 1994, 1995; Terrell & Terrell, 1993). First, child socialization practices and children's play characteristics should be considered. For example, children who typically utilize peers as conversational partners might be less comfortable interacting in play situations with adults. In terms of the assessment process, the SLP would want to use peers (or perhaps siblings) to interact with the client in order to obtain a language sample. Second, family characteristics also need to be taken into account, including factors such as country of birth, degree of acculturation into American society, knowledge of the United States of America's education system, family attitude toward English and English speakers, family structure, geographic location (e.g., urban versus rural), religious beliefs, social status, and socioeconomic status. For example, Heath (1983) found that narratives varied according to socioeconomic level. Thus, SLPs should elicit the narrative type that is characteristic of individuals from the client's speech community. Finally, in assessing clients from culturally and linguistically diverse populations, SLPs must also consider individual differences. For example, not all African Americans speak AAE, and speakers of AAE are not all African Americans.

BILINGUALISM AND DIALECTS

In providing assessment and intervention services to individuals from culturally and linguistically diverse populations, you undoubtedly will encounter individuals who either speak more than one language (i.e., bilingual) or speak a dialect of English (in this case, we are focusing on dialects of English, although there is no doubt that there are dialects of all languages). We first discuss bilingualism and then turn our attention to dialects.

Bilingualism

Speaking only one language is the exception to the norm if we take a world perspective. According to the Linguistic Society of America (1996), the majority of the world's countries are at least bilingual, and many are multilingual. For example, the European Union has more official languages than the United Nations, and nearly 60% of Europeans have learned a second language (Sollors, 1998). The United States of America, although officially not bilingual, is home to more than 30 million speakers of languages other than English. According to the U.S. Bureau of the Census (1995), there are 26 languages spoken in the United States of America with more than 100,000 speakers, ranging from Gujarathi with 102,000 speakers to Spanish with more than 17 million speakers. Spanish, French, German, Italian, and Chinese are each spoken by more than 1 million individuals.

Bilingualism should be viewed as a continuum. At the two extremes of the continuum are monolingual individuals raised and living in monolingual environments (e.g., Spanish-speaking children raised and living in Mexico). Bilingual individuals fall between the ends of the continuum and will differ from monolingual speakers of each language across phonological, semantic, morphosyntactic, and pragmatics areas. The degree of bilingualism achieved by an individual will be dependent on linguistic, social, emotional, political, demographic, and cultural factors (Hakuta, 1986; Pease-Alvarez, 1993). In addition, studies in bilingualism suggest that the degree of bilingualism depends on such factors as generational level, age, occupation, opportunities for contact with speakers of English, exposure to English media, and the nature of the bilingual speaker's interactions with members of his or her community.

Bilingual speakers demonstrate various degrees of proficiency in either language depending on the situation, topic, interactants, and context. Impressionistically, many bilingual individuals appear indistinguishable in normal social interactions in what Cummins (1984) referred to as possessing *basic interpersonal communication skills (BICS)*. Differences are evident, however, in cognitively demanding, decontextualized interactions in what Cummins referred to as having *cognitive academic language proficiency (CALP)*.

Let us return to the previous example of the Latino child being evaluated for a possible language delay. In the first interaction between the mother and the child, both interactants were speaking in Spanish, whereas in the second interaction the mother used English and Spanish. The child–child interaction was all in English. The first interaction could be classified as one in which the child was relying heavily on his BICS to communicate with his mother. The second interaction was more cognitively demanding and required the child to understand and use more cognitively demanding language, although the mother used contextualization to facilitate the conversation. The use of both languages by the mother is typical of that seen when both interactants are bilingual. The peer–peer interaction was all in English and required the child to further use more cognitively and academically demanding language. As a result of the situation, the interactants and the topic on which the child was being evaluated demonstrated different proficiencies in the two languages.

Although there are many specific definitions of bilingualism, most people accept Grosjean's "holistic" view of bilingualism (Grosjean, 1989, 1992, 1997). This view posits that the languages of bilinguals are an integrated whole that cannot be easily separated into the component languages. According to Grosjean, bilinguals have one linguistic system that results in different surface structures. This interdependence between the two languages allows for the transfer of skills across languages. From the standpoint of an SLP, adopting this view of bilingualism means that the communication assessment of bilinguals will necessitate 1) studying bilinguals without comparison to monolinguals, 2) examining both of the bilingual's languages, and 3) investigating how bilinguals organize and use both languages.

Dialects

There are many dialects spoken in the United States of America, including Southern White Standard, Appalachian English, Caribbean English, African American Vernacular English, and General American English. A **dialect** is a rule-governed variety of a language characterized by social, ethnic, and geographical differences in its speakers. Dialects are mutually intelligible forms of a language associated with a particular region, social class, or ethnic group. Dialects may differ across all areas of language—phonology, syntax, morphology, lexicon, and pragmatics. In fact, every person has his or her own unique way of speaking, termed an **idiolect.** Varieties of a language that depend on the context and conversational participants are called **registers.** Registers change depending on the participants, setting, and topic. For example, a person would usually use one register when talking to a potential employer and another variety when speaking to friends at a club. The terms dialect and **accent** are often used interchangeably. Although the term *dialect* refers to all aspects of a language, *accent* refers only to the pronunciation of a language variety. Accent does not take into account lexical, syntactic, morphological, and pragmatic aspects of the variety.

One dialect of a language is not superior to another dialect. This is not to say that all varieties of a language are equally prestigious. Some varieties of a language, specifically those used by dominant groups in any socially stratified society, will be considered to have higher prestige (Wolfram, 1986), will be preferred in the educational system (Adler, 1984), and will be valued by the private sector of the society (Terrell & Terrell, 1983). General American English is considered the prestige dialect in the United States of America and is preferred in the educational system. Because of mass media saturation, there has been some decreased differences between dialects and greater acceptance of others. There has also been increasing differences between dialects, however, because of the isolation of some groups, especially those of low socioeconomic status (Wolfram & Schilling-Estes, 1998). The increased immigration and ethnic isolation that has occurred among some subgroups has further increased the number of ethnic dialects. At least in terms of dialects, the "melting pot" hypothesis appears to be a myth for certain segments of our society.

COMPLETING APPROPRIATE ASSESSMENTS

SLPs will need to use information on communication and culture, bilingualism, and dialects to complete reliable and valid assessments. The goal of an assessment with an individual from a culturally and linguistically diverse population is to conduct a *least-biased assessment*. This means that you understand the person's culture and language (and/or dialect) and understand how the factors cited previously might impact the diagnostic process. The goal of a least-biased assessment is to differentiate typically developing individuals who may have a **language difference** (i.e., expected community variations in syntax, semantics, phonology, pragmatics, the lexicon) from those with **language disorders** (i.e., communication that deviates significantly from the norms of the community; Taylor & Payne, 1994). So, why is it necessary to make adjustments in the way that individuals from culturally and linguistically diverse populations are assessed? Historically, individuals from culturally and linguistically diverse populations have not been assessed appropriately. In the case of school-age children, this has meant an over-referral of all children from culturally and linguistically diverse populations to special education despite a recognition of cultural differences and their impact on linguistic development. That is, many children from culturally and linguistically diverse backgrounds were placed in special education because of a language difference not a language disorder. It has also meant, in some cases, an under-identification due to the assumption that any variation from what is expected is due to cultural and linguistic differences.

Many laws have been passed and lawsuits have been filed to help ensure that children are placed appropriately into special education. For example, public laws such as the Individuals with Disabilities Education Act (IDEA) of 1990 (PL 101-476) and the Individuals with Disabilities Education Act (IDEA) Amendments of 1997 (PL 105-17) mandate that a child's native language must be used in all direct contact with the child. Thus, SLPs must find means to conduct assessments employing the language that the child normally uses in the home or learning environment. Lawsuits such as *Larry P. v. Riles* (1972) nullified the use of standardized IQ tests in California to place African American children in special education. Thus, society at large and the courts have acknowledged the rights of linguistic minority populations. This acceptance has resulted in greater acceptance of the variety of dialects and languages that are spoken in the United States of America. Although General American English is the most common and dominant language variety spoken in the United States of America, there has been a realization that other varieties have a right to exist in our linguistically plural society. These laws have a definite impact on conducting least-biased assessments.

To diagnose individuals who truly have a communication disorder, the communicative standards of one group cannot be imposed on another. By analogy, you cannot determine what is typical about whales by studying dolphins, even though both swim in the water. Thus, operationally, a communication disorder is defined as different from the norm. That norm has to be, among other things, culturally based (Taylor & Clarke, 1994). To be certain that least-biased assessments take place, you should take into account the factors that may influence the assessment process (Kayser, 1993, 1995a; Roseberry-McKibbin, 1995; Terrell & Terrell, 1993; Toliver Weddington, 1981).

Clinician Factors

Prior to conducting an assessment, clinicians must assess their cultural and linguistic competence. Your attitudes, knowledge, and actions have an impact on the quality of the services that you provide. To respond optimally to the children and families that you serve, you must have 1) a positive attitude toward family values and beliefs, even if they are significantly different from yours; and 2) an understanding of typical and nontypical language development, including an understanding of what is considered to be a disorder. As you gain a better understanding and an appreciation of the families that you serve, your intervention goals and approaches will be congruent with those of the families.

You must also assess the extent to which your linguistic skills in a language other than English are sufficient to evaluate your assessment tools and to carry out your assessment. Although some working knowledge of a language is helpful, clinicians should be aware that less-than-native or near-native proficiency in a language will not be sufficient to carry out a proper assessment. In the case of a bilingual child, the clinician must not only be proficient in both languages but also should be able to create an environment where the clients can freely code-switch or mix, thus using their full linguistic repertoire. In preparing to complete a least-biased assessment, you should conduct an attitudinal self-assessment (i.e., know your own culture and worldview), have a solid understanding of variations across and within cultural-linguistic groups and an acceptance of a range of human behavior, and determine whether you have the language skills and training to assess and treat bilingual individuals (responsibilities and roles of the monolingual SLP will be covered later in the chapter). According to ASHA (1989), an SLP or audiologist may be considered bilingual if he or she speaks one native language and a second language with native or near-native proficiency in lexicon, semantics, phonology, morphology, and pragmatics. To provide bilingual clinical services in the client's language, the bilingual SLP should be able to

- Describe typical speech and language development using contemporary data and theory

- Possess knowledge of dialects in the child's home language

- Use least-biased evaluation tools to gauge speech and language development

- Administer and interpret formal and informal evaluation tools

- Apply treatment strategies in the child's language

- Recognize cultural factors that affect assessment and treatment

- Aid parents and other professionals in understanding the child's diagnosis, assessment results, and treatment options and approaches

General Assessment Factors

During the assessment process, you can increase the likelihood of an appropriate diagnosis in a number of ways. First, you should administer several formal (i.e., standardized) and informal (i.e., nonstandardized) measures. Using both types of measures will allow for a more representative sample of the individual's abilities. Moreover, you should choose the test with the most valid items for the skills to be assessed. Second, assess skills in all languages/dialects. It is common for individuals to exhibit some skills in one language/dialect and other skills in the other language/dialect. For example, some bilingual Latino children first learn the names of colors in preschool. The names of colors will be produced in English by their English-speaking teacher. Thus, the children will know the names of colors in English only and not in Spanish. If bilingual children were tested in Spanish only, they might not label colors in Spanish, leading the clinician to mistakenly believe that the child did not know color names. Also, observe whether the disorder exists in all languages/dialects; it should. Finally, recognize that different modes of communication may be in effect and that performance may vary because of those factors rather than the person's abilities. Remember that rules are in effect during all communicative events; there may be a mismatch of communicative style between the family and SLP.

Assessment Tool Factors

Most SLPs administer formal (i.e., standardized) assessment tools to their clients. Not all formal assessments, however, will be appropriate for all clients. In administering formal assessments to your clients, you should take into account the following issues (Erickson & Iglesias, 1986; Kayser, 1989, 1995a; Roseberry-McKibbin, 1995; Toliver Weddington, 1981):

- Examine each item before administering the test to determine whether the client may have had access to the information and if failure should be considered a disorder.

- Determine whether modification of specific test items can reduce bias.

- Have families complete case history information, permission forms, and release of information documents in person.

- Make an effort to identify those measures that include individuals from culturally and/or linguistically diverse populations in the normative sample.

- Modify the items before administering the test.

- Observe **code-switching** (alternations between languages at the word, phrase, or sentence levels; e.g., an individual may start a sentence in one language and finish it in another; Mattes & Omark, 1991) and **language interference** (the influence of one language on another; e.g., a native speaker of Japanese may pronounce English with a Japanese accent; Roseberry-McKibbin, 1995).

- Report all modifications of standardized administration procedures.

- Report norms only if they are valid for the population being assessed.

- Select a test that examines those aspects of language that need to be assessed.

- Use a variety of elicitation procedures.

ALTERNATIVE METHODS OF ASSESSMENT

Just as you would alter the assessment process if you were evaluating someone with a language disorder versus a voice disorder, you will also need to tailor the assessment of individuals from culturally and linguistically diverse populations to their specific language and culture. That is, you are designing your assessment to fit the specific needs of the client. In this case, one size clearly does *not* fit all. Alternative methods of assessment also need to be used in order to make a proper differential diagnosis. Without using modifications, there is a chance for either **overdiagnosis** or **underdiagnosis.** Overdiagnosis may occur because the individual will be labeled with a communication disorder using a test standardized on a different population. It is as if your score on a test assessing your knowledge of the English monarchy was compared with individuals born and raised in Great Britain. Underdiagnosis may occur because the assessment does not take into account the individual's linguistic features, or the SLP may not understand how the individual's language or dialect differs from General American English. For example, assume you are assessing a 5-year-old child who speaks AAE. You collect a language sample and note the morphological and syntactic forms produced by the client. There may be some errored forms (e.g., "he eated the doughnut") that you erroneously label as a dialect feature ("eated" is ungrammatical in AAE).

A number of suggestions in completing alternative methods of assessment have been given by many researchers (compiled from Cheng, 1993; Erickson & Iglesias, 1986; Kayser, 1989, 1993, 1995a; Langdon, 1992; Norris, Juarez, & Perkins, 1989; Roseberry-McKibbin, 1994; Taylor & Payne, 1983; Terrell & Terrell, 1993; Toliver Weddington, 1981; Van Keulen, Weddington, & DeBose, 1998; Vaughn-Cooke, 1986). Existing tests should be standardized on individuals from culturally and linguistically diverse backgrounds and/or new tests should be developed. Also, administer standardized tests in nonstandardized ways. Given that many standardized tests have not included individuals from culturally and linguistically diverse populations in their standardization sample, the validity of those tests must be questioned. Thus, many standardized assessments must be developed or administered in alternative ways. If you use an alternative format, you must indicate in your report that you made adjustments to the administration. For example, you might alter the test by giving individuals credit if they change their mind, especially when clearly demonstrating that they know the correct answer, repeating and/or rewording instructions, providing additional time for the individual to respond, testing beyond the ceiling of the assessment, adding practice items, and asking individuals to explain their answers. Standardizing existing tests on individuals from culturally and linguistically diverse backgrounds requires the development of **local norms.** That is, administer the test to typically developing individuals in the community in which you are working and note the scores that they receive and the quality of their responses.

It may be difficult and time consuming to restandardize existing tests or develop new tests. Thus, the use of alternative testing formats (i.e., other than standardized tests) is also recommended. Alternative testing formats might include

- **Criterion-referenced tests:** These are tests that specify the linguistic behaviors to be tested, establish criteria for acceptable responses, and do not compare the child's responses against some other standard. One disadvantage is that they still assume a developmental framework.

- **Dynamic assessment** (Peña, 1996): Assessment is gauged by examining **modifiability** (i.e., change through mediation or teaching). Examiners can determine how a child learns and what is needed for that child to learn and generalize the task to new situations. Modifiability involves three factors: 1) child responsiveness (how the child responds to and uses new information), 2) examiner effort (quantity and quality of effort needed to make a change), and 3) transfer (generalization of new skills).

- **Portfolio assessment:** Collect a student's work over time representing a variety of tasks and assignments; assignments might include writing samples; observations from teachers, parents, and so forth; language samples; and tapes of performance.

- **Ethnographic assessment** (Heath, 1982, 1983): Observe the client in many contexts with many conversational partners. Ask the family about their own culture, their attitudes about the host culture, and their communication in the home and with their family members. Interact with clients, being sensitive to their culture, their frame of reference, and their view of what is important. Describe clients' communicative abilities during genuine communication in a naturalistic environment with low anxiety and high motivation.

- **Probe techniques:** Assess a small amount of information over a short period of time (weekly or biweekly) to gauge rate and amount of learning.

If a school-age child is being evaluated, the SLP might also obtain academic information from teachers and school records in addition to utilizing the alternative testing formats described previously. Damico (1993) suggested observing in the classroom and analyzing academic tasks—interactions with the curriculum, conversational tasks, literacy-related tasks, and test-taking abilities—during structured activities and actual conversations.

There are also some testing "don'ts" that you should follow to decrease the possibility of misdiagnosis (Kayser, 1993; Roseberry-McKibbin, 1995):

1. Do not use norm-referenced tests only.

2. Do not use only a language sample to qualify someone for services.

3. Do not use multiple assessments in order to get low scores so that someone will be qualified for services.

4. Do not translate tests (Roseberry-McKibbin, 1994). First, there are differences in structure and content in each language. The same translated item may differ in structure and difficulty across the two languages. Second, it mistakenly implies that children acquiring English proficiency and English-speaking children receive similar socialization, life experiences, language input, academic instruction, and so forth. Third, differences in the frequency of target words vary from one language to the next. Fourth, grammatical forms may not be equivalent between the languages. Finally, translated tests do not tap a child's ability to acquire language.

5. Do not use only one elicitation technique.

6. Do not use tests administered in English only if the individual is bilingual.

7. Do not assume that features of a second language or a dialect of English are characteristics of a disorder.

8. Do not assume that support personnel are automatically trained to aid in the diagnostic process.

RESPONSIBILITIES AND ROLES OF THE MONOLINGUAL SPEECH-LANGUAGE PATHOLOGIST

Given the demographic changes occurring in the United States of America and the fact that most SLPs are monolingual and English-speaking, ASHA has developed guidelines regarding the responsibilities of monolingual SLPs relative to individuals who are bilingual. According to ASHA (1985), monolingual SLPs may test, perform the oral-peripheral examination, conduct hearing screenings, complete nonverbal assessments, and conduct the family interview (with appropriate support personnel) in English. In preparing to assess an individual whose language they do not speak, monolingual SLPs should research the culture, language, and dialect of the person that they are going to assess and apply contemporary data and theory to the assessment using least-biased assessment tools. They should also be prepared to ask for help if necessary, advocate for the individual, and be willing to refer the client, if necessary.

Monolingual SLPs might also consider (ASHA, 1985) 1) establishing contacts and hiring bilingual SLPs as consultants or diagnosticians to provide clinical services; 2) establishing cooperative groups in which groups of school districts or programs might hire an itinerant bilingual SLP; 3) establishing networks, such as forging links, between university settings and work settings to help recruit bilingual speakers into the work force; 4) establishing Clinical Fellowship Year and graduate student practica sites; 5) establishing interdisciplinary teams in which monolingual SLPs are teamed with bilingual professionals from other fields; and 6) training support personnel such as bilingual aides, students, family members, or members of the community. You should be aware that there is a limit as to the types of tasks that support personnel can complete (ASHA, 1996b). Although support personnel can conduct tasks such as speech-language screenings, following documented treatment plans or protocols, documenting patient/client progress, and assisting during assessment, there are also other tasks that support personnel should not complete. These include tasks such as performing standardized or nonstandardized diagnostic tests; conducting formal or informal evaluations; interpreting test results; participating in parent conferences; taking part in case conferences; participating in any interdisciplinary team without the supervising SLP present, or writing, developing, and modifying a patient/client's individualized treatment plan.

INTERVENTION

Intervention is a process by which a clinician deliberately sets out to systematically change the course of an ongoing behavior. This process always involves an expert who has an awareness of what is appropriate behavior (intervention goal) and what to do to achieve this goal (intervention approach). The specific goals and approaches selected are driven by the clinician's values, beliefs, and knowledge. As clinicians, it is your ethical responsibility to examine how your own biases and the limits of your knowledge base influence the direction and outcome of your intervention. To achieve this, you must engage in consciousness-raising experiences that bring to the forefront your biases and assist you in overcoming them, as well as in activities that expand your conceptual perspective of sociocultural and linguistic factors that have an impact on intervention. You must be aware that in many cases you will be implementing interventions based on very limited empirical research. The majority of your intervention programs will be based on this limited knowledge coupled with logic and experience. Ongoing evaluation of your goals, intervention approaches, and outcomes will be a source for your ongoing decision-making process.

Let us assume that the results of the evaluation indicated that the client needed to receive intervention in order to facilitate her language acquisition. Based on the results of the assessment, the clinician decides that one of the goals of the intervention is to increase the use of questions, commands, and statements that the child is using. The rationale used by this clinician is that greater use of these communicative functions would increase the child's communication skills necessary to function in school. Unfortunately, the child's parents were not co-equal in the decision-making process. On the surface, the goal appears to be appropriate. The clinician should have noted, however, that this goal shifts child-rearing practices—a child is to view an adult as an equal partner. Does it create new adjustment problems for the family? The mother came back 3 weeks later to complain about the child's disrespectful behavior toward adults. A better intervention strategy, assuming the same goal, would have been to discuss with the parents the need to achieve this goal and to ask the parents for optional ways to achieve it. Perhaps the parents would have suggested that the clinician explicitly state that this type of communication is only to be used in the classroom, or perhaps the intervention should have been carried out in a group situation where peers would interact with one another. Perhaps the parents would have agreed to change their own rules of who talks to whom about what. Any or all of these strategies would have avoided the negative side effects of the intervention.

Providing appropriate intervention services to individuals from culturally and linguistically diverse populations has often proved to be difficult. There is a severe lack of research into effective intervention strategies. We have provided you with general intervention guidelines, however, for providing intervention to individuals from culturally and linguistically diverse populations with communication disorders (compiled from Beaumont, 1992; Cheng, 1989, 1996; Damico & Hamayan, 1992; Damico, Smith, & Augustine, 1996; Kayser, 1995b; Seymour, 1986).

General Considerations

There are a number of general considerations you should take into account in providing intervention services to individuals from culturally and linguistically diverse populations. First, assess continually. Each session should be a mini-assessment, helping you to plan for the next session. Complete comprehensive re-evaluations periodically (every 3–6 months or so). Second, set up natural opportunities for language to be used in natural interactions, utilize natural language-learning activities, and interrelate activities. We acquire new knowledge by being in situations that require us to use multiple bases of knowledge; that is why driver's education is not confined solely to the classroom. You should also utilize meaningful and interesting materials and activities. Third, consider a holistic strategies approach by encouraging students to 1) explain new information in their own words, 2) summarize information, 3) generalize information to new contexts, and 4) analyze new information (Roseberry-McKibbin, 1995). SLPs should focus on meaning rather than structure; have students relate new information to information that has already been learned; teach strategies for learning and remembering new content; and use an intervention strategy of teaching the "whole," breaking it down into its "parts," and reconstructing it into a "whole" again (Roseberry-McKibbin, 1995). Fourth, allow students to think, to discuss options, to make decisions, to establish accountability, and to show knowledge both verbally and nonverbally. Emphasize printed material to build a literacy-rich environment. These considerations will empower individuals as learners and teachers. Fifth, use a variety of social organizations (e.g., large-group projects, small-group projects, peer–peer projects), and use individual, peer–peer, and group work. Sixth, if appropriate, use a bidialectal/bilingual approach. That is, incorporate the individual's home language and/or dialect into the intervention process. Research has shown that individuals acquire knowledge better in the second language if it is presented in the first language initially (e.g., Perozzi & Sanchez, 1992). Finally, use all of the resources that are available to you (e.g., if you are working in a school, get help from English as a second language teachers, classroom teachers, reading teachers).

Family-Centered Intervention

It is likely that nobody knows your client better than his or her family members. It is imperative to involve your client's family in the intervention process (Lynch & Hanson, 1992). The family's involvement, however, must be at a level in which they are most comfortable. Some families may be comfortable actually participating in the intervention process by being in the room with you, whereas other families may wish to observe the intervention sessions and ask questions after the session.

There are some specific ways in which you ought to work with families in the intervention process. First, alert the family to the purpose of the sessions and who will be present. Second, attempt to involve the family in decision making, if appropriate. Third, match your client's goals to the family's concerns and needs. Fourth, allow time for questions, but also be prepared to answer questions that other families have asked before. Finally, utilize practices that are culturally appropriate. These strategies include checking often for comprehension, emphasizing key words continually, reviewing previously learned material on a daily basis, including literacy activities, rephrasing information, teaching concepts in naturalistic situations, teaching strategies so that students can monitor their own learning activities, using all modalities, and using stories and narratives. These strategies have been shown to be effective for individuals from culturally and linguistically diverse populations (Roseberry-McKibbin, 1995).

CONCLUSION

Providing appropriate assessment and intervention services to individuals from culturally and linguistically diverse populations is, no doubt, challenging. Before the assessment even takes place, you will probably have to gather information on your client's language, dialectal variety, verbal and nonverbal communication styles, and so forth. This information will have to be applied to the specific person you are evaluating/treating. It may be necessary for you to employ support personnel to aid in the clinical management process, particularly if you do not speak the client's language. You may also have to alter your typical assessment protocol in order to ensure that you are making a valid diagnosis. That accurate diagnosis will lead to intervention approaches and techniques that are suited to your particular client.

REFERENCES

Adler, S. (1984). *Cultural language differences: Their educational and clinical-professional implications.* Springfield, IL: Charles C. Thomas.

American Speech-Language-Hearing Association. (1985). Clinical management of communicatively handicapped minority language populations. *ASHA, 27*(6), 29–32.

American Speech-Language Hearing Association. (1989). Definition: Bilingual speech-language pathologists and audiologists. *ASHA, 31,* 93.

American Speech-Language-Hearing Association. (1996a). *Accreditation manual: Council on academic accreditation in audiology and speech-language pathology.* Rockville, MD: Author.

American Speech-Language-Hearing Association. (1996b, Spring). Guidelines for the training, credentialing, use, and supervision of speech-language pathology assistants. *ASHA, 38*(Suppl. 16), 21–34.

Beaumont, C. (1992). Language intervention strategies for Hispanic LLD students. In H. Langdon (Ed.), *Hispanic children and adults with communication disorders: Assessment and intervention* (pp. 272–333). Gaithersburg, MD: Aspen Publishers.

Cheng, L.R.L. (1989). Intervention strategies: A multicultural approach. *Topics in Language Disorders, 9,* 84–91.

Cheng, L.R.L. (1993). Asian-American cultures. In D. Battle (Ed.), *Communication disorders in multicultural populations* (pp. 38–77). Boston: Andover Medical Publishers.

Cheng, L.R.L. (1996). Enhancing communication: Toward optimal language learning for limited English proficient students. *Language, Speech, and Hearing Services in Schools, 27,* 347–354.

Cummins, J. (1984). *Bilingualism and special education: Issues in assessment and pedagogy.* San Diego: College Hill Press.

Damico, J. (1993). *Appropriate speech and language assessment for bilingual children.* Presented at Bilingualism: What Every Clinician Needs to Know conference, Alexandria, VA.

Damico, J., & Hamayan, E. (1992). *Multicultural language intervention.* Buffalo, NY: Educom Associates, Inc.

Damico, J., Smith, M., & Augustine, L. (1996). Multicultural populations and language disorders. In M. Smith & J. Damico (Eds.), *Childhood language disorders* (pp. 272–299). New York: Thieme Medical Publishers.

Erickson, J., & Iglesias, A. (1986). Assessment of communication disorders in non-English proficient children. In O. Taylor (Ed.), *Nature of communication disorders in culturally and linguistically diverse populations* (pp. 181–217). San Diego: College Hill Press.

Grosjean, F. (1989). Neurolinguists, beware! The bilingual is not two monolinguals in one person. *Brain and Language, 36,* 3–15.

Grosjean, F. (1992). Another view of bilingualism. In R. Harris (Ed.), *Cognitive processing in bilinguals* (pp. 51–62). Amsterdam: Elsevier.

Grosjean, F. (1997). Processing mixed languages: Issues, findings, and models. In A. de Groot & J. Kroll (Eds.), *Tutorials in bilingualism: Psycholinguistic perspectives* (pp. 225–254). Mahwah, NJ: Lawrence Erlbaum Associates.

Hakuta, K. (1986). *Mirror of language: The debate on bilingualism.* New York: Basic Books.

Heath, S. (1982). What no bedtime story means: Narrative skills at home and school. *Language in Society, 11,* 49–76.

Heath, S. (1983). *Ways with words: Life and work in communities and classrooms.* New York: Cambridge University Press.

Individuals with Disabilities Education Act (IDEA) of 1990, PL 101-476, 20 U.S.C. §§ 1400 *et seq.*

Individuals with Disabilities Education Act (IDEA) Amendments of 1997, PL 105-17, 20 U.S.C. §§ 1400 *et seq.*

Iglesias, A., & Quinn, R. (1997). Culture as a context for early intervention. In S.K. Thurman, J.R. Cornwell, & S.R. Gottwald (Eds.), *Contexts of early intervention: Systems and settings* (pp. 55–71). Baltimore: Paul H. Brookes Publishing Co.

Kayser, H. (1989). Speech and language assessment of Spanish-English speaking children. *Language, Speech, and Hearing Services in the Schools, 20,* 226–244.

Kayser, H. (1993). Hispanic cultures. In D. Battle (Ed.), *Communication disorders in multicultural populations* (pp. 114–157). Boston: Andover Medical Publishers.

Kayser, H. (1995a). Assessment of speech and language impairments in bilingual children. In H. Kayser (Ed.), *Bilingual speech-language pathology: An Hispanic focus* (pp. 243–264). San Diego: Singular Publishing Group.

Kayser, H. (1995b). Intervention with children from linguistically and culturally diverse backgrounds. In M. Fey, J. Windsor, & S. Warren (Eds.), *Language intervention: Preschool through the elementary years* (pp. 315–331). Baltimore: Paul H. Brookes Publishing Co.

Langdon, H. (1992). Speech and language assessment of LEP/bilingual Hispanic students. In H. Langdon (Ed.), *Hispanic children and adults with communication disorders: Assessment and intervention* (pp. 201–271). Gaithersburg, MD: Aspen Publishers.

Larry P. vs. Riles, 343 F. Supp. 1306.502F 2d 963 (1972).

Linguistic Society of America. (1996). *Statement on language rights.* Washington, DC: Author.

Lynch, E.W. (1992). Developing cross-cultural competence. In E.W. Lynch & M.J. Hanson (Eds.), *Developing cross-cultural competence: A guide for working with young children and their families* (pp. 35–62). Baltimore: Paul H. Brookes Publishing Co.

Lynch, E.W., & Hanson, M.J. (1992). Steps in the right direction: Implications for interventionists. In E.W. Lynch & M.J. Hanson (Eds.), *Developing cross-cultural competence: A guide for working with young children and their families* (pp. 355–370). Baltimore: Paul H. Brookes Publishing Co.

Mattes, L., & Omark, D. (1991). *Speech and language assessment for the bilingual handicapped* (2nd ed.). Oceanside, CA: Academic Communication Associates.

Norris, M., Juarez, M., & Perkins, M. (1989). Adaptation of a screening test for bilingual and bidialectal populations. *Language, Speech, and Hearing Services in the Schools, 20,* 381–389.

Pease-Alvarez, L. (1993). *Moving in and out of bilingualism: Investigating native language maintenance and shift in Mexican-descent children.* Santa Cruz, CA: National Center for Research on Cultural Diversity and Second Language Learning.

Peña, E.D. (1996). Dynamic assessment: The model and its language applications. In K.N. Cole, P.S. Dale, & D.J. Thal (Eds.), *Assessment of communication and language* (pp. 281–307). Baltimore: Paul H. Brookes Publishing Co.

Perozzi, J., & Sanchez, M. (1992). The effect of instruction in L1 on receptive acquisition of L2 for bilingual students with language delay. *Language, Speech, and Hearing Services in the Schools, 23,* 348–352.

Peters-Johnson, C. (1998). Action: School services. *Language, Speech, and Hearing Services in the Schools, 29,* 120–126.

Roseberry-McKibbin, C. (1994). Assessment and intervention for children with limited English proficiency and language disorders. *American Journal of Speech-Language Pathology, 3,* 77–88.

Roseberry-McKibbin, C. (1995). *Multicultural students with special language needs.* Oceanside, CA: Academic Communication Associates.

Roseberry-McKibbin, C., & Eicholtz, G. (1994). Serving children with limited English proficiency in the schools: A national survey. *Language, Speech, and Hearing Services in the Schools, 25,* 156–164.

Seymour, H. (1986). Clinical principles for language intervention among nonstandard speakers of English. In O. Taylor (Ed.), *Treatment of communication disorders in culturally and linguistically diverse populations* (pp. 115–133). San Diego: College Hill Press.

Sollors, W. (1998). Introduction: After the culture wars; or, from "English only" to "English plus." In W. Sollors (Ed.), *Multilingual America: Transitionalism, ethnicity, and the languages of American literature* (pp. 1–13). New York: New York University Press.

Taylor, O., & Clarke, M. (1994). Communication disorders and cultural diversity: A theoretical framework. *Seminars in Speech and Language, 15,* 103–113.

Taylor, O., & Payne, K. (1983). Culturally valid testing: A proactive approach. *Topics in Language Disorders, 3*(8), 8–20.

Taylor, O., & Payne, K. (1994). Language and communication differences. In G. Shames, E. Wiig, & W. Secord (Eds.), *Human communication disorders: An introduction* (4th ed., pp. 136–173). Upper Saddle River, NJ: Prentice Hall.

Terrell, S., & Terrell, F. (1983). Effects of speaking Black English upon employment opportunities. *ASHA, 25,* 27–29.

Terrell, S., & Terrell, F. (1993). In D. Battle (Ed.), *Communication disorders in multicultural populations* (pp. 3–37). Boston: Andover Medical Publishers.

Toliver Weddington, G. (1981). *Valid assessment of children.* San Jose, CA: San Jose State University.

U.S. Bureau of the Census. (1995). *Statistical abstract of the United States: 1995* (115th ed.). Washington, DC: U.S. Department of Commerce.

U.S. Department of Education. (1998). *Digest of Education Statistics, 1998.* Washington, DC: Author.

Van Keulen, J., Weddington, G., & DeBose, C. (1998). *Speech, language, learning and the African American child.* Needham Heights, MA: Allyn & Bacon.

Vaughn-Cooke, F. (1986). The challenge of assessing the language of nonmainstream speakers. In O. Taylor (Ed.), *Treatment of communication disorders in culturally and linguistically diverse populations* (pp. 23–48). San Diego: College Hill Press.

Washington, J., & Craig, H. (1994). Dialect forms during discourse of poor, urban African American preschoolers. *Journal of Speech and Hearing Research, 37,* 816–823.

Wolfram, W. (1986). Language variation in the United States. In O. Taylor (Ed.), *Treatment of communication disorders in culturally and linguistically diverse populations* (pp. 73–116). San Diego: College Hill Press.

Wolfram, W., & Schilling-Estes, N. (1998). *American English: Dialects and variation.* Oxford, England: Blackwell Publishers.

FURTHER READING

Baetens-Beardsmore, H. (1986). *Bilingualism: Basic principles* (2nd ed.). San Diego: College Hill Press.

Battle, D. (Ed.). (1993). *Communication disorders in multicultural populations.* Boston: Andover Medical Publishers.

Brice, A. (1994). Spanish or English for language impaired Hispanic children? In D. Ripich & N. Creaghead (Eds.), *School discourse problems* (2nd ed., pp. 133–153). San Diego: Singular Publishing Group.

Cheng, L.R.L. (1991). *Assessing Asian language performance: Guidelines for evaluating limited-English-proficient students* (2nd ed.). Oceanside, CA: Academic Communication Associates.

Coleman, T. (2000). *Clinical management of communication disorders in culturally diverse populations.* Needham Heights, MA: Allyn & Bacon.

Gutierrez-Clellen, V., Restrepo, M.A., Bedore, L., Peña, E., & Anderson, R. (2000). Language sample analysis in Spanish-speaking children: Methodological considerations. *Language, Speech, and Hearing Services in the Schools, 31,* 88–98.

Harris, G. (1993). American Indian cultures: A lesson in diversity. In D. Battle (Ed.), *Communication disorders in multicultural populations* (pp. 78–113). Boston: Andover Medical Publishers.

Iglesias, A., & Goldstein, B. (1998). Language and dialectal variations. In J. Bernthal & N. Bankson (Eds.), *Articulation and phonological disorders* (4th ed., pp. 148–171). Needham Heights, MA: Allyn & Bacon.

Kayser, H. (1998). *Assessment and intervention resource for Hispanic children.* San Diego: Singular Publishing Group.

Langdon, H. (Ed.). (1992). *Hispanic children and adults with communication disorders: Assessment and intervention.* Gaithersburg, MD: Aspen Publishers.

Quinn, R., Goldstein, B., & Peña, E. (1996). Cultural/linguistic variation in the United States and its implications for assessment and intervention in speech-language pathology: An introduction. *Language, Speech, and Hearing Services in the Schools, 27,* 345–346.

Stockman, I.J. (1996). Phonological development and disorders in African American children. In A.G. Kamhi, K.E. Pollock, & J.L. Harris (Eds.), *Communication development and disorders in African American children: Research, assessment, and intervention* (pp. 117–153). Baltimore: Paul H. Brookes Publishing Co.

Taylor, O., & Leonard, L. (Eds.). (1999). *Language acquisition across North America: Cross-cultural and cross-linguistic perspectives.* San Diego: Singular Publishing Group.

Van Kleeck, A. (1994). Potential cultural bias in training parents as conversational partners with children who have delays in language development. *American Journal of Speech-Language Pathology, 3,* 67–78.

1. Describe your own culture, language, and dialect. How have aspects of each one changed since high school? How do your culture, language, and dialect compare with the group you think is most different from you? How might your culture, language, and dialect influence assessment and intervention of an individual not from your cultural and/or linguistic group?

2. How do culture and communication relate? Consider three ways in your own experience that culture and communication are interrelated.

3. Describe four ways that you would use alternative methods of assessment in the diagnosis of communication disorders of individuals from culturally and linguistically diverse populations.

4. What is the relationship between child socialization practices and language development? In an assessment, how might you determine that a child's linguistic performance was due to his or her socialization versus characteristic of a communication disorder?

5. Define bilingualism. How might monolingual SLPs assess and treat bilingual individuals?

6. Do you think immigrants to the United States of America should maintain their native/home language? Provide a rationale for your response. How would their maintenance or loss of their home language influence your selection of an intervention approach and intervention goals?

7. Using data from the U.S. Census Bureau (http://www.census.gov), determine the racial/ethnic composition of your community.

8. Go to the grocery store, department store, or airport (or anywhere diverse groups of individuals congregate) and describe the different ways that individuals interact with one another. You might compare how adults interact with other adults, how adults interact with children, and how children interact with other children.

Technology and Communication Disorders

Douglas Martin
Ann K. Lieberth

The 1990 annual convention of the American Speech-Language-Hearing Association (ASHA) included hands-on computer workshops as a component of the educational program for the first time. These sessions met with overwhelming and somewhat unexpected success as speech-language pathologists (SLPs) and audiologists recognized the emerging importance of computer technology in all aspects of their professional practice. Ten years later at the 2000 annual ASHA convention, the computer workshops continued to be a popular and important component of the educational program. This enduring popularity reinforces the simple truth that computer technology will continue to play a major role in our lives, both professional and personal.

The pace at which computer technology is evolving is nearly staggering. The technologies that were demonstrated or taught in the computer workshops at the 2000 convention—inexpensive and accessible **digital photography,** full-motion/full-screen **digital video, real-time** Internet-based transmission of speech and video signals, voice controlled computer application, and complex **data modeling** applications—had barely escaped the realm of science fiction a mere 10 years ago. Given these rapid changes, one might be reluctant to forecast the future in terms of technological applications. History does allow us, however, to make some fairly safe predictions. Costs of technology are expected to continue to decrease while ease of use, power, and number of applications are expected to increase. **Universal design** (e.g., built-in design that makes the software accessible to the greatest number of individuals) will lead to greater accessibility for professionals and consumers.

Concurrent with the evolution of computer technology, there continue to be changes in the professional field of communication sciences and disorders that affect how professionals are trained, how services are delivered, and how consumers will gain access to the services. With increased emphasis on managed care and accountability, clinicians will see more clients and, in the process, assume greater responsibility for documenting the need for services, tracking progress, and justifying service delivery. Now and in the future, SLPs and audiologists will be asked to work more efficiently and more effectively. In order to do that, they will need to take advantage of the support that technology can and will be able to provide.

Technology has always been an integral part of the service delivery of audiologists. The very nature of the tools of the trade demands that the audiologist integrate technology into all aspects of service delivery. Audiologists working within medical environments have used technologically intensive diagnostic tools since 1980. Hearing aids, which represent an important part of the rehabilitative audiologist's treatment process, have also benefited from the technology explosion with the introduction of **digitally programmable** and fully digital systems. Audiologists must develop skills to use this wide range of technology tools effectively in order to fully serve their consumers' needs. In addition to audiometers and other computer-driven equipment, audiologists need to evaluate and tap technology to make what they do to support the assessment and rehabilitation of hearing loss in individuals easier and more cost effective without sacrificing quality. The following information highlights some specific technology applications in the field of audiology.

The field of audiology has a long history of integrating technology into all aspects of clinical practice. Examples can be cited from both diagnostic and rehabilitative areas of the field.

Diagnostic Applications

All modern *audiometers* (the instruments used to measure basic aspects of hearing) are examples of dedicated, stand-alone, hardware-based solutions. Essentially, an audiometer is a computer designed specifically to generate test signals (i.e., pure tones, various types of noise) and present them to a client under a very controlled condition. Many audiometers connect to a desktop computer to ease the process of record keeping.

- Auditory brainstem response (ABR) is a diagnostic test designed to assess both basic hearing capabilities and to determine the presence of lesions (e.g., tumors) in the VIII cranial nerve or lower brain stem. This task is accomplished by using electrodes applied on the client's scalp to measure electrical activity in the cochlea, VIII nerve, and brain stem in response to a specific type of auditory stimulus. This test involves a very sophisticated analysis of the electrical activity resulting from the auditory stimulus and was not possible prior to the availability of digital signal processing. The test did not become clinically feasible until the late 1970s and early 1980s when the computer power necessary for the test could be housed within a "portable" cabinet. In 2001, standard desktop or laptop computers are used along with special signal processing and delivery "cards" for administering these tests.

- *Otoacoustic emissions (OAE)* are very faint sounds that a typical inner ear produces in response to specific types of stimuli. The presence of OAEs is a very strong indicator of a typically functioning inner ear. These signals produced by the ear are very difficult to measure. A sophisticated signal processing program is necessary in order to measure an OAE in the presence of environmental or bodily noises that are often significantly louder than the OAE. Indeed, as with the ABR test described previously, measurement of OAEs without the availability of desktop or laptop computers would be impossible.

- *Universal newborn hearing screening* is a program that has received a lot of attention since the late 1990s. These programs are designed to help professionals identify infants with hearing impairments and begin intervention prior to 6 months of age. The tools of choice for completing the screenings are ABR and OAE, which were described previously. Although the advantages of these screening programs for the infant and his or her family has long been recognized, the opportunity to implement such programs could not be realized until the technology—in the form of portable desktop or laptop computers—was widely accessible and affordable to audiologists.

REHABILITATIVE APPLICATIONS

The impact of computer technology on the field of audiology may be most obvious in the area of hearing aids. Hearing aids are the most commonly employed rehabilitative technique in the audiologist's rehabilitative repertoire. Since the late 1990s, there have been dramatic advances in the integration of sophisticated signal processing technologies into hearing aids. The audiologist now has access to hearing aids ranging from those that use standard electrical components that are programmed by a desktop computer to hearing aids that are fully digital signal processors. The incorporation of fully digital processors into wearable hearing aids provides the promise for extremely sophisticated amplification systems that can be precisely matched to a given individual's hearing loss and hearing needs. This area of audiology is very exciting for practitioners in the field. It also demands, however, that the audiologist establish a firm understanding in basic computer technology, in general, and digital signal processing, in particular.

SLPs have been slower to embrace technology and integrate it into service delivery. The profession itself has long been considered to be "high touch," not "high tech." The broad spectrum of **technology-based** or **technology-enhanced** applications, however, that have evolved since 1990—many of which are briefly addressed in this chapter—have proven that "high tech" does not eliminate the "high touch" in the assessment and treatment of individuals with communication disorders. Indeed, with the assistance of technology, most tasks that the SLP performs on a daily basis can be done faster and, perhaps, more effectively than using paper and pencil. Technology will not replace the skills of a clinician, but it can enhance the service delivery process.

Technology has also affected clients and their families as they seek an assessment or treatment. Consumers are becoming more savvy about communication disorders and their treatment, thanks in part to gaining access to information on the Internet. They are demanding "the latest" in treatment (whether it is appropriate). The latest treatment, with increasing frequency, involves treatment materials that are used with a home computer allowing the patient to either self-deliver the treatment or practice outside of the clinical setting. At the same time, laws such as the Education for All Handicapped Children Act of 1975 (PL 94-142) and the Individuals with Disabilities Education Act (IDEA) Amendments of 1997 (PL 105-17) continue to mandate that clinicians provide services in the form of **assistive technology** devices to individuals with disabilities, including those people with communication disorders.

This chapter focuses on a general description of some of the technology available to assist the professional in speech-language pathology and audiology. Examples of applications of technology are discussed in the traditional areas of clinical practice; namely, assessment and intervention. The applications of so-called **productivity technology** to the support of daily practice and administrative needs is delineated. The potential impact that evolving **multimedia/hypermedia** and Internet-based technologies will have on our fields is also addressed. Before any of these issues can be discussed, however, a discussion of basic computing competencies is in order.

Finally, a warning: Just like anything involving technology, product development and resources are moving at the speed of sound. As a result, the day that this book goes to print, much of the product-specific information included in this chapter will be out of date. One of the many responsibilities facing the professional is to stay current with the technology applications available for the field. A number of resources are provided throughout this chapter to help with this task. The reader is encouraged to explore many of these resources on a regular basis.

BASIC COMPUTING COMPETENCIES

As computer technology continues to evolve to the point of being seamlessly integrated into all aspects of service delivery, professionals in communication sciences and disorders will, at the very least, need the basic skills and knowledge necessary to select and use technology in their practice with a variety of clients. Specifically, clinicians must have basic computer skills, understand the basics of operating a computer chip-driven device, be able to assess the needs of the client in light of the technology available, recommend or use the appropriate technology, and train the client and his or her family to use the technology. In 1993, a group of professionals in communication disorders with experience in clinical, administrative, and research applications of computer technology developed a list of basic computer competencies (Cochran et al., 1993) representing the most basic level of performance that practitioners must be able to comfortably demonstrate. These competencies assume a basic level of **computer literacy** on the part of the practitioner. Students lacking basic computer literacy skills are strongly encouraged to seek out classes or other resources for developing these skills. One key to the future of our field and your future as a contributing practitioner within the field lies in the ability to master the technology of today.

COMPUTING COMPETENCIES FOR COMMUNICATION SCIENCES AND DISORDERS

Computing competencies that support program administration and development

1. *Use of a computer as a productivity tool*

   Broad goal: The clinician will increase and maintain personal productivity by using a computer for administrative purposes.

2. *Awareness of technology-related ethical issues*

   Broad goal: The clinician will demonstrate familiarity with ethical considerations that apply to the use of computers in the management of communication disorders and will adhere to appropriate ethical standards.

3. *Awareness and use of computer-related resources*

   Broad goal: The clinician will demonstrate awareness of the resources that are available to inform professionals about the availability and efficacy of software and hardware products and sources of technical support.

4. *Basic computer operations*

   Broad goal: The clinician will demonstrate the ability to complete basic computer operations and troubleshoot common problems.

Computing competencies that support delivery of speech-language services

5. *Using a computer as a diagnostic tool*

   Broad goal: The clinician will make appropriate use of computer-based instruments designed to assist in the evaluation or diagnosis of communication disorders.

6. *Using computer-based materials as a context for conversation*

   Broad goal: The clinician will demonstrate the ability to use computer-based materials (or other new technology such as video, CD-ROM, photo CD) to form a shared context for communication.

7. *Using a computer as an instructor*

   Broad goal: The clinician will demonstrate the ability to choose, configure, and evaluate appropriate computer-assisted instruction activities for independent use by clients.

8. *Using a computer as a clinical data recorder/analyzer*

   Broad goal: The clinician will demonstrate the ability to use the computer-assisted data tracking and analysis during speech and/or language therapy session.

9. *Using a computer as a biofeedback device*

   Broad goal: The clinician will demonstrate the ability to plan and implement activities in which performance feedback to the client from the clinician is supplemented by biofeedback (visual and/or auditory) from the computer.

10. *Using a computer as a clinical materials generator*

    Broad goal: The clinician will take advantage of computer capabilities to generate personalized clinical materials to enhance intervention with specific clients.

11. *Using a computer as a resource for information*

    Broad goal: The clinician will be able to search for information on the Internet, use a listserv, and locate sources of continuing education on the World Wide Web.

CASE EXAMPLE 1

Susie has just graduated from a graduate program in speech-language pathology. She is ready to start her Clinical Fellowship Year (CFY). For graduation, she received a computer. She wants to use the computer in her clinical work and has a limited budget both from her CFY site and her personal budget to purchase software. She wants to get the most software for the least amount of money. As she begins deciding what to buy, she finds that this will be a difficult decision due to the wide range of software solutions that are available.

Of the many competencies discussed previously, one of the more complex involves selecting appropriate hardware or software applications for clinical or administrative use. Before beginning a discussion of the hardware and software available, a discussion of some general principles involved in evaluating products is necessary. Learning a method for evaluating software allows comparison of programs with similar, stated objectives to determine what might work most effectively in a particular setting. A software review methodology also allows the user to determine if the software program might be used in ways other than those stated by the manufacturer, thus expanding the utility of the program. Errors in allocating scarce resources might be reduced in this way. Software review systems help to organize information about a particular program. The review should provide a checklist of important criteria to be evaluated when using the program. Ideally, the software review system should correlate with a facility's needs assessment in which important tasks that might be done by computer are identified and prioritized. Thus, when a particular software program is evaluated, the review system would focus on the specific factors expected from that particular application in light of the needs of the user. If more than one software program exists that might meet that particular need, then these programs can be efficiently compared on similar criteria.

Most commercially available software programs have stated learning objectives. A software review system offers the opportunity to validate these objectives through systematic assessment. With a software review system, the user can look at important questions quickly and make educated decisions as to what should be purchased and what should not (Scherz, 1993). A software evaluation guideline developed and described by Scherz follows.

SOFTWARE EVALUATION GUIDELINES

1. **DETERMINE YOUR REQUIREMENTS.**

   A. IMPORTANT QUESTION #1: "What do I want this software application to do?"

      1. Administrative tasks (e.g., test scoring, language sample analysis)?

      2. Materials preparation (e.g., individualized education programs [IEPs], communication board overlays)?

      3. Clinical tasks (e.g., cognitive retraining, concept development, language stimulation)?

   B. IMPORTANT QUESTION #2: "Who will use this software application?"

      1. Children? Adults?

      2. Novices? Experienced users?

      3. People with physical challenges?

      4. Clients? Staff?

   C. IMPORTANT QUESTION #3: "How much does it cost?"

      1. What are the direct/indirect costs?

      2. Is there a cost-savings benefit?

      3. How much staff time does it take to learn how to use the program?

2. RULE OUT PROGRAMS THAT WILL NOT MEET YOUR REQUIREMENTS.

    A. Consult published reviews.

    B. Contact manufacturers. (Are demo disks available?)

    C. Consult other users.

3. CONDUCT A SYSTEMATIC REVIEW. USE THESE GENERIC QUESTIONS.

A. TASK PERFORMANCE

    1. Does this software application do things faster?

    2. More thoroughly?

    3. Accurately?

    4. Does the "teaching" in the application follow sound principles?

        a. Are a range of concepts covered?

        b. Is the difficulty and rate of presentation appropriate? Modifiable?

        c. Does the program provide a way to track client performance?

        d. Is there appropriate feedback/help offered?

        e. Does the program promote creative problem-solving responses?

        f. If the program provides drill and practice, are the repetitive responses varied enough to maintain the client's interest?

B. EASE OF USE

    1. Is the program "user friendly"?

    2. Is it menu driven?

    3. Does it contain error trapping?

    4. Does it require multiple keystrokes? Frequent disk switching?

    5. Is it easy to quit?

C. DOCUMENTATION

    1. Is there a tutorial?

    2. Is there a reference card for frequent, time-saving keystrokes?

    3. Is the manual well organized?

    4. Is important information highlighted?

    5. Are there illustrations?

D. DEALER SUPPORT

    1. Is there a realistic preview/return policy?

    2. Is there a policy for back-up/replacement disks?

    3. Are upgrades made available at no or low cost?

    4. Is there a customer service hotline?

E. OTHER REQUIREMENTS

    1. Is the operating system used compatible with your computer?

    2. How much memory is needed for the application?

    3. Are peripheral devices required or can they be used?

        a. Speech synthesizer?

        b. Power pad? Touch window?

        c. Joystick? Switches?

F. OTHER CONSIDERATIONS

    1. Are the graphics easily identifiable? Do they require a color monitor?

    2. Are the sound effects appropriate? Distracting?

    3. Is there a sourcebook of suggested activities to use with the program?

    4. Is the program modifiable? Can individualized vocabulary be programmed in?

    5. Is the application usable with a variety of clients?

4. CONDUCT YOUR SOFTWARE REVIEW FROM THE PERSPECTIVE OF THE POTENTIAL CLIENTS WITH WHOM YOU HOPE TO USE THE APPLICATION.

A. How difficult is it to boot up and start the program independently?

B. Make creative responses or try to make mistakes, like hitting the "return" key when it says to "press the space bar," or answer something that is not in the array of choices offered. What happens?

C. Sample each major aspect of the program, then try skipping around in the program or quitting in the middle of an activity. Can you do that?

D. Try to observe similar types of clients using the program. How well do they do?

CASE EXAMPLE 2

Susie is ready to use the software review checklist to help her choose what she needs. She has decided to purchase at least one assessment and four intervention software products—two for children and two for adults—as her caseload is heterogeneous. She already has an integrated software package (spreadsheet, draw, paint, word processing, and database program) and an internet service provider.

BASIC COMPUTER TECHNOLOGY APPLICATIONS

Hardware-Based Applications

Before describing some of the specific applications commonly used in the field of communication disorders, a brief overview of the more common types of computer technology solutions is in order. Computer technology solutions can typically be defined as either software based or a hardware/software combination. The software-based solutions are designed to run on a typically configured desktop personal computer platform. This typical configuration includes the main computer processor (including a hard drive storage device), a color monitor, a keyboard, and a mouse. More and more computers are now commonly equipped with a CD-ROM drive and a sound system including a sound card, speakers, and a microphone.

Although this typical hardware configuration provides enough computing power to run many of the computer solutions available for our field, some applications require more specialized hardware components to accomplish the desired task. These applications may involve the use of a special "card" that is added to the desktop computer to expand its processing capabilities. Alternatively, these applications may be configured as a stand-alone instrument. The Visi-Pitch is a common example found in speech-language pathology clinics. These specialized hardware solutions tend to be somewhat more expensive to implement and may be more complicated to operate than more common software solutions. As such, they may be more commonly found in specialized clinics or research laboratories. As clinicians become more technologically savvy, however, and the cost of technology continues to decrease, use of these more sophisticated hardware-based solutions will become more widespread.

Software-Based Applications

In contrast to hardware-based applications, most typical computer applications involve a software package that is designed to be loaded and run from a desktop personal computer. These programs are designed to operate using the basic computing power and capabilities found in desktop computer systems. Unfortunately, a standard desktop computer configuration does not exist yet. Clinicians must have the means of determining whether a software package is compatible with their computer system's basic capabilities. Because of this lack of standardization across computer systems, the clinician should have a method of evaluating the software prior to purchase.

In general, software programs can be classified into one of five different application types: dedicated, educational, entertainment, productivity, and clinician authored. Each type is described in more detail and within the context of service delivery solutions. Examples from each of these categories can be found in common use in our field. It is important to recognize before going any further that, in all cases, the software serves only to reinforce the efforts of the client, supported and guided by the clinician.

Multimedia Software Applications

Pick up any computer magazine published since 1995 and you can see the evolution and the explosion of a new computer application: multimedia. Actually, we have used the term *multimedia* in the past to describe the presentation of material in many forms: auditory, visual, and tactile. SLPs have recognized the advantages and the disadvantages of presenting stimuli to clients in multiple forms. For example, we have long used pictured or written stimuli to accompany auditory stimuli. Although this approach is beneficial in many applications, we have found that children and adults can be overstimulated by stimuli in multiple forms. We also acknowledge that this presentation of material can confuse some clients. The use of multimedia computer interfaces in our practices, however, may hold additional benefits for our clients—benefits not apparent or available in traditional static pencil, paper, or pictured form.

Multimedia (sometimes referred to as *new media, hypermedia,* and *integrated media*), when used in conjunction with computers, refers to the presentation of virtually any combination of media on the computer screen. It is not a new technology but rather a combination of existing technologies. A multimedia document can contain sound, motion, and video, as well as traditional text and graphics. These features are controlled, coordinated, and delivered on the computer screen. The information may be stored on a CD, a **laser video disc,** or the user's hard disk.

Multimedia also implies **interactivity;** the user is actively involved with the information. The user can control the pace of learning and ask for repetitions of or additional information on a topic. The information presented is controlled by the learner's responses and requests. Individualized teaching/learning is not only a possibility but a reality. Multimedia technology has been used to prepare interactive textbooks, to create simulations, to enliven lectures or presentations, and to create electronic books (with sound, video clips, animations or additional information to supplement the text).

Multimedia certainly fits the bill when we are talking about intervention. The stimuli can be presented to the client in multiple forms: visual, auditory, graphic, text, and animation. The learning of a new skill can be individualized, something that clinicians with their heterogeneous case loads appreciate. The learning of most skills can be monitored by the either the computer or the clinician. With increasing costs of services, decreasing reimbursement, and increasing numbers of clients to be served, computer-assisted drill and practice may be a practical solution.

Although multimedia can be a valuable tool for drill and practice for your clients, *it is not a replacement for the clinician or the clinician–client interaction.* It is an extension of the possibilities for drill and practice in a variety of situations and with a variety of people. It affords an individualized, self-paced approach to clinical intervention. "Computers should be used to enhance, not replace, the teacher and supplement, not supplant, traditional teaching methods. Computers should be used for the things they're good at, and people should be used for the things they're good at" (Reinhardt, 1995, p. 70).

COMPUTER TECHNOLOGY APPLICATIONS IN ASSESSMENT

As outlined previously, assessment applications in the field of communication disorders can involve both hardware- and software-based solutions. The majority of these solutions are **dedicated applications** in that they were developed to serve a particular assessment purpose. A number of these solutions, however, also have an intervention component to them.

Computer-based scoring software allows the clinician to input data or raw scores following an assessment using a standardized test. The client's standardized scores, percentile ranks, and so forth are generated by the computer, which saves the clinician time spent looking up information in a manual. As with any software, the accuracy of the output depends on the accuracy of the input. Also, the clinician should evaluate if the time saved by using the computer-based scoring software justifies its cost. If the clinician is using a test only occasionally and/or only has to use one table to derive the score needed, then the investment in the software may not justify the cost. Table 11.1 provides examples of three software products that can be used for scoring commonly used clinical tests.

CASE EXAMPLE 3

Susie realizes that some of the assessment tools that she will be using, at least for now, have computerized scoring systems. She believes, however, that the use of these scoring systems will not save her any time. She has decided that she can do the same thing

Table 11.1.   Computer-based scoring software

Test	Web address	Description
Woodcock-Johnson Tests of Academic Achievement and Cognitive Ability	http://www.riverpub.com/products/clinical/wjr.htm	This software calculates standardized scores from raw data on these tests for measuring cognitive abilities and academic achievement.
Peabody Picture Vocabulary Test Computer ASSIST from American Guidance Systems	http://www.agsnet.com	This program converts raw data from the Peabody Picture Vocabulary to derived scores, identifies strengths and weaknesses, and suggests remediation techniques.
Oral Written Language Expression test (OWLS): Written Expression Scale Computer ASSIST from American Guidance Systems	http://www.agsnet.com	When used with the OWLS test, this program converts raw data into derived scores, identifies strengths and weaknesses, and suggests remediation strategies.

the computerized scoring does by hand in nearly the same time. She also believes that she can design a spreadsheet template for each assessment tool. Thus, she decides not to spend additional money to purchase the computerized scoring systems.

Computerized phonological and language sample analyses are available to facilitate the analysis of a client's speech and language by comparing it to normative values (see Table 11.2). The advantages of these programs are speed and detail of analysis. These programs do not allow direct input of the speech or language of the client. The clinician must learn the keystrokes or input codes required by the computer program and input the data accurately if it is to be usable. The clinician must also be familiar with the method of analysis of the software chosen. For example, if the clinician is not familiar with phonological processes, then categorization and input of the data will be in error and the computer-produced analyses will be in error. Is the time saved (or used) in inputting the data worth the investment? Does the software do what you ordinarily do by hand faster without compromising accuracy? As with any software program, the clinician should look at the documentation to see if it is readable and understandable. The availability of technical support is also a plus when evaluating software.

CASE EXAMPLE 4

Susie has chosen to purchase the Systematic Analysis of Language Transcripts (SALT) program after attending a workshop at ASHA where she learned the methods for inputting language samples. She also attended a workshop at her state association convention in which she had further practice in data entry. She can use this tool for language sample analysis for a variety of clients. She felt that it was backed up with research and that upgrades and technical support were readily available.

Assessment and quantification of aspects of *speech and voice* have been facilitated due to advancements in technology. Measures of respiration, resonance, phonation, and articulation can be completed using a personal computer as an **instrumentation interface.** These objective measures can be used to document

Table 11.2.   Computerized phonological and language sample analyses

Test	Web address	Description
Automatic Articulation Analysis Plus, Parrot Software, State College, Pennsylvania	http://www.parrotsoftware.com	This software provides the clinician with a complete phonological articulation analysis consisting of a listing of the patterns of misarticulation.
SALT: Systematic Analysis of Language Transcripts	http://www.waisman.wisc.edu/salt	This software aids in analyzing English and Spanish language samples, compare to referenced databases (conversation and narratives), and identifies and describes disordered language performance.

Table 11.3.   Hardware-based examples of speech and voice analysis

Product	Web address	Description
Nasometer, Kay Elemetrics	http://www.kayelemetrics.com	The nasometer quantifies air flow from the nasal cavity. It is used to evaluate patients who have voice qualities described as *hypernasal* or *denasal*.
AeroPhone II, Kay Elemetrics	http://www.kayelemetrics.com	This hardware and its accompanying software allows the clinician to measure airflow and respiratory function in speech and nonspeech tasks.
Cafet, Cafet, Inc., Annandale, Virginia	http://www.mankato.msus.edu/ dept/comdis/kuster/Therapy WWW/intensive/cafet.html	A computer-aided fluency establishment trainer aids clients in establishing six target behaviors necessary to achieve fluency in speech.

changes from pretherapy to posttherapy, from presurgery to postsurgery, need for further treatment, verification of treatment outcomes, and so forth. Commercial hardware-based products are also available for physiologic analysis of speech and voice (see Table 11.3). This instrumentation can be expensive, complex, and not easily used by the practicing clinician. These devices do, however, provide quality, accurate, and detailed analyses. Therefore, the cost, the ease of use, the percentage of time used by the clinicians, and the different types of analyses possible should be considered prior to purchasing stand-alone instrumentation.

The number of computer programs available to analyze the various parameters of voice production is increasing as the capability of the basic computer system to process and analyze voice input has increased. Software programs are available that perform an acoustic analysis of voice production from which the physiological parameters can be inferred (see Table 11.4). Some of these programs can also be used during intervention (see the intervention section of this chapter).

As with the other areas, cost, ease of use, usability of the results, and technical support should be evaluated prior to the clinician ordering the software and/or the instrumentation. A beginning clinician needs to be familiar with the parameters involved in the acoustic and physiologic analysis of speech so that the choice of a product can be geared toward an environment in which it is to be used; who will be using it, for what purpose (versatility), and how often should also be considered.

CASE EXAMPLE 5

Susie has been asked by her CFY supervisor to research and recommend a speech and voice analysis system to be used by the facility—a rehabilitation center where both children and adults are seen. Susie chose the Computerized Speech Lab (CSL) and Dr. Speech Science. The CSL requires a bit more hardware at start up but for research and accountability the data is superior. Dr. Speech Science is less expensive and requires less hardware but the results are less precise.

Table 11.4. Software-based examples of speech and voice analysis

Product	Web address	Description
Visi-Pitch, Kay Elemetrics	http://www.kayelemetrics.com	An integrated hardware/software system that provides simple and innovative real time displays of important speech/voice parameters for visual feedback and for tracking progress.
Computerized Speech Lab (CSL), Kay Elemetrics	http://www.kayelemetrics.com	The CSL allows analysis of speech and voice of a client including measurement of pitch and intensity.
Dr. Speech Science, Tiger Electronics	http://www.asha.org/professionals/buyers_guide/slp.htm	This software is a collection of programs that when combined with special hardware enables the clinician to measure the parameters of voice (resonance, nasality, etc.)
IVANS, AVAAZ Innovations, Inc.	http://www.avaaz.com	Interactive Voice ANalysis System provides the clinician with tools for objective, noninvasive, and acoustic analytical vocal function assessment.
SoundScope, GW Instruments	http://www.gwinst.com	This allows you to record, view, analyze, play, store, and print sound waveforms for speech and voice analysis

The bottom line for choosing hardware and software for assessment purposes is the same as that used in choosing any technology: *If you do not have the knowledge base in each area (if you do not know what you are measuring), then the time you save in applying technology will be lost in inaccuracy.*

COMPUTER TECHNOLOGY APPLICATIONS IN INTERVENTION

There are a variety of programs available to support and facilitate intervention in speech and language across a variety of clients manifesting a variety of disorders. Most of the solutions useful for intervention are software-based, although a few hardware-based solutions are discussed. Although most of the software applications discussed for assessment purposes involve dedicated programs, applications useful within the intervention venue come from each of the five software categories.

CASE EXAMPLE 6

Susie was overwhelmed when she started to look for software for intervention and treatment. She knew that she wanted something that was versatile and flexible, and she knew she did not have a lot of money to spend. She needs guidelines or an evaluation system to use before she purchases anything.

Dedicated software applications are solutions written and designed for SLPs to use in intervention. Because it is designed specifically for use with clients with

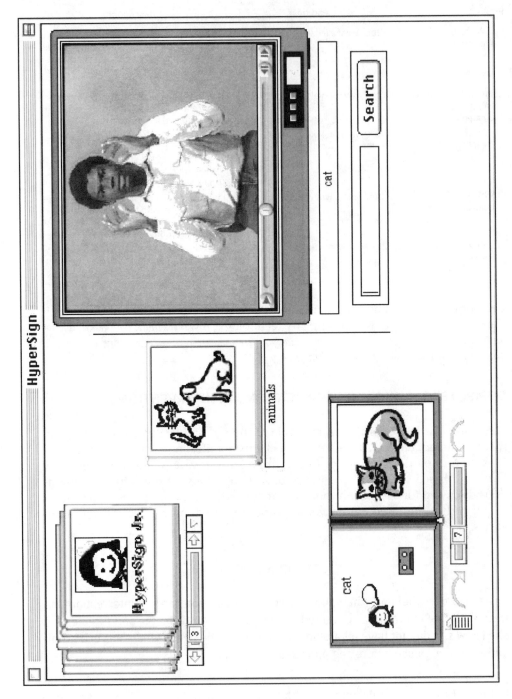

Figure 11.1. The children's dictionary window from HyperSign: An Interactive Dictionary of American Sign Language. (Courtesy of Trinity Software.)

speech-language disorders, dedicated software is organized around the order of acquisition of skills. This makes this software particularly useful but not versatile; that is, dedicated software can often only be used for disorders for which it was written. Again, the clinician should evaluate the software in light of needs, use, and clients served prior to purchase.

Educational software refers to software programs written for educational purposes (i.e., to improve or reinforce reading skills, to provide drill and practice in following directions, to practice writing skills; see Figure 11.1). These products have the advantage of focusing on academic information. Although the efficacy of the use of educational software in speech-language intervention has not been widely researched, the vocabulary and language contained therein are age-appropriate, academically oriented, and designed around educational objectives and learning strategies. The software can be used to reinforce the language and speech used in the classroom. The versatility of the software in intervention with children with speech and language disorders is limited only by the creativity of the clinician using it. Table 11.5 provides a number of software packages that can be adapted for clinical use. For example, the vocabulary in the Reader Rabbit Reading program can be used as a basis for vocabulary drills, expanded language activities in which the concepts and vocabulary introduced in the program can be put into different contexts, and sequencing activities that can be drilled in speech therapy based on the stories presented in the program.

Entertainment software describes programs designed for fun (see Table 11.6). These programs can be used as a substitute for the manipulatives that are traditionally used in therapy. The software chosen should allow the client several opportunities for practicing the target structure. Sometimes, the games or activities included in entertainment software may distract the client from the goal or objective of the session. At the same time, the action of the activity and its accompanying sounds and movement may overstimulate the client. Entertainment software, however, can provide a wealth of activities for drill and practice of targeted speech and language structures. Entertainment software can be used by the clinician to replace the board game or the activity used to reinforce correct responses in the clinic. For example, Wheel of Fortune and Hangman can be used effectively as rewards following correct responses.

Table 11.5.   Education software

Product	Web address	Description
Jump Start Programs, Davidson and Associates	http://www.knowledge-adventure.com /home	This is a series of games and learning activities to accompany a variety of subjects and a variety of age levels.
HyperSign: An Interactive Dictionary of American Sign Language, Trinity Software	http://www.trinitysoftware.com	This is an interactive multiage level dictionary of 2000 American Sign Language signs presented in full motion video clips complete with games and practice activities.
Reader Rabbit, The Learning Company	http://www.mattelinteractive. com	This is a series of software providing drill and practice on basic reading and phonics skills for beginning readers.

Table 11.6.   Entertainment software

Product	Web address	Description
Arthur Talking Book Series, Broderbund	http://www.mattelinteractive. com	This is a series of interactive books for children. The words in the story can be highlighted and read to the child. There are hidden pictures that can be activated with the mouse.
Kid Pix, Brøderbund	http://www.mattelinteractive. com	This is paint, draw, and animation software allowing children to prepare a variety of projects
Interactive Stories, Softdisk	http://www.softdisk.com	This software allows a child to write a story, make the choices for what actions are taken, and determine how his or her story ends.

CASE EXAMPLE 7

Susie decided to purchase a dedicated software program called Picture Gallery. She felt that she could use this program to generate materials for both children and adults. She also chose one educational program, Reader Rabbit, because of its emphasis on phonics and its user-friendliness for young children. Finally, she chose one entertainment program, Interactive Stories, because this could be used with children, teenagers, and adults.

Productivity software is the generic term used to categorize software applications designed to facilitate common everyday tasks. Word processing software would fall into this category. Other examples of productivity software include **databases, spreadsheets,** and basic **graphics programs.** Many publishers provide suites of productivity applications that are designed to share data between the various software programs within the suite. Microsoft Office is perhaps the most widely recognized productivity suite of this type. AppleWorks is another widely used product primarily for the Macintosh platform. Both of these products include a complete word processor package along with database, spreadsheet, and basic drawing or painting programs. Productivity software sees its greatest utility to the clinician outside of the actual clinical assessment or intervention venue. Resourceful clinicians, however, can incorporate capabilities of productivity software (e.g., spelling or grammar checkers in a word processing program, data organization and manipulation in a database or spreadsheet program) into their clinical protocols.

Clinician-authored software represents specific software applications that are actually created by the clinician. This is not a commonly encountered software solution as the development of effective software applications involves well-developed programming or **authoring** skills. This has become an even greater issue as more commercially published software incorporates multimedia components into the applications. These commercially developed multimedia packages set a high standard for clinical software.

A number of applications are available, however, to help ambitious clinicians in developing their own software solutions. These applications are referred to as *authoring packages.* The more commonly encountered authoring programs include HyperCard and HyperStudio for the Macintosh platform and Assymetrix ToolBook for the Windows-based platforms. Macromedia Director is an authoring tool that is available for both the Macintosh and Windows platforms. These authoring packages typically involve an actual authoring component and some form of a playback engine. The authoring component allows the author to build the basic program components. A scripting language is also available to allow the author to program specific tasks for the program to perform. Once the authoring of the program is completed, the program is run on the user's computer using the playback engine. The playback engine is a small program that runs the completed program by incorporating the various interface elements and scripts constructed by the author.

For the ambitious clinician, authoring provides a potential solution for computer solutions that are not available commercially. A number of clinicians within the field of communication disorders have successfully used authoring tools to create useful clinical computer solutions. Although a more detailed discussion of this topic is beyond the scope of this chapter, the interested reader is encouraged to consult the authoring resources pertaining to the previously listed programs.

Biofeedback software refers to dedicated, computer-based instrumentation that provides the user with real time displays of physiologic activities in the production of speech and voice. Other software and its accompanying hardware have been designed for clinical measurements and research. Using these programs, the clinician does not have to subjectively evaluate the client's performance. With many biofeedback software packages, the computer compares the production of the client to normative data contained in the program. With other biofeedback

Table 11.7. Biofeedback computer applications

Product	Web address	Description
Computerized Speech Lab, Kay Elemetrics	http://www.kayelemetrics.com	This provides tools for the clinician to analyze and measure voice parameters: pitch, frequency, spectrograms, and so forth.
SpeechViewer, IBM	http://www.ibm.com	This provides user-friendly computer feedback for loudness, pitch, and other parameters of voice production as well as voice analysis, and so forth.
The Indiana Speech Training Aid, Communication Disorders Technology, Inc.	http://www.comdistec.com/	This is a computer-based speech training program integrating speech recognition with speech drill and practice material.
Video Voice, Micro Video	http://www.videovoice.com	This is a visible speech training aid with a wide variety of entertaining and motivational graphic displays that have many applications for developing speech skills.
Cafet, Cafet, Inc.	http://www.mankato.msus.edu/ dept/comdis/kuster/Therapy WWW/intensive/cafet.html	This computerized fluency trainer aids clients in establishing six target behaviors necessary to achieve fluency in speech.

programs, the computer simply analyzes and displays the acoustic features of the production of the client. Determination of the adequacy of the speech production is left to the clinician. Biofeedback software programs, a number of which are shown in Table 11.7, are available for use with both children and adults.

CASE EXAMPLE 8

Although Susie really liked what some of the biofeedback programs had to offer, the cost of most of these programs was prohibitive. She decided to wait and try to get the IBM SpeechViewer II funded at a later date.

COMPUTER TECHNOLOGY APPLICATIONS IN AUGMENTATIVE AND ALTERNATIVE COMMUNICATION

Individuals who are unable to speak; have mobility, hearing, or vision impairments; or limitations in cognition and perception have benefited tremendously from the invention of the computer chip. It is now possible for those individuals unable to produce spoken language to speak for themselves through the interface of a computer. Behrmann (1998) called technology the "great equalizer" for individuals with disabilities, assisting them in fully participating in school, work, or community.

Assistive technology refers to "any item, piece of equipment, or product system whether acquired commercially off the shelf, modified, or customized, that is used to increase, maintain, or improve functional capabilities of individuals with disabilities" (Behrmann, 1998, p. 3). This definition encompasses both high-tech devices such as **communication boards** and eye movement or breath-controlled computers, to low-tech devices such as switches, joy sticks, tape recorders, mouth sticks, or pencil grips.

Clinicians have many options when recommending assistive technology for individuals with communication disorders (see Table 11.8). The choices range from basic communication boards to sophisticated voice input communication aids. Clinicians need to understand the equipment and what it does or may be able to do and then match it with the client's abilities and needs. For example, the clinician can make personalized communication boards using software for that purpose or a client may need an alternate **input system** for a computer such as a switch or a touchscreen. **Input devices,** such as track balls and joy sticks, may need to be larger or slower in responding than in their traditional form in order to accommodate a given client's capabilities. For some patients with significant motoric constraints (e.g., quadriplegia) a completely different method of input into the computer may be necessary. For instance, input devices are available that respond to eye blinks or eye movements, a suck or a puff on a straw-like control, or a pointer that is worn on a special headband. Consideration can also be given to the use of handheld or portable devices instead of, or in addition to, communication aids designed to be used with a laptop or a desktop computer.

Table 11.8. Augmentative and alternative communication devices

Title	Web address	Description
Speaking Dynamically and BoardMaker, Mayer-Johnson	http://www.mayer-johnson.com	Speaking Dynamically Pro is a speech output communication program. It allows you to use your computer as a communication device. BoardMaker is software that allows the user to create communication boards.
Speaking Academically and Language Exercises for You and Me, Mayer-Johnson	http://www.mayer-johnson.com	This provides more than 180 interlinking school curriculum and communication boards designed to help nonvocal students communicate in the classroom. Language exercise software includes a set of over 190 fun and engaging language activity boards allowing students to practice vocabulary, listening skills, and language expression.
Storytime Tales, Mayer-Johnson	http://www.mayer-johnson.com	This software acts like an animated picture book to introduce beginning literacy activities to young children.
DynaVox, Sentient	http://www.sentient-sys.com	This is a self-contained computerized communication board.
Dynamo, Sentient	http://www.sentient-sys.com	This is a stand-alone computerized communication board with easy-to-understand graphics and interface. A good first device for those who cannot talk.

CASE EXAMPLE 9

Susie decided to purchase Board Builder and the Picture Exchange Communication System from Mayer Johnson. These items would enable her to prepare communication boards for adults and children.

COMPUTER TECHNOLOGY APPLICATIONS IN RECORD KEEPING

With the increased emphasis on accountability, clinicians will be asked to keep accurate, up-to-date records on their clients. Productivity software, as described previously, provides the tools for assisting the clinician in these tasks. Many of these productivity tools such as word processors, spreadsheets, and databases can be purchased in application suites such as Microsoft Office or AppleWorks. The advantage of the use of an **integrated software** package is that data, text, and graphics can easily be shared by each or all of the component programs. In addition, each program has the same windows, menu "looks," and commands, easing the use of the entire suite of programs.

The clinician can use integrated software for many purposes. Unfortunately, a detailed examination of the productivity enhancement possible with the use of these software tools is beyond the scope of this chapter. Numerous books and classes are available to guide the beginning—or even advanced—computer user in realizing the potentials of productivity software. A sample of some of the clinical tasks made easier or possible with productivity software are as follows.

- Prepare templates for form letters, progress reports, IEPs, and similar items using the word processing program.

- Use a spreadsheet to track progress by entering the client's performance percentages for each session. That data could be charted and then merged into a word processed progress report or template.

- Prepare a database for keeping records for billing purposes.

- Create word and picture drill and practice materials for clients using the graphics program.

- Create your own pictures using clip art or graphics programs to illustrate stories.

- Prepare a database of clients and then merge the information (e.g., addresses of clients) into a form letter.

- Maintain a list of personal books, journals, or journal articles in a database.

- Track your materials budget or supplement a child's math instruction using the spreadsheet program.

- Use the communication tool to connect to the Internet; make your own web page.

CASE EXAMPLE 10

Susie found out that her computer came with Microsoft Office already loaded. She used the database program to enter names of publishers of materials. When it came time to order the materials, she typed a form letter to the publishers and used the mail merge function in the word processing program to import those addresses for the letters and the envelopes. She also used this software to prepare an individualized education program (IEP) template.

A commonly encountered task by SLPs working with school-age children and their families involves the generation of IEPs. These IEP documents contain a great deal of information regarding the client and can be a somewhat cumbersome task to create. Numerous computer-based solutions for generating IEP documents have been proposed. One of the simplest involves the development of a word processing document IEP template. In use, the relevant information for a client is simply typed into the template to create the custom report for the child. Although an IEP template can be made using any word processing software program, the documents produced using a template may sound stereotypic and choppy. The programs may not allow the modification or addition of goals. As an alternative, there are dedicated IEP generator software programs available. The software generates an IEP based on the information entered by the clinician: background information, test results, goals, and other information about clients. As with a word processing template prepared by the clinician, however, IEPs generated using the commercially produced software all appear to be similar.

CLINICIAN COMMUNICATION AND THE INTERNET

One could easily argue that no technological innovation has influenced the melding of the computer into all aspects of our culture more than the emergence and evolution of the Internet. The Internet has opened up entire new avenues of communication, established new entertainment media, and changed the way that many individuals shop for nearly anything one could want to purchase. Perhaps most importantly, however, the Internet has provided instant access to information on virtually any topic. With a click of the mouse, one can research a syndrome a new client presents with, look up side effects of a medication that a patient may be taking, leave an e-mail requesting information on therapy techniques, download an article on promising treatments, get on a **listserv** of clinicians working with similar patients, consult a **newsgroup** to follow a discussion surrounding a new and controversial intervention technique, order office supplies, or download a variety of therapy materials. All of this can be done from the comfort of your own home or office in a relatively short time. No longer do we have to go to the library and look in our "old" college texts for information.

Clinicians have found many innovative ways to use this new communication medium. E-mail has become an immensely popular means of communicating within professional communities. This communication often takes the form of individual e-mail message exchanges between practitioners. Another common means of using e-mail technology involves subscribing to a special topic listserv. A *listserv* is essentially a community of individuals interested in a particular topic who exchange e-mail messages as a means of discussing topics of interest. Within a listserv community, all of the messages sent to the listserv are distributed to all community members. Individuals wishing to join a listserv community simply subscribe to the listserv by e-mailing a subscription request to the list manager. (Be aware, however, that membership in many listservs is limited to members of some other related community. For instance, ASHA maintains an audiology listserv that is available only to members of ASHA.) Once subscribed to a listserv, an individual will receive all e-mail messages that are sent to a central mailbox location for the list and can participate in the community conversation by simply sending e-mail messages of their own to the list. There exists an amazingly large number of listserv communities covering an equally large number of specific topics. A sampling of listservs of interest to communication disorder professionals can be found in the resources section of this chapter. The interested student is encouraged to subscribe to a listserv of interest, even if on a trial basis, to experience the opportunities available within a listserv community. Beware, however, that with some lists the amount of e-mail coming to your computer from the listserv can overwhelm your system.

Closely related to listserv are Internet newsgroups. Newsgroups work in much the same way as listservs with two important differences. First, the individual does not need to subscribe to the newsgroup in order to participate. One simply uses a software program called a **newsgroup reader** to gain access to the messages posted to the newsgroup. (Newsgroup reader software is now a bundled component of all major web browser software packages such as Netscape Communicator and Internet Explorer so that there is little need to obtain a stand-alone newsgroup reader program.) Secondly, newsgroups use a threaded structure to organize the messages posted to the group. Within a newsgroup lexicon, a **thread** is a series of messages relating to a single topic. Thus, a reader can submit (or post) a message to the newsgroup and other readers may choose to respond to that particular message. The newsgroup reader software will present the listing of the initial message and the subsequent replies to the initial message in an organized structure that will allow the reader to easily follow and read the series of messages pertaining to the particular topic (see Figure 11.2). A given newsgroup can have any number of threads going at any given time. This is a significant difference from a simple listserv because with a listserv the messages are simply forwarded to your e-mail box in the order that they are sent to the list and not organized by message topic. As with listservs, a multitude of newsgroups are available that discuss topics relative to the field of communication disorders. The resources section of this chapter lists a number of newsgroups of potential interest to practitioners within our field. Again, students are encouraged to visit a number of these newsgroups to experience the types of interaction that occur within these communities.

There are also a large number of listservs and newsgroups that could be of interest to your clients and/or their families. These client- and family-centered newsgroups and listservs serve much the same function of face-to-face support groups and can be immensely beneficial to patients for whom access to a local support group is compromised by any number of circumstances. Referring your patients or their families to these newsgroups/listservs can be a very effective adjunct to your intervention program. The clinician must also be aware, however, of potential problems that exist within these communities. These consumer/client oriented newsgroups or listservs can serve as an outlet for useful support information for your clients. Unfortunately, they can also serve as a means of easily circulating inaccurate, inappropriate, controversial, or even dangerous information to individuals who may not have the necessary background to evaluate the validity of the information. It is a good idea for the clinician referring clients and their families to these newsgroups or listservs to regularly monitor the communities in order to stay current with the information that is being circulated.

The Internet technology that may be most responsible for accelerating the computer revolution is the World Wide Web or simply "the web." The web began as a network that allowed military and physics researchers to easily interchange information using a simple to use hypertext format. From these fairly simple beginnings, the web has continued to grow to the point that it permeates all aspects of recreation, commerce, and educational environments with millions of individuals regularly accessing the web each day.

The basic technology underlying the web involves documents written in a language called *HyperText Mark-up Language* or **HTML.** These documents are

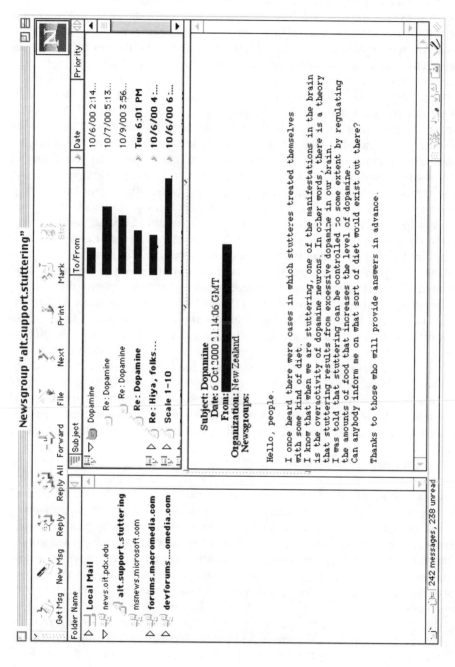

Figure 11.2. A sample newsgroup reader window.

made available on a computer designated as a web server. The function of the web server is to send these HTML documents to a remote computer via the Internet when a request for the document is sent from a user's desktop computer. A special program called a *web browser* runs on the user's desktop computer and is capable of interpreting the HTML code from the requested document into a readable format. A hallmark of the HTML format is the inclusion of **hyperlinks** within HTML documents. Hyperlinks (any text that is underlined in color) provide a means of linking one document to another by way of a mouse click.

The power of the web evolves from a number of characteristics inherent in its basic design and organization. The hyperlink function within HTML documents provide the user the opportunity to follow links in a manner that suits his or her needs. Second, the nature of the HTML language makes it a fairly straightforward task to create and publish web documents. The widespread availability of HTML editing programs such as Adobe PageMill and Netscape Composer allows for the creation of basic web documents as easily as creating a word processing document. Finally, the HTML language and all of the commonly used web browsers allow for the display of not only text information but also various other media such as graphics, sound, and digital movies. As a result, the web has matured into a very effective multimedia delivery system.

As web technology continues to evolve, the opportunities presented by this multimedia delivery system will continue to impact many aspects of the clinician's practice. Most home-based users of the web continue to connect to the web via a conventional modem. This conventional modem technology places some significant limitations on the transmission of sound and digital movie files due to the size of these files. For instance, a digital movie file with a playing time of 1 minute can easily take more than 30 minutes to load via a conventional modem. Over the next few years, connection technologies utilizing digital cable, fiber optics, and satellite transmission will become widely available to home-based users. These technologies will significantly reduce the transmission time for these large format files making the real-time delivery of many different media types a reality.

As the barriers to transmission of large sound and video files continue to be overcome, the utility of the web to the practitioner in communication disorders will increase dramatically. The web has the potential to become a useful means of delivering assessment or intervention services to patients located at a distance from the clinician. This aspect of service delivery has already begun to impact other areas of health care. In much the same manner, web technology will impact the delivery of both preprofessional and continuing education services. Many institutions are already using technology-enhanced courses as part of their training program. Current and future practitioners can also anticipate completing continuing education activities using this distance-based technology.

With all of its advantages, however, using the web presents some problems. The primary problem for consumers and professionals alike is that anyone can publish anything without peer review. The quality and accuracy of the information you get on the web is, therefore, questionable. Yet, for students, our clients, and professionals alike, the temptation is to "get on the net" to gather informa-

Table 11.9.   Web site evaluation guidelines

Who is the author or institution?
- If an individual has written the resource, is there biographical information available?
- If an institution has produced the resource, does it give information about itself?
- Have you seen the author's or institution's name cited in other sources or bibliographies?

How current is the information?
- Is there a date on the web page that indicates when the page was placed on the web?
- Is it clear when the page was last updated?
- Is some of the information obviously out-of-date?

Who is the audience?
- Is the web page intended for the general public, or is it meant for scholars, practitioners, children, and so forth?
- Is the audience clearly stated?
- Does the web page meet the needs of its stated audience?

Is the content accurate, objective, and supported by other sources?
- Are there political, ideological, cultural, religious, or institutional biases?
- Is the content intended to be a brief overview of the topic or an in-depth analysis?
- If the information is opinion, is this clearly stated?
- If there are facts and statistics included, are they properly cited?
- What is the purpose of the information?

Is the purpose of the information to inform, explain, persuade, market a product, or advocate a cause?
- Is the purpose clearly stated?
- Does the resource fulfill the stated purpose?

Source: Hartman and Ackerman, 1999.

tion, trusting that the information they get is accurate because it is convenient and fast. Table 11.9 presents some suggestions on evaluating a web site.

A way of verifying the accuracy and objectivity of published information is to use the triangulation process: find at least three sources that agree with the opinion or findings that the author of the web page presents as fact. Books and journals and other materials in libraries may contain more comprehensive information than is on the Internet. You can use the resources in the library to verify or expand information found on the web. A good guideline in evaluating the information you get from a search or a web site is to revert back to journalism practices: the 5-wh questions.

1. *Who* else might speak knowledgeably on this subject? Enter that person's name into a search engine.

2. *What* event might shed more information on your topic? Is there a group or organization that represents your topic? Do they hold an annual conference? Are synopses of presentations posted on the sponsoring organization's web site?

3. *When* do events happen?

4. *Where* might you find this information? Remember, web search engines are fallible; they don't find every site you need (Leeper & Gotthoffer, 2000).

5. *Why* is the information being searched for important and why does a particular site address this topic?

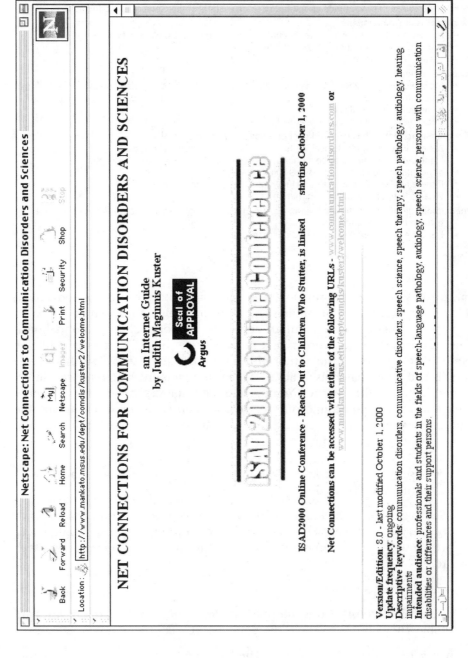

Figure 11.3. The home page for Net Connections for Communication Disorders and Sciences." (Courtesy of Dr. Judith Kuster.)

RESOURCES

As discussed previously, the Internet has opened up numerous opportunities for widespread distribution of information. In pre-Internet days, distribution of information often required the use of either a broadcast (i.e., television, radio) or print (i.e., newspapers, leaflets, brochures) media channel. Achieving widespread distribution of information using these distribution channels can be quite expensive and time consuming. The ease with which information can be posted to various types of Internet communication channels and the ease with which consumers can gain access to these channels has allowed for a proliferation of readily available information resources. Although there are many useful Internet-based information sites of interest to the professional in communication sciences and disorders, two are highlighted here.

The first is a site that represents the efforts of a committee sponsored by ASHA to investigate the impact of technology on our field in the coming years. The report from this committee is available at the following address: http://www.asha.org/tech_resources/tech2000/index.htm. This site is structured around a so-called FAQs format. **FAQ** stands for *frequently asked questions* and is a common format for presenting information within a web site. This site expands on some of the topics addressed in this chapter and could be of value for the student or professional in investigating the technology question in a more in-depth manner.

The second site is entitled "Net Connections for Communication Disorders" and can be found at the following address: http://www.communicationdisorders.com. This site represents the work of Dr. Judith Kuster from Mankato State University in Mankato, Minnesota (see Figure 11.3). This comprehensive site lists hundreds of communication disorders–related Internet resources of potential interest to students, professionals, and consumers. A small sampling of the types of resources available from this site is listed in the appendix at the end of this chapter.

CONCLUSION

Since 1980, computer technology has played an ever-increasing role in the field of communication disorders. Early in this process, technology was often viewed as an intrusion into the practitioner's realm or at the very least a necessary evil. As the technology has continued to evolve and has impacted all aspects of society, clinicians and patients have come to accept and even embrace computer solutions as a regular and expected part of the professional process. One can only anticipate that this infusion of technology will continue to the point where computer technology becomes such an integral part of all activities that it becomes transparent to all involved. Hopefully, future editions of this textbook will not include a chapter devoted to computer technology as the information would, by necessity, be infused into the other chapters of the text.

REFERENCES

Behrmann, M. (1998, Summer). Assistive technology for young children in special education. *Edutopia*, 3–5.

Cochran, P.S., Masterson, J.J., Long, S.H., Katz, R., Seaton, W.H., Wynne, M., Lieberth, A., & Martin, D. (1993). Computing competencies for clinicians. *ASHA, 35*(8), 48–49.

Education for All Handicapped Children Act of 1975, PL 94-142, 20 U.S.C. §§ 1400 *et seq.*

Hartman, K., & Ackerman, E. (1999). Finding quality information on the Internet: Tips and guidelines. *Syllabus, 13*(1), 52–54.

Individuals with Disabilities Education Act (IDEA) Amendments of 1997, PL 105-17, 20 U.S.C. §§ 1400 *et seq.*

Leeper, L.H., & Gotthoffer, D.. (2000). *Quick guide to the Internet.* Needham Heights, MA: Allyn & Bacon.

Reinhardt, A. (1995, March). New ways to learn. *Byte,* 50–72.

Scherz, J. (1993, November) *The computer's great: How's the software.* Computer Instructional Lab presented at the annual meeting of the American Speech-Language-Hearing Association, Anaheim, CA.

1. *Identify two changes in computer technology that can reasonably be anticipated in the near future.*

2. *Identify two aspects of clinical practice in speech-language pathology that will affect the way that computer technology is integrated into the day-to-day activities of clinicians.*

3. *Identify and discuss the significance of three computing competencies that support program administration and three that support the delivery of speech-language services.*

4. *Identify and discuss the four steps in evaluating software. Include a discussion of the important questions to be asked during each step.*

5. *Differentiate hardware-based from software-based computer applications.*

6. *List three types of computer applications useful in treating communication disorders. List two computer applications that can be used in record-keeping tasks.*

7. *Differentiate a listserv from a newsgroup, identifying basic differences in operation and in usefulness for both the clinician and his or her patient.*

8. *Discuss ways in which web resources can be integrated into the daily practice of SLPs.*

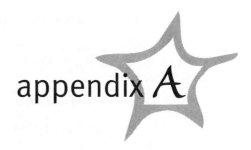

appendix A

Internet Resources

WEB PAGES[1]

The following list of web pages provides a sampling of the available information sources on the web. Many of these web sites provide links to additional related sites. As a warning, however, one must recognize that the web is a constantly evolving environment and there are no guarantees that a particular web page will always be available. Thus, there is no guarantee that the sites listed will be available in the future; however, it is safe to assume that many of them will. Dr. Kuster attempts to keep her resource site up-to-date to the extent possible. Due to this characteristic of the web, it is strongly recommended that students learn how to use web search resources to help stay current with the resources available on the web.

What Is Attention Deficit Disorder—from the ERIC Clearinghouse:

> http://www.kidsource.com/kidsource/content3/ADD.ERIC.html

Great Connections One ADD Place—attempts to consolidate in one place information and resources on the Internet relating to attention-deficit/hyperactivity disorder:

> http://www.oneaddplace.com/

Is it Alzheimer's Disease?—10 warning signs:

> http://gator.naples.net/presents/Alzheimer/isitalz.html

---

[1]These examples have been taken from the "Net Connections for Communication Disorders" web site and are used with the permission of Dr. Judith Kuster.

Dementia Web—a source of information, advice, education, research findings, and support for patients, caregivers, doctors, and other professionals:

> http://dementia.ion.ucl.ac.uk/

Caroline Bowen's Questions and Answers—about speech sound disorders:

> http://members.tripod.com/Caroline_Bowen/phonol-and-artic.htm

Wide Smiles—a private, nonprofit corporation providing information and networking among families of children with cleft lip/palate and craniofacial anomalies:

> http://www.widesmiles.org/

Center For Voice Disorders of Wake Forest University, by James A. Koufman—contains information on voice disorders:

> http://www.bgsm.edu/voice

Crossing the Communication Bridge: Speech, Language and Brain Injury—from the Brain Injury Association's seven-part document online information about treatment and rehabilitation:

> http://www.biausa.org/road05.htm

LISTSERVS

As discussed previously, the only software necessary to participate on a listserv is an e-mail reader. The listserv resources described include the necessary information to allow you to subscribe to the particular list.

CDMAJOR@LISTSERV.KENT.EDU is a forum for students and faculty in speech-language pathology, audiology, speech science, or hearing science programs. To subscribe, send the following message to listserv@listserv.kent.edu:

> **subscribe CDMajor firstname lastname**

The list owner is Antony Caruso (acaruso@kentvm.kent.edu)

COMMDIS@CIOS.LLC.RPI.EDU is part of Comserve, a service of the Communication Institute for Online Scholarship, established for students and professionals interested in the study of human communication. It provides a variety of services, including e-conferences, an e-journal of communication, a resource library, and so forth. Comserve is available at no charge to the general public for certain services. There are several affiliated institutions, and associate membership is also available for a fee. Commdis is the hotline service set up to facilitate communication on the topic of communication disorders. It is designed in a digest format. To subscribe, send the following message to comserve@cios.llc.rpi.edu:

> **join commdis firstname lastname**

The list moderator is C. Richard Dean (hssdean@ouaccvmb.cats.ohiou.edu)

GRNDRNDS@WVNVM.WVNET.EDU is a forum that discusses all aspects of the clinical process with respect to the evaluation and treatment of communication disorders. To subscribe, send the following message to listserv@wvnvm.wvnet.edu:

subscribe grndrnds firstname lastname

The list owner is Karen McComas (mccomas@marshall.edu)

PARENTS-W@F-BODY.ORG is a mailing list for parents concerned about stuttering behaviors in children. Professionals, students, and others interested are also welcome to join. To subscribe send the following message to majordomo@f-body.org:

subscribe parents-w

LATETALKERS is a list about children who talk late. A web-based subscription form is available. Those without web access can subscribe by sending a blank message to subscribe-latetalkers@onelist.com

LD-LIST@CURRY.EDU is a forum that provides an information exchange network for individuals interested in learning disabilities, including persons with learning disabilities, family members and friends, educators and administrators, researchers and others. To subscribe, send the following message to majordomo@curry.edu:

subscribe ld-list (no name is necessary)

NEWSGROUPS

To access these newsgroups, follow your news reader software instructions for subscribing to newsgroups. When asked to enter the name of a news group to subscribe to, enter one or more of the newsgroup names listed. The newsgroup will then be listed as one of your subscribed groups. You will be able to read the various postings to the group by selecting the group namealt.support.attn-deficit

alt.support.stuttering	alt.education.disabled
alt.support.ataxia	bit.listserv.down-syn
alt.support.cerebral-palsy	bit.listserv.tbi-support
alt.support.hearing-loss	alt.support.mult.sclerosis
alt.support.epilepsy	
alt.society.deaf	
alt.human.brain	

Family-Centered Practice

Denise LaPrade Rini

Many clinicians who are first entering home- and family-based work situations experience some trepidation. Although they feel prepared to provide treatment and have a wide range of techniques to utilize, they often feel overwhelmed when faced with the multiple demands of the family context. Traditional service delivery methods have centered around the needs of the individual client. Clinicians have typically worked with an individual or small group within a clinical setting, such as a speech center, a hospital, or a school. Increasingly, though, services are being provided within the contexts natural to the client, such as their homes, vocational settings, or recreational settings. A number of federal and state legislative provisions, as well as certain insurers, mandate that services be provided through a family-centered, natural environment framework. The increasing rate of an aging population predicts that the incidence and prevalence of communication disorders will increase, as will the need to provide services through a family-centered framework. It is likely that, in the near future, the family milieu will be second only to school settings, in terms of frequency, as a site for practice of communication disorders.

Daughters and sons, wives and husbands, sisters and brothers—all clinicians are family members as well as professionals. To what extent can we draw upon our own experience in the family role in order to deliver services successfully in a family-centered context? What roles do family members assume when one of them is involved in treatment for communication disorders? How does this impact the manner in which the clinician provides the treatment? In order to answer these questions, the clinician needs to know something about the concepts of family systems and family-centered practice and must be familiar with

The author wishes to acknowledge the invaluable assistance, materials, support, and input from Grace Caruso-Whitney, Southern Connecticut State University colleagues Jane Hindenlang and Mary Purdy, and Early Stimulation Program (ESP) colleague Talia Luck. Special thanks goes to Rhea Paul for her extremely gracious and patient editorial input and to colleagues at Birth to Three/ESP who exemplify the concept of true family-centered practice in their work with young children and their families every day.

clinical tools and resources to draw upon in order to implement family-centered practice effectively.

FAMILY SYSTEMS THEORY

When we prepare to work with clients, both directly and through their families, we need to understand what families are and how they function. Rosin et al. (1996) discussed the range of diversity among contemporary American families and the impact that this diversity has on professionals and educators who inter-act with them. They listed four sources of diversity that present particular challenges for clinicians:

1. The growing number of families whose ethnic and cultural backgrounds are different than those of service providers

2. The differences in family structure (i.e., decrease in traditional two-parent homes)

3. The increase in the number of infants and toddlers who are living in poverty

4. The increase in the number of families that have parents/adults with disabil-ities

In addition, it is important to be aware that the family as a unit is not a static entity but rather a dynamic and complex system. The family may include primary relatives and secondary people, such as more distant relatives (grandparents, aunts, and uncles) or friends and neighbors who fulfill family roles. *Family* refers to those people who live with the client and provide financial, physical and/or financial support, as well as affect the quality of life and well-being for the client. Families change and develop over time. Major life experiences, such as new part-nerships, the birth of a child, children leaving the home, aging, illness, and death, create changes. Many other situations also create similar challenges for families: a change in an economic situation, a change in employment, a household move, an acute or chronic illness, or an accident. Often, the clinician does not enter the family system during its typical functioning, but during one of these challenge stages. It is important to be aware that the family may be in flux at this time and that roles and responses to illness, disability, and developmental delay may be dif-ferent than usual.

Specific reactions related to the age and role of the family member affected may also occur. A family with an infant or a child in early development may react to the loss of their dreams for the child and their loss of hope regarding future experiences that they believe the child may never have. There may also be an awareness of the demands of life-long care that family members may be respon-sible for if the disability is serious. When an adult family member experiences ill-ness or a condition resulting in communication disorder, the impact is different because that person has held certain roles in the family that may no longer be possible to carry out. The economic status of the family may be directly and sig-nificantly affected and caregiver roles may require reversal due to the disability.

The concomitant communication disorder itself further creates frustration, difficulty coping, negotiating, and exchanging important information.

THE KEY CONCEPTS OF A *Family Systems* PERSPECTIVE (Begun, 1996)

The family as a whole is greater than the sum of its parts. This concept reflects that each family has its own patterns, rules, behaviors, and boundaries. The family as a whole has meaning and its preservation may transcend the goals and interests of any one member.

Change in one part of the family affects the whole family system. The interdependence among family members will cause any change or experience that occurs to any one member to affect the entire family (e.g., member illness and concomitant communication disruption).

Subsystems are embedded within the larger family system. Different family members have their own particular relationships/systems (e.g., siblings, spouses, parent–child).

The family system exists within a larger social and environmental context. The family is a component of larger systems, such as extended families, neighborhoods, religious communities, and political and economic communities.

Families are multigenerational. Most family systems of multiple generations are also interwoven with members and ideas of past generations, along with future anticipated generations.

What implications do these concepts have for professionals in the field of communication disorders? If we acknowledge and act on these concepts, our approach to the family and the information that we will obtain from them will be different than if we hold a more traditional client-centered approach. For example, in a traditional approach, the clinician might consider how a specific therapeutic intervention will affect the client. In a systems approach, however, the clinician will also consider how therapy approaches may affect the other members of the family and their relationships to one another. In a traditional approach, a clinician might make assumptions about a family member's role based on his or her position (e.g., parent, sibling), but in a systems approach, each family member's true role would be deduced through interview and observation of how members interact and how that interaction may change over time with new experiences (Begun, 1996).

Each clinician brings to the experience his or her own beliefs about what families are and how they "should" function, as well as the roles that all members, including the clinician, should assume. The clinician needs to place these beliefs aside in order to be effective and clear-sighted in the service delivery process, through a family-centered approach.

DEFINING FAMILY-CENTERED PRACTICE

Many authors have discussed and defined the term *family-centered practice*. One definition generated by the Beach Center on Families and Disability states,

Family centered service delivery, across disciplines and settings, recognizes the centrality of the family in the lives of individuals. It is guided by fully informed choices made by the family and focuses upon the strengths and capabilities of these families. (1997, p. 1)

This change in approach to service delivery has constituted a significant and important shift in professional orientation. The focus from client-centered to family-centered treatment has occurred parallel to the emergence of the family support and family empowerment movement. Representing both a set of beliefs about children and families as well as an approach to working with them, the family support movement acknowledges and builds on the many strengths and resources of families and communities (Rini & Whitney, 1999). The Beach Center lists key components of family-centered service delivery (see Table 12.1). In addition, key concepts of family-centered care indicated by the Institute for Family-Centered Care (1998) include respect, support, choice, flexibility, collaboration, information, and identification of family strengths.

Family *empowerment* extends beyond support by systematically assisting family members to direct their strengths and resources toward meeting the present and future needs of their members, themselves, and their communities. Thus, it is now accepted as best practice that the client's relations to both family and community should be explored when formulating an intervention and that these relations should be actively integrated into the course of treatment.

Even though every family-centered intervention cannot address the full range of a complex set of systems, an acceptance of the family context as part of the individual's treatment has become a standard of family-centered practice. Family-centered practice necessitates that the full context of the family, assessed *with* the family, is taken into consideration whenever an intervention occurs (see Table 12.2).

Table 12.1.   Principles of family support

Staff and families work together in relationships based on equality and respect.

Staff embrace families' capacity to support the growth and development of all family members—adults, youth, and children.

Families are resources to their own members, to other families, to programs, and to communities.

Programs affirm and strengthen families' cultural, racial, and linguistic identities and enhance their ability to function in a multicultural society.

Programs are embedded in their communities and contribute to the community-building process.

Programs advocate with families for services and systems that are fair, responsive, and accountable to the families served.

Practitioners work with families to mobilize formal and informal resources to support family development.

Programs are flexible and continually responsive to emerging family and community issues.

Principles of family support are modeled in all program activities, including planning, governance, and administration.

Source: Beach Center on Families and Disability, 1997.

Table 12.2. Premises of family support

The primary responsibility for the development and well-being of children lies within the family, and all segments of society must support families as they rear their children. The systems and institutions on which families rely must effectively respond to their needs if families are to establish and maintain environments that promote growth and development. Achieving this requires a society that is committed to making the well-being of children and families a priority and to supporting that commitment by allocating and providing necessary resources.

Assuring the well-being of all families is the cornerstone of a healthy society and requires universal access to support programs and services. A national commitment to promoting the healthy development of families acknowledges that every family, regardless of race, ethnic background, or economic status, needs and deserves a support system. Because no family can be self-sufficient, the concept of reaching families before problems arise is not realized unless all families are reached. To do so requires a public mandate to make family support accessible and available, on a voluntary basis, to all.

Children and families exist as part of an ecological system. An ecological approach assumes that child and family development is embedded within broader aspects of the environment, including a community with cultural, ethnic, and socio-economic characteristics that are affected by the values and policies of the larger society. This perspective assumes that children and families are influenced by interactions with people, programs, and agencies, as well as by values and policies that may help or hinder families' ability to promote their members' growth and development. The ecological context in which families operate is a critical consideration in programs' efforts to support families.

Child-rearing patterns are influenced by parents' understanding of child development and of their children's unique characteristics, personal sense of competence, and cultural and community traditions and mores. There are multiple determinants of parents' child-rearing beliefs and practices, and each influence is connected to other influences. For example, a parent's view of his or her child's disposition is related to the parent's cultural background and knowledge of child development and to characteristics of the child. Because the early years set a foundation for the child's development, patterns of parent–child interaction are significant from the start. The unique history of the parent–child relationship is important to consider in programs' efforts.

Enabling families to build on their own strengths and capacities promotes the healthy development of children. Family support programs promote the development of competencies and capacities that enable families and their members to have control over important aspects of their lives and to relate to their children more effectively. By building on strengths rather than treating impairments, programs assist parents in dealing with difficult life circumstances as well as achieving their goals, and in doing so, enhance parents' capacity to promote their children's healthy development.

The developmental processes that make up parenthood and family life create needs that are unique at each stage in the life span. Parents grow and change in response to changing circumstances and the challenges of nurturing a child's development. The tasks of parenthood and family life are ongoing and complex, requiring physical, emotional, and intellectual resources. Many tasks of parenting are unique to the parent's point in her or his life cycle. Parents have been influenced by their own childhood experiences and their own particular psychological characteristics, and are affected by their past and present family interactions.

Families are empowered when they have access to information and other resources and take action to improve the well-being of children, families, and communities. Equitable access to resources in the community—including up-to-date information and high-quality services that address health, educational, and other basic needs—enables families to develop and foster optimal environments for all family members. When families have meaningful experiences, participate in programs, and influence policies it strengthens existing capabilities and promotes the development of new competencies, such as the ability to advocate on their own behalf.

Source: Family Resource Coalition, 1996.

There are legal provisions that mandate family primacy in communication assessment and intervention of family members. The Individuals with Disabilities Education Act (IDEA) Amendments of 1997 (PL 105-17), with its birth-to-3 component, require that parents or guardians direct the contents of the individualized family service plan (IFSP), including outcomes for the child and family, and a statement of family needs and resources around which intervention must be designed. For children ages 3–21, IDEA '97 requires family input for permission to assess and to develop the individualized education program (IEP). Although school-based services are less likely to be fully family-centered, many school systems require clinicians to have contact with family on a regular basis to discuss the course of treatment, to integrate family goals, and to share ideas for both school- and home-based intervention. For adults in many hospitals, rehabilitation centers, or long-term care settings, there is the Patient Bill of Rights, which ensures family notification and patient/family input and/or attendance at all case conferences. A patient and his or her family may also partner with professionals to set short- and long-term plans of care, as well as to formulate statements of family expectations and need.

Cultural Considerations

When there is a discrepancy between the linguistic/ethnic/cultural background of a family and client and their service providers, these differences can impede the development of a positive, family-centered intervention program if a clinician brings his or her own belief and value expectations into the therapeutic situation and imposes them onto the family. It is critically important for the clinician to be aware of the many areas affected by culture and tradition and to understand how those values impact communication behavior, both at the level of clinician–family information exchange and at the level of client–clinician therapy interaction (see Chapter 10).

Poverty and Families

Rini and Whitney (1999) surveyed a number of studies that illustrate the deleterious effect poverty has on families and children in particular. Poverty is often accompanied by a host of other deficits in family resources: inadequate food and housing (which may include toxins such as lead paint and asbestos that are directly dangerous to health); restricted access to medical care, medications and equipment; lack of transportation; and below-standard education. Chronic illness of family members may be more common than in families of high socioeconomic status. If further complicated by substance use (i.e., alcohol, legal and illegal drugs), environmental or domestic violence, and/or mental illness, the family of low socioeconomic status experiences multiple stressors that threaten family function.

In her discussion of family-centered services among the chronically impoverished, Humphry (1995) described issues that affect parents' and clinicians' views of each other and that threaten the effectiveness of the intended partnership. She noted the influences of poverty on parenting and pointed out that demographics between those of low socioeconomic status and the clinician are often radically different. If different cultural backgrounds are also involved, then the number of obstacles between the members of this intervention team increase greatly. Humphry stressed the importance of understanding these factors in order to create an environment for more open communication between the clinician and the families who exhibit these differences. When families are experiencing multiple stressors, additional resources, besides those directed at remediating a communication disorder in one family member, are needed. It becomes important for interventionists to work with families to identify their wider range of strengths and needs, to know the resources in their communities, and to effectively link to them for the benefit of the client and family.

FAMILY-CENTERED PRACTICE IN COMMUNICATION DISORDERS

Traditionally, service delivery in communication disorders has followed a model in which the professional is viewed as the authority in the field who identifies behaviors that might indicate possible communication disorders and subsequently determines the degree of severity of the disorder and appropriate recommendations. Intervention would include modeling interactive intervention behaviors that family members were expected to imitate. Family members, particularly parents of children with communication disorders, were often perceived as being unsophisticated or too subjective to adequately observe or delineate the aspects of their children's communication. Links with children and parents were forged through a counseling relationship revolving around the communication issues (Crowe, 1997). During the 1990s, particularly with the initiation of birth-to-3 services across the country (IDEA '97) and the expansion of home health care services for adults, there has been an increasing movement toward true inclusion of parents and other significant family members in the decision-making process. Families are now involved in planning and conducting assessment tasks and approaches, identifying and prioritizing desired intervention outcomes if delays are diagnosed, developing intervention objectives, and implementing intervention activities.

Family-Centered Assessment Procedures

Best practice suggests that we view assessment as a dynamic process that should be completed over time and in a variety of contexts in order to sample a representative set of communication behaviors (Lidz & Pena, 1996). The importance of using naturalistic contexts is also emphasized (Lund & Duchan, 1993). These contexts include the places where clients are comfortable and familiar, places that contain objects that are salient and immediate for them, and places in which typical social and communication exchanges occur. Linder (1993) discussed the limitations of traditional assessment in communication disorders, which has often required that the client be evaluated out of context (e.g., in an unfamiliar office or clinic setting, separated from family, seen individually rather than in a setting with peers or siblings) and presented with tasks that are often unrelated to any immediate activity, interest, or communication exchange. Federal and state birth-to-3 guidelines ensure that developmental assessment takes place within a natural environment and with family members as key team members.

Using intensive parent–family interviews and observation of family–client interaction are aspects of family-centered assessment. There is a difference, though, between applying these techniques in such a way that family members feel as though they are being assessed themselves for their adequacy rather than engaging in a dialogue to obtain valid information about the client's behavior (Hanson, 1998). Several assumptions that should be made in implementing a true family-centered approach to communication assessment and intervention for clients are as follows.

FAMILY-CENTERED ASSESSMENT AND INTERVENTION ASSUMPTIONS

1. Any circumstance that affects one family member (the client) affects other members, as well as the family as a whole.

2. The family has a right to establish its own priorities.

3. The family must be accepted as being the experts concerning their family member.

4. The clinician must evidence genuine listening in collaborating with family members to obtain assessment information and in developing intervention goals.

5. The family must be acknowledged as having the right to form their own approach to raising their child or caring for an older family member, as long as health and safety are not at issue.

6. The clinician must acknowledge any personal bias regarding preconceived notions of expected role behavior in approaching a family and must place these notions aside in order to assess the function of the specific family and client.

7. In situations in which a family report appears to differ significantly from a clinician's observation (particularly in situations in which communication behaviors are underreported), it is the responsibility of the clinician to explore with the family the situations in which they may perceive the client differently or to assist them in identifying behaviors that help them become aware that the client may have expanded skills.

A number of family factors must be included in the assessment process. Knowledge of the cultural and linguistic contexts and characteristics of the family are primary in developing a preliminary understanding of the communication expectations and style of the environment (Halpern, 1993; Lund & Duchan, 1993). Size of the family, educational and socio-economic backgrounds, and family members' expectations of each other and of their children all have an impact on what clinicians will see and what parents and family perceive as areas of competence and need. One of the greatest challenges involves obtaining a representative sample of child and family communication behavior within the constraints of time and materials set by the agencies that govern the provision of services. A clinician must also conduct a comprehensive family assessment in such a way that the family does not feel that their privacy is violated (Donahue-Kilburg, 1992). The evaluation session(s) should present several questions to be answered by the clinician and family.

Family-Centered Assessment Questions

1. Is there a communication difference in this client in comparison to peers of his or her chronological and/or mental age and linguistic/cultural community?

2. Is this difference interfering with daily interactions within the family unit?

3. Is the client's communication functional for the purposes of attending to safety issues, expressing needs, negotiating, coping, planning, and developing literacy skills?

4. If the client's communication appears adequate within the immediate family context, is it sufficient for the larger context of the world outside of the family and for purposes that the family and the client intend (school, work, social settings)?

5. Do issues with the client's communication indicate areas of need, such as medical, economic, or mental health, to be addressed by and for the entire family?

Family and/or caregiver interviews are the typical means by which much of this information is obtained, often in the absence of an already established relationship between the clinician and the family members. It is obviously important for the clinician to be perceived as trustworthy and responding to the concerns voiced by the family. At times, these concerns may go beyond communication to include illness, housing, coping issues, education, domestic issues, substance abuse, and so forth. At other times, the family may need to focus on communication problems; in this case, trust revolves around the clinician's ability to hone in on what is important to the family and to place the client's communication issue in that context. The following information presents Donahue-Kilburg's (1992) listing of the issues inherent in traditional ways of conducting family interviews, and the skills that must be developed by clinicians to foster a truly family-centered interview that creates greater balance and equality between both parties in the dialogue.

Family-centered Interviewing

1. Observation of the client in a natural environment with family members

2. Direct task presentation with family member assistance and interaction

3. Parent/family description of client communicative behavior relative to specific speech and language components

4. General behavioral profile

For children younger than age 3, there are a number of instruments and procedures that enable the clinician to obtain information regarding areas of language development from the parent (Dale, 1996). The parent may then provide both binary responses concerning specific areas of inquiry, as well as elaborate information regarding circumstances and situations in which specific communication abilities and impairments may come to light. The *Vineland Adaptive Behavior Scale* (Sparrow, Balla, & Ciccetti, 1984) includes a communication scale that provides information regarding receptive and expressive language. The *MacArthur Communicative Development Inventories* (Fenson et al., 1993) assesses receptive and expressive vocabulary size and early grammatic production. These two instruments provide results in terms of standard scores, which are often required to provide documentation criteria to determine eligibility for intervention services. Among other available parent-report format instruments are the *Receptive-Expressive Emergent Language Scale-2* (Bzoch & League, 1991), *The Rossetti Infant-Toddler Language Scale* (Rossetti, 1990), and the *Early Language Milestone Scale* (Coplan, 1987). These scales include areas of specific language milestones by age level to which a parent responds; results are reported in terms of language age-equivalents or language quotients. In addition, the *Rossetti Infant-Toddler Language Scale* provides information on gesture, play, and interaction to provide additional communication information. Wetherby and Prizant's (1990) *Communication and Symbolic Behavior Scales* provide for direct parent–child interactions revolving around a number of structured and unstructured tasks that are videotaped and then observed, analyzed, and scored by the clinician. Results are provided in terms of normative scores according to three developmental levels. This instrument provides for a more comprehensive and dynamic family-centered assessment; however, it may require more time to conduct and analyze because of the components and method of collecting the required data. Family interactions and child play can provide excellent opportunities for assessment. Linder (1993) provided suggestions for organizing and utilizing play for assessment purposes.

There are few tools for assessment of older children that rely heavily on parent report or parent implementation. Several assessment tools for specific communication areas include parent interview forms that become part of the final body of information used to analyze diagnostic data. Particularly, when assessments are completed within the school system, it is easy for the family to become separated from the assessment experience. Special education laws require that parents be notified in writing and give signed consent for assessment to take place, so that, presumably, parents are aware of the upcoming evaluation and have the opportunity to initiate input into the process. It is incumbent on the clinician to obtain information from family members regarding aspects of communication being assessed and to verify results with perceptions and observations that the family has made concerning the functional aspects of any communication differences. The child's wishes, perceptions, and input are critical components in this process.

For adults, there are several interview scales such as the *Analysis of Nonlinguistic and Linguistic Behaviors of an Adult Aphasic Patient from His Child's Perspective* (Chapey, 1981), *The Aphasic Impact Rating Scale for Children and Spouses* (Chwat & Gurland, 1981), and the *Independent Rater Questionnaire: Behavioral Assessment of the Dysexecutive Syndrome* (Wilson, Alderman, Burgess, Emslie, &

Evans, 1996) that can be completed by family members to provide pertinent communication information.

Family-Centered Intervention

As with assessment, family-centered intervention implies that family members have key decision-making power in all aspects of intervention, and that their personal styles of child rearing, as well as linguistic, cultural, and traditional values, will be respected and incorporated into the intervention. Styles of interaction between the family and the client may dictate, to a large extent, how directly involved with intervention the family may actually be. Intervention also includes type of service delivery (e.g., direct, indirect, consultative), personnel involved, and location of treatment.

IDEA '97 provides mechanisms for parents and other family members to have direct input into the intervention process for children. From ages birth to 3 years, the document that is collaboratively developed between parents and providing professionals is the IFSP, which when developed as intended is family directed. The family indicates information regarding family structure and needs and states the specific outcomes that they feel are the priority issues that they wish to have addressed by the entire team, including themselves. Issues related to economic circumstance such as education, employment, child care, respite, and housing, or medical issues such as health of the child or other family members, substance abuse, or mental health issues may be addressed on the IFSP. Communication outcomes are expected to project long-term goals and are generated by parents in their own words. Interim objectives for a specific period of time (3–6 months) are developed by parents and the providing professionals. The materials and techniques included are chosen for their desirability and comfort for the parents as well as appropriateness for the child.

For school-age children (ages 3–21), the planning and placement team is the mechanism that provides for parent input. Intervention is outlined through the IEP, which should be developed by all team members, including parents (IDEA '97). Within the public schools, however, family-centered intervention may be difficult to achieve. Service delivery is provided through the academic setting and with a focus on literacy goals. Issues of parent access to classrooms, availability of school staff and activities to working parents, and school accessibility to parents without transportation or with child care needs provide obstacles to family-centered practice in this setting. Ongoing contact needs to be established and maintained so that family-centered needs can be heard and addressed. Flexibility of professionals and systems is key in achieving this responsiveness to family needs.

Although there is no legislated mechanism to ensure family input to intervention plans for adults with disabilities, many facilities follow a Patient Bill of Rights in administering adult care. This document provides for the patient's right to have his or her family involved with every case conference and aspect of planning, as well as family input as to services to be provided. A central issue relative to family involvement with an adult with disabilities is the willingness of the patient to have that involvement. This will be partially dependent upon preexisting family relationships, the degree of independence the patient has previously had in self-care, and medical determination of whether the patient is capable of being responsible for his or her own decisions and future care. Family involvement cannot be mandated because the integrity of the adult's right to decide must be protected. This can present a challenge for the clinician when there is a disagreement between patient and family members about who is "in charge" of the patient's care. Often, when such conflicts exist, mediation may be needed to explore possible resolutions, and special personnel (e.g., social worker) may need to take the lead in the situation.

Within the framework of family-centered practice there is a spectrum of family involvement with intervention. On the one end is the model in which family's and client's targeted goals for communication are the focus and the mode of service delivery is also chosen by them, but intervention is provided by designated professionals or team members while family members focus indirectly on communication goals through modeling and daily family interactions. On the other end is the model in which parents or other family members function directly as interventionists, assuming responsibility for designing intervention strategies and selecting techniques and materials to implement these strategies according to collaboratively selected communication goals. For example, for one 33-month-old boy with developmental apraxia of speech, the goal of the family was for him to use family names, say *yes* and *no,* and attempt to repeat some words of other family members. Through consultation with the clinician, the child's mother constructed specific pictorial material and games that were of particular interest to the child (his favorite animals and characters), and they reviewed these daily. After 3 months, the established objectives were achieved.

Not all families are able and willing to assume this role, however. Some clients resist their families' efforts to assume the role of instructor. Some clients reject any activities that are structured and perceived as focusing directly upon their own difficulty. Between these two poles is a range of family involvement that includes both family-directed and client-directed activities along with clinician input. There are a number of "parent programs" for communication skills available commercially, including "Hickory Dickory Talk" (Johnson & Heinze, 1990), "HELP...at Home" (Parks, 1990), "Parent Articles" (Schrader, 1988), and "Help Me Talk" (Eichten, 1993). Paul (2001) included an extensive list and descriptions of programs, materials, and videos that can be used by parents of infants, toddlers, and preschoolers in implementing family-directed intervention. These tools provide family members with suggestions for activities and materials that can be adapted to suit the family's needs. Many families are eager to learn about various intervention approaches and techniques. Curricula and materials devised for overall early childhood education, such as that included in *The Crosscultural, Language, and Academic Development Handbook* (Diaz-Rico & Weed, 1995), can also provide ideas and sequences of activities that parents can implement and that incorporate themes that are salient for each individual family.

In providing support for the older child or adult with communication disorders, families and clinicians have developed materials and approaches that can include family members. For example, in areas of articulation and fluency, family members can review lists of specific practice materials with the client. Carryover activities require the involvement of the family to provide contexts in which the client can practice new communication behaviors. Specific contracts or procedures to implement this aspect of therapy may be devised jointly by client, family, and clinician. For higher level language skills, a number of commercially available workbooks can provide basic stimuli for client–family work sessions; clinician, client, and family can collaborate on choosing specific stimuli and methods of creating a session.

The individual who experiences significant communication loss due to neurological illness or trauma presents a different challenge to the family. As an adult, the client has held a specific position and role in the family. A style of communication and interaction has developed between him and his family, friends, and social/work associates. Loss of communication is devastating because it affects all of these areas. In addition, the client often is experiencing other medical difficulties, which may include loss of mobility, decrease in sensory or cognitive function, coronary and vascular fragility, and so forth. Communication disorders superimposed on preexisting medical conditions will significantly affect the person's overall function and degree of independence, which has consequent impact on the family. Still, much can be done to facilitate and broaden communication among the client, the family, and the community. Participation in client-directed group therapy situations and working toward specific goals for each client within a social context with SLP support and with parallel group support for spouses is often also an invaluable intervention experience. (Johannsen-Horbach, Crone, & Wallesch, 1999). In her chapter regarding caregiver training, Bourgeois (1997) listed the relative benefits and limitations of various intervention models for adults.

Professional Collaboration

To achieve a more comprehensive and family-centered approach, there are a number of areas in which collaboration is necessary. First, it is important that professionals become familiar with the cornerstones of each other's disciplines and how these relate to family-centered and transdisciplinary practice. Typically, when one discipline learns the language of the other, the opportunities to collaborate expand. Second, it is helpful when each discipline is able to incorporate a broader perspective into evaluations and treatments. For example, the SLP who recognizes that there may be sensory issues with her client that impact overall development and communication can call upon the expertise of her colleague in occupational therapy to assist with this issue. A psychologist may recognize that a client or his family experience presents challenges in treatment sessions because of hearing impairments and will therefore consult with the audiologist. Collaborating professionals can offer a broader spectrum of insight and support to the family being served. This is particularly important when service is provided through a single transdisciplinary professional who must address a range of needs within the family as well as the client himself.

Another area of collaboration is in identifying the range of community needs and resources. Professionals can work together to assess the level and types of needs that exist in their community. They can also work together to develop a familiarity with whatever additional resources exist that they may need to call upon to assist families comprehensively, and they can share information on how to effectively gain access to these resources. In addition, they may find opportunities to partner with families to advocate for additional resources as a result of their joint assessment of the community.

Family-Centered Service Provision in Natural Environments

There are many strengths to family-centered service provision in natural environments. Providing communication services in the home, in child or adult care centers, in the classroom, or in a work environment serves to immediately address the specific communication requirements of that context and to choose appropriate objectives and stimuli for those contexts; to involve family members and colleagues who are a part of that environment; to facilitate carryover by placing the client directly in those settings in which he or she needs to use his or her specific new skills. There are also challenges that the clinician may face, however, in working toward achieving established goals. Distractions of a typical environment, such as noise, extraneous activity, and the comings and goings of the family or others in the environment, may be a factor. Natural environments may not always be safe, secure, healthy, supportive, or facilitative of development or habilitation. As the clinician–family relationship develops, it is natural for the family to confide in the clinician, at times revealing highly sensitive or complex situations and emotions. The clinician may also be affected by organizational/administrative issues. For example, best practice in assessment and intervention that recommends evaluation over time may be obstructed by the demands of time management, commuting from site to site, medical managed care, and economic realities such as quotas of client contacts that clinicians must meet or maximum amounts of time clinicians are limited to in assessment, treatment, or family conferencing. In many states, consultation (i.e., the time spent conferring with other professionals, the family, or physicians that is not direct treatment time) is not compensated by insurance. Flexibility, creativity, and the ability to adapt quickly are critical survival skills.

CONCLUSION

Family-centered practice is not merely a theoretical construct or philosophical position. Its practical implementation dictates that the family, the client, and professionals will interface and collaborate in ways that are based on the needs and wishes of the family, community makeup, and complexity of the issues involved. For the clinician who embraces the notion that communication assumes immersion in human interactions, a family-centered approach to service provision will prove to be a vital element of practice.

REFERENCES

Allen, R.I., & Petr, C.G. (1995). *Family-centered service delivery: A crossdisciplinary literature review and conceptualization.* Lawrence: University of Kansas.

Alper, S., Schloss, P., & Schloss, C. (Eds.). (1994). *Families of students with disabilities.* Needham Heights, MA: Allyn & Bacon.

Anderson, W., Chitwood, S., & Hayden, D. (1990). *Negotiating the special education maze.* Bethesda, MD: Woodbine House.

Andrews, M., & Andrews, J. (1993). Family-centered techniques: Integrating enablement into the IFSP process. *Journal of Childhood Communication Disorders 15,* 1.

Bayley, N. (1993). *Bayley Scales of Infant Mental Development—Revised* (2nd ed.). New York: Psychological Corporation.

Beach Center on Families and Disability. (1997). *Families and disability newsletter, 8*(2), 1. Lawrence: University of Kansas.

Begun, A.L. (1996). Family systems and family-centered care. In P. Rosin, A.D. Whitehead, L.I. Tuchman, G.S. Jesien, A.L. Begun, & L. Irwin (Eds.), *Partnerships in family-centered care: A guide to collaborative early intervention* (pp. 33–63). Baltimore: Paul H. Brookes Publishing Co.

Behrman, R.E. (Ed.). (1997). Children and poverty. *The Future of Children, 7.*

Bourgeois, M. (1997). Families caring for elders at home: Caregiver training. In P. Shaddon & M. Toner (Eds.), *Aging and communication* (pp. 227–250). Austin, TX: PRO-ED.

Bradley, R.H., Whiteside, L., & Mundfrom, D.J. (1994). Early indications of resilience and their relation to experiences in the home environments of low birthweight, premature children living in poverty. *Child Development 65,* 346.

Brinker, R.P., Seifer, R., & Sameroff, A.J. (1994). Relations among maternal stress, cognitive development, and early intervention in middle and low SES infants with developmental disabilities. *American Journal of Mental Retardation 98,* 463.

Bromwich, R. (1978). *Working with parents and infants.* Baltimore: University Park Press.

Bronfenbrenner, U. (1979). *The ecology of human development: Experiments by nature and design.* Cambridge, MA: Harvard University Press.

Bronfenbrenner, U. (1995). Developmental ecology through space and time: A future perspective. In P. Moen, G.H. Elder, Jr., & K. Luscher (Eds.), *Examining lives in context, perspectives on the ecology of human development.* Washington, DC: American Psychological Association.

Brooks-Gunn, J., & Duncan, G.J. (1997). The effects of poverty on children. *The Future of Children, 7,* 55.

Buzzell, J.B. (1996). *School and family partnerships.* Albany, NY: Delmar.

Bzoch, K., & League, R. (1991). *The Receptive-Expressive Emergent Language Scale* (2nd ed.). Austin, TX: PRO-ED.

Cambourne, B. (1995). Toward an educationally relevant theory of literacy learning: Twenty years of inquiry. *The Reading Teacher 49,* 3.

Caruso Whitney, G. (1997). Early intervention for high-risk families: Reflecting on a 20-year-old model. In G.W. Albee & T.P. Gullotta (Eds.), *Primary prevention works.* Thousand Oaks, CA: Sage Publications.

Chapey, R. (1981). The assessment of language disorders in adults. In R. Chapey (Ed.), *Language intervention strategies in adult aphasia* (pp. 81–140). Baltimore: Lippincott Williams & Wilkins.

Chwat, S., & Gurland, G.B. (1981). Comparative family perspectives on aphasia: Diagnostic, treatment, and counseling implications. In R.H. Brookshire (Ed.), *Clinical Aphasiology Conference Proceedings* (p. 212). Minneapolis: BRK.

Clark, L. (1997). Communication intervention for family caregivers and professional health care providers. In P. Shaddon & M. Toner (Eds.), *Aging and communication* (pp. 251–274). Austin, TX: PRO-ED.

Cole, K.N., Dale P.S., & Thal D.J. (1996). *Assessment of communication and language.* Baltimore: Paul H. Brookes Publishing Co.

Connecticut Birth to Three. (1996). *Service coordination training.* Division of Child and Family Studies: University of Connecticut Health Center.

Coplan, J. (1987). *Early Language Milestone Scale.* Austin, TX: PRO-ED.

Crockenberg, S., Lyons-Ruth, K., & Dickstein, S. (1993). The family context of infant mental health: II. Infant development in multiple family relationships. In C.H. Zeanah (Ed.), *Handbook of infant mental health* (pp. 38–55). New York: The Guilford Press.

Crowe, T.A. (1997). Counseling: Definition, history, rationale. In T.A. Crowe (Ed.), *Applications of counseling in speech-language pathology and audiology* (pp. 3–29). Baltimore: Lippincott Williams & Wilkins.

Dale, P.S. (1996). Parent report assessment of language and communication. In K.N. Cole, P.S. Dale, & D.J. Thal (Eds.), *Assessment of communication and language* (pp. 161–182). Baltimore: Paul H. Brookes Publishing Co.

Diaz-Rico, L.T., & Weed, K.Z. (1995). *The Crosscultural, Language, and Academic Development Handbook.* Needham Heights, MA: Allyn & Bacon.

Donahue-Kilburg, G. (1992). *Family-centered early intervention for communication disorders.* Gaithersburg, MD: Aspen Publishers.

Dougherty, D.M., Saxe, L.M., Cross, T., et al. (1987). Children's mental health: Problems and services. Durham, NC: Duke University Press.

Duncan, G.J., Brooks-Gunn, J., & Klebanov, P.K. (1994). Economic deprivation and early childhood development. *Child Development, 65,* 283.

Eichten, P. (1993). *Help me talk: Parent's guide to speech & language stimulation techniques for children 1–3 years.* VA: Pi Communication Materials.

Erichson, J.G., & Omark, D. (1981). *Communication assessment of the bilingual bicultural child.* Baltimore: University Park Press.

Family Resource Coalition. (1996). *Guidelines for family support practice.* Chicago: Author

Fenson, L., Dale, P., Reznick, J.S., Thal, D., Bates, E., Hartung, J., Pethick, S., & Reilly, J. (1993). *Macarthur Communicative Development Inventories.* San Diego: Singular Publishing Group.

Forman, E.A., Minick, N., & Stone, C.A. (1993). *Contexts for learning: Sociocultural dynamics in children's development.* New York: Oxford University Press.

Garbarino, J. (1992). *Children and families in the social environment* (2nd ed.). New York: Aldine de Gruyter.

Garcia Coll, C., Lamberty, G., Jenkins, R., et al. (1996). An integrative model for the study of developmental competencies in minority children. *Child Development, 67,* 1891.

Gombay, D.S., & Larson, C.S. (Eds). (1993). Homevisiting. *The Future of Children, 3,.*

Greenspan, S. (1995). *The challenging child.* Reading, MA: Addison-Wesley.

Halpern, R. (1993). Poverty and infant development. In C.H. Zeanah (Ed.), *Handbook of infant mental health* (pp. 73–86). New York: The Guilford Press.

Hanson, M.J. (1998). Ethnic, cultural, and language diversity in intervention settings. In E.W. Lynch & M.J. Hanson (Eds.), *Developing cross-cultural competence: A guide for working with children and their families* (2nd ed., pp. 3–22). Baltimore: Paul H. Brookes Publishing Co.

Hashima, P.Y., & Amato, P.R. (1994). Poverty, social support, and parental behavior. *Child Develooment, 65,* 394.

Haynes, W. (1994). *Caretaker–child interaction communication development.* Englewood Cliffs, NJ: Prentice Hall.

Heller, R., & McKlindon, D. (1996). Families as "faculty": Parents educating caregivers about family-centered care. *Pediatric Nursing, 22,* 5.

Hooper, C. (1996). Forming a therapeutic alliance with older adults. *ASHA,* 43–45.

Hulit, L., & Howard, M. (1993). *Born to talk.* Upper Saddle River, NJ: Prentice Hall.

Huston, A.C., McLoyd, V.C., & Garcia Coll, C. (1994). Children and poverty: Issues in contemporary research. *Child Development, 65,* 275.

Humphry, R. (1995). Families who live in chronic poverty: Meeting the challenge of family-centered services. *American Journal of Occupational Therapy, 49,* 7.

Individuals with Disabilities Education Act (IDEA) Amendments of 1997, PL 105-17, 20 U.S.C. §§ 1400 *et seq.*

Johannsen-Horbach, H., Crone, M., & Wallesch, C. (1999). Group therapy for spouses of aphasic patients. *Seminars in Speech and Language, 20*(1), 73–82.

Johnson, K., & Heinze, B. (1990). *Hickory Dickory Talk: A family approach to infant and toddler language development.* East Moline, IL: LinguiSystems.

Kelly, E. (1995). Parents as partners: Including mothers and fathers in the treatment of children who stutter. *Journal of Communication Disorders, 28,.*

Lewis, M., & Volkmar, F. (1990). *Clinical aspects of child and adolescent development* (3rd ed.). Philadelphia: Lea & Febiger.

Lidz, C., & Pena, E. (1996). Dynamic assessment: The model, its relevance as a nonbiased approach, and its application to Latino American preschool children. *Language, Speech, and Hearing Services in Schools, 27*, 367–384.

Linder, T.W. (1993). *Transdisciplinary play-based intervention: Guidelines for developing a meaningful curriculum for young children.* Baltimore: Paul H. Brookes Publishing Co.

Locke, J. (1993). *The child's path to spoken language.* Cambridge, MA: Harvard University Press.

Lund, N., & Duchan, J. (1993). *Assessing children's language in naturalistic contexts* (3rd ed.). Englewood Cliffs, NJ: Prentice Hall.

Lynch, E.W. (1998). Developing cross-cultural competence. In E.W. Lynch & M.J. Hanson (Eds.), *Developing cross-cultural competence: A guide for working with children and their families* (2nd ed., pp. 47–89). Baltimore: Paul H. Brookes Publishing Co.

Lynch, E.W., & Hanson, M.J. (1998). *Developing cross-cultural competence: A guide for working with children and their families* (2nd ed.). Baltimore: Paul H. Brookes Publishing Co.

Lyons-Ruth, K., & Zeanah, C. (1993). The family context of infant mental health: I. Affective development in the primary caregiving relationship. In C.H. Zeanah (Ed.), *Handbook of infant mental health* (pp. 14–37). New York: The Guilford Press.

Minami, M., & Kennedy, B. (Eds.). (1991). *Language issues in literacy and bilingual/multicultural education.* Cambridge, MA: Harvard Educational Review.

Owens, R. (1992). *Language development: An introduction* (3rd ed.). Upper Saddle River, NJ: Prentice Hall.

Parks, S. (Ed.). (1990). *HELP...at Home.* Palo Alto, CA: VORT.

Paul, R. (2001). *Language disorders from infancy through adolescence* (2nd ed.). St. Louis: Mosby.

Prizant, B., Wetherby, A., & Roberts, J. (1993). Communication disorders in infants and toddlers. In C.H. Zeanah (Ed.), *Handbook of infant mental health* (pp. 260–279). New York: The Guilford Press.

Rini, D., & Whitney, G. (1999). Family-centered practice for children with communication disorders. In R. Paul (Ed.), *Child and adolescent psychiatric clinics of North America: Language disorders* (pp. 153–174). Philadelphia: W.B. Saunders.

Rosin, P., Whitehead, A.D., Tuchman, L.I., Jesian, G.S., Begun, A.L., and Irwin, L. (1996). *Partnerships in family-centered care: A guide to collaborative early intervention.* Baltimore: Paul H. Brookes Publishing Co.

Rossetti, L. (1990). *The Rossetti Infant-Toddler Language Scale.* East Moline, IL: LinguiSystems.

Rossetti, L. (1993). Enhancing early intervention services to infants/toddlers and their families. *Journal of Childhood Communication Disorders, 15,*(1), .

Sameroff, A.J. (1993). Models of development and developmental risk. In C.H. Zeanah (Ed.), *Handbook of infant mental health* (pp. 3–13). New York: The Guilford Press.

Schrader, M. (1988). *Parent articles: Enhance parent involvement in language learning.* Tucson, AZ: Communication Skill Builders.

Schwab, W.E. (1998, May 5). *Family-centered care: From principles to practice.* Materials presented at the University of Wisconsin, Department of Family Medicine, Madison.

Scott, A. (1998). Calling the shots: Parents take the lead in family-centered early intervention. *Advance, 6,* 6.

Seifer, R., & Dickstein, S. (1993). Parental mental illness and infant development. In C.H. Zeanah (Ed.), *Handbook of infant mental health* (pp. 120–142). New York: The Guilford Press.

Sparrow, S., Balla, D., & Ciccetti, D. (1984). *Vineland Adaptive Behavior Scales.* Circle Pines, MN: American Guidance Service.

Sroufe, L.A., Cooper, R.G., DeHart, G.B., et al. (1996). *Child development, its nature and course* (3rd ed.). New York: McGraw-Hill.

Stern, D. (1985). *The interpersonal world of the infant.* New York: Basic Books.

Taylor, O. (1994). Communication and communication disorders in a multicultural society. In F. Minifie (Ed.), *Introduction to communication sciences and disorders* (pp. 43–76). San Diego: Singular Publishing Group.

Turnbull, A., & Turnbull, H.R. (1996). *Families, professionals and exceptionality* (3rd ed.). Englewood Cliffs, NJ: Prentice Hall.

Walker, D., Greenwood, C., Hart, B., et al. (1994). Prediction of school outcomes based on early language production and socioeconomic factors. *Child Development, 65,* 606.

Wetherby, A., & Prizant, B. (1990). *Communication and Symbolic Behavior Scales.* Chicago: Riverside Publications.

Williams, F. (Ed.). (1973). *Language and poverty.* Chicago: Rand McNally.

Wilson, B., Alderman, N., Burgess, P., Emslie, H., & Evans, J. (1996). *Behavioral assessment of the dysexecutive syndrome: Independent rater questionnaire.* Bury St. Edmonds, England: Thomas Valley Test Co.

Winton, P. (1988). Effective communication between parents and professionals. In *Family assessment in early intervention* (pp. 207–228). Columbus, OH: Charles E. Merril.

Yoshikawa, H., & Knitzer, J. (1997). *Lessons from the field: Head start mental health strategies to meet changing needs.* New York: National Center for Children in Poverty, Columbia School of Public Health.

Zeanah, C. (Ed.). (1993). *Handbook of infant mental health.* New York: The Guilford Press.

1. *What is family-centered practice?*

2. *What are the key concepts of a family system theory?*

3. *In what ways is family-centered practice different than traditional practice?*

4. *What are some ways in which assessment and treatment services can be provided in a family-centered manner?*

5. *What role does collaboration have in family-centered practice?*

Glossary

Accent   The pronunciation of a language variety.

Acute care hospital   A facility to which an individual is admitted for immediate medical management.

Adaptation   The reduction or increase in the amount of stuttering between successive readings of the same information.

Advocacy   Steps taken by individuals or groups to understand, implement, or influence public policy.

Age equivalent   A derived score that expresses an individual's performance as the average performance for that age group. It is interpreted to mean that the individual's performance is equal to the average performance of an X-year old.

Alternate form reliability   Two forms of a test that measure the same skills and are standardized on the same population (also called *equivalent form reliability*).

Alternative and augmentative communication device (AAC)   A system used for communication when oral communication is limited.

Alzheimer's disease   A progressive disease of the brain that affects the ability to think, remember, and perform everyday activities.

American Sign Language   A symbolic communication system making use of manual signs; used by deaf people to communicate.

Americans with Disabilities Act (ADA)   United States law enacted to provide equal access for individuals with disabilities.

Aphasia   A language disorder resulting from brain damage and characterized by impairment of comprehension, formulation, and language use.

Appraisal   The process of collecting observations and measurements of a client's performance during assessment.

Apraxia   A disorder characterized by difficulty in performing voluntary motor acts in the absence of paralysis.

Apraxia of speech   Inability to produce intelligible speech in the absence of any paralysis or paresis of the speech mechanism.

ASHA Board of Ethics; AAA Ethical Practice Board   Centralized committees that address ethical situations, including ethical position statements, adjudication processes when violations are alleged, and professional education.

Assessment   The process of collecting and analyzing data about an individual in order to make clinical decisions.

Assistive technology   Any piece of equipment or product that is used to increase, maintain, or improve functional abilities of individuals with disabilities.

Asymmetry   Lack of symmetry: disproportion between two normally alike parts.

Atrophy   A wasting of tissues, organs, or the entire body; decreased cellular volume.

Auditory brainstem response (ABR)   An electrophysiologic response to sound, consisting of five to seven peaks that represent neural function of auditory pathways.

Augmentative and alternative communication (AAC)   An area of practice that attempts to compensate temporarily or permanently for the impairment and disability patterns of individuals with severe communication disorders.

Authoring   Writing a program for the computer.

Baseline   Rate or frequency of a behavior or level of functioning prior to the initiation of treatment.

Behavior modification specialist   The professional responsible for analysis and intervention surrounding the antecedents, responses, and reinforcement associated with challenging behavior.

Behavioral audiologic tests   Measures that pertain to the observation of the activity of a person in response to some stimuli.

Behavioral objective   An intervention goal that specifies an action a client is to perform, specifies the conditions under which the action will be performed, and specifies how well the action must be performed for the objective to be achieved.

Beneficence   The promotion of interests and welfare of others.

Benefit period   Time defined by policy during which certain provisions of a policy are in force.

Bifid   Split or cleft into two parts.

Biofeedback software   Dedicated, computer-based instrumentation that provides the user with real-time displays of physiologic activities in the production of speech and voice.

Blissymbols   A set of visual symbols developed to serve as an alternative communication system for individuals with severe speech disorders.

Block   A complete stoppage of the flow of speech, including air, voice, and articulators. One of the core behaviors in stuttering.

Bound morphemes   Units of meaning that do not appear unless attached to another morpheme (e.g., plural /s/, past tense -ed).

Capitated finance structure   System in which a health management organization pays the service provider a set amount of money per enrollee per month for a defined set of medical services.

Case conferences   Formal meetings involving service providers, clients, and family members in which evaluation findings, treatment outcomes, and necessary support services are discussed.

Case history questionnaire   A written set of questions used as a tool to gather and organize information regarding the nature of a person's speech, language, and hearing concerns; his or her general developmental and health history; educational background; and history of related support services.

Case law   Court decisions regarding disputed interpretations of laws that influence how policies are implemented in the disputed case and that also set a precedent for future practice.

Central auditory processing disorder   Disorder in function of central auditory structures, characterized by impaired ability of the central auditory nervous system to manipulate and use acoustic signals, including difficulty understanding speech in noise and localizing sounds.

Cerebral palsy   A neuromotor disorder caused by injury to the brain, often acquired before birth; often characterized by involuntary movements or difficulty in control of voluntary movements.

Cerumen   Earwax; the waxy secretion in the external auditory meatus.

Chaplain   A professional who addresses the spiritual needs of patients.

Clinical service delivery model   Direct intervention by an SLP.

Closed questions   Questions that elicit only a yes–no or one-word answer (e.g., "Do you have a dog?" "What did you eat for lunch?").

Cochlear implant   Device that enables people with profound hearing loss to perceive sound, consisting of an electrode array surgically implanted in the cochlea, which delivers electrical signals to the eighth cranial nerve, and an external amplifier, which activates the electrodes.

Code of Ethics   ASHA and AAA guidelines that define clinically acceptable conduct and conscientious judgment that members are expected to internalize and apply into clinical settings.

Code-switching   Alternations between languages at the word, phrase, or sentence levels.

Cognition   The collection of mental processes and activities used in perceiving, remembering, thinking, and understanding.

Cohesive ties   Linguistic markers used to achieve structural coherence among parts of a text (e.g., pronouns, conjunctions).

Commission on the Accreditation of Rehabilitation Facilities   A regulatory body that oversees the quality of care provided to patients in rehabilitation facilities.

Communication boards   Pictures or symbols that allow the client who cannot speak to communicate by pointing.

Comorbidity   The co-occurrence of two disorders.

Compensatory strategy   A method of intervention that provides clients with skills and tools for improving their own performance, eventually without the support of a clinician.

Competent practice   Clinician actions, including effective diagnostic procedures, accurate prognosis, appropriate therapy strategies for the particular disorder, and ongoing analysis of client outcomes.

Complex sentences   Sentences that contain more than one main verb phrase; these include sentences containing conjoined, embedded, and subordinate clauses.

Computer literacy   Indicating a basic understanding of computer technology and the ability to use basic computer technology.

Concurrent validity   The relationship between an individual's performance on a test and performance on a criterion measure.

Confidence interval   The range of scores within which a person's true score will fall with a given probability.

Confidentiality   The act of taking privileged client information and sharing it only with people directly responsible for client management and care and only for purposes related to client welfare.

Conflict of interest   A compromise in professional judgment in which a clinician loses his or her sense of objectivity because of personal or financial gifts from clients or manufacturers.

Conjunctions   Linking words that tie ideas within and across sentences; both coordinate (*and, but, or*) and subordinate (*when, if, because*) are included in this category.

Consistency   The percentage of words that are stuttered on in a subsequent reading that were also stuttered on during a previous reading.

Construct validity   The way in which a test measures the theoretical trait or construct that it purports to measure.

Consultation   The provision of communication services through both direct and indirect formats.

Content   Semantics; one aspect of language development.

Content validity   A measure of the extent to which a test represents an adequate sample of the domain being assessed.

Continuing education   The act of updating clinical skills and keeping current of the latest trends and advances; achieved through reading textbooks and journal articles, attending workshops, shadowing professional colleagues, and participating in research activities.

Continuum of care (COC)   Levels of rehabilitation through which patients pass based on need and intensity of services.

Continuum of naturalness   The range of intervention activities, from the most highly structured to the most naturalistic, that are available for use by clinicians.

Conversation analysis   A type of qualitative research methodology used to analyze social interactions through conversation.

Craniofacial anomalies   Disorders that affect the structure and/or function of the head and face (e.g., cleft palate, cleft lip).

Criterion-referenced tests   Tests or procedures that measure a person's performance in terms of absolute levels of mastery.

Criterion-related validity   A measure of the extent to which performance on a test can be correlated with performance on another instrument believed to measure the same skill or behavior.

Cronbach's coefficient alpha   A statistical procedure for calculating internal reliability of a test.

Crossbite   When a single tooth or the entire arch of the maxillary (upper) teeth overlap the mandibular (lower) teeth.

Cut-off score   A predetermined score used to make pass/fail decisions in a screening.

Cyst   A small sac or pouch that contains fluid or semi-solid material.

Data modeling   The mathematical representation of data describing a process or concept often implemented by a computer program (e.g., a spectrogram representing the frequency and intensity characteristics of a spoken utterance).

Database   A software program used to store and organize sets of related information.

Decontextualized   Tasks, such as tests, that require language comprehension or formulation out of the context of naturally occurring events or activities.

Dedicated applications   Computer applications designed for one purpose.

Dementia   Organically based deterioration of mental processes.

Descriptive developmental model of assessment   An approach to assessment that emphasizes the client's current communication status.

Developmental scale   Assessment instrument that samples behaviors from developmental stages.

Developmental scores   Test scores that have been transformed into age or grade equivalents.

Deviated   Turning away or aside from the normal point or course.

Diagnosis   Identification of a disease or disorder based on symptoms presented.

Diagnostic   Synonym for evaluation.

Diagnostic evaluation reports   Written reports used to summarize information obtained in both audiological and speech and language evaluations. These reports serve as legal records of assessment findings, diagnoses, and recommendations.

Dialect   Rule-governed and mutually intelligible forms of a language characterized by social, ethnic, and geographical differences in its speakers.

Dietician   A professional who evaluates the nutritional needs of the patients and sets up a plan to meet those needs.

Differential diagnosis   The process of distinguishing a disorder or condition from others with similar symptoms.

Digital   Representation of information in a format understandable by computers (i.e., binary numbers).

Digital photography   Still photographic images converted into a digital format for editing and/or display on a computer monitor.

Digital video Full motion video that has been digitized for playback on a computer screen.

Digitally programmable A computer or computer-driven device that can be programmed using a software program.

Direct services Working with a client in a hands-on format.

Disability The loss of function or inability to perform certain activities as a result of an impairment.

Discharge summary A written report of a client's cumulative progress from the initiation of therapy to his or her discharge from service.

Due process Provisions in law or regulation that outline the legal rights of those affected to question interpretations or implementation of the law or regulations.

Dynamic assessment Assessment process in which the examiner modifies interactions in order to achieve success for the client. The client is seen as an active participant in the process.

Dysarthria Motor speech disorder resulting from nervous system impairment.

Dysfluency An interruption in the smoothness of the flow of speech (e.g., stuttering).

Dysphagia Disorder of swallowing.

Dysprosody Disorders that affect the rate, loudness, intonation, and stress used in speech to modulate and enhance the meaning of words and sentences.

Educational software Written for educational purposes (reading skill development, writing skill practice, etc.).

Electronystagmography (ENG) A method of measuring eye movements, especially nystagmus, to assess the integrity of the vesitibular mechanism.

Electrophysiologic testing Audiological testing procedures that measure involuntary responses to sound within the auditory nervous system.

Electrophysiological Refers to measuring the electrical activity of the brain and body.

Endoscopic observation A procedure in which a device (endoscope) is used for observing a bodily function through a body opening. The device contains an optic device and a tube that can be inserted into the opening in order to view movements or structures otherwise not viewable.

Entitlement program Program of expected government benefits for selected groups who meet eligibility criteria defined by Congress, such as age, income, retirement, disability, or unemployment.

Equivalent form reliability Two forms of a test that measure the same skills and are standardized on the same population (also called *alternate form reliability*).

Ethics The moral and/or civil codes of conduct for a particular person, situation, community, religious group, organization, or society that evolve from a philosophy of human interaction that values behaviors that are personally or collectively regarded as good, honest, proper, and respectable.

Ethics Calibration Quick Test A series of questions to enable clinicians to analyze the ethical propriety of a situation.

Ethnographic assessment Assessment process in which the examiner observes the client in many contexts with many conversational partners.

Ethnography A qualitative method that provides an analytical description of a cultural scene.

Etiology Cause of a disorder or condition.

Evaluation The formal and informal procedures conducted as part of an assessment.

Facilitative play A client-centered method of intervention in which the clinician provides indirect language stimulation by modeling language forms that are related to client-initiated actions.

FAQ (Frequently Asked Questions) A commonly encountered section of a web site that provides answers to commonly asked questions.

Fee-for-service finance structure   System in which service providers are paid a fee for each service provided.

Fistula   An abnormal passage from one epithelialized surface to another; congenital, caused by disease or injury, or created surgically.

Fluency   The smooth, uninterrupted flow that is typical of speech.

Fluency induction   A technique that is likely to significantly decrease stuttering behaviors. These techniques are used as probes to identify whether a person who stutters can speak fluently under optimal conditions.

FM amplification system   An assistive listening device designed to enhance signal-to-noise ratio, in which a remote microphone/transmitter worn by a speaker sends signals via FM to a receiver worn by a listener.

Focused stimulation   A hybrid method of intervention that provides numerous models of target forms in response to client-initiated targets and activities. Clients are invited, but not required, to use the models to form their own utterances.

Follow-up letters   Letters written to referral sources discussing the status of the individual referred for clinical services, evaluation finding, and/or treatment outcomes.

Form   An aspect of language development that includes syntax, word order, morphology, phonology, and prosody.

Formant analysis   Analysis of an acoustic signal through studying concentrated frequency bands of energy caused by resonance patterns produced by the speech production mechanism.

Frenulum   Fold of mucous membrane extending from the floor of the mouth to the midline of the undersurface of the tongue.

Fundamental frequency   The tone produced by cyclic movements of the vocal folds, measured in cycles per second (Hz).

Gag reflex   Reflex triggered when contact of a foreign body with the mucous membrane of the fauces causes retching or gagging.

Generalization   Carryover of trained behavior into settings other than the training context.

Gloss   A clinician's interpretation of the intended meaning of a client's word or utterance.

Grade equivalent   A derived score that expresses an individual's performance as the average performance for a particular grade. It is interpreted to mean that the individual's performance is equal to the average performance of a student in X grade.

Graphics program   A software program designed for creating pictures or other graphic elements for printing and/or display on a computer screen.

Grass roots advocacy   Steps taken by individuals affected by a policy to influence its development or implementation.

Group services   Working with two or more clients, most of whom are working on similar speech-language skills.

Guidelines   Suggestions for implementing and monitoring public policies that do not have the weight of law.

Handicap   The negative effect that an impairment or disability has on an individual.

Health maintenance organization (HMO)   A type of managed care organization that provides a range of care on a prepayment basis.

Hearing Conservation Program   A program designed to protect the ears from hearing loss due to exposure to noise.

Home care services   Nursing and rehabilitation services provided to patients confined to their homes.

HTML   (HyperText Markup Language) The "language" used for developing pages for the World Wide Web.

Hyperlinks   Underlined text in a web page; by clicking on the text, the web page user is taken to the another web site for further information about the underlined text.

Hypernasality   Speech produced with excessive resonance in the nasal cavity, often due to dysfunction of the soft palate.

Idiolect   Every person's unique way of speaking.

Immittance   An audiological procedure for assessing the mobility of the eardrum.

Impairment   A disruption or abnormality in physiologic structure or function.

Indirect services   Consultation with family members, teachers, and/or medical personnel about a client's communication needs.

Individual services   Frequent and often one-to-one treatment.

Individualized education program (IEP)   A federally mandated written program developed by an interdisciplinary educational team identifying services and supports for children ages 3–21 who have been determined eligible for special education services.

Individualized family service plan (IFSP)   A written plan outlining family-centered supports and services for children from birth to 3 years old who have been determined eligible for early intervention services based on the presence of significant developmental delays or disabilities.

Individualized transition plan (ITP)   An integrated component of an IEP for students 14 years and older, developed to facilitate their transition from an educational environment to an appropriate vocational or supported adult service setting.

Infection control   The safeguarding of clients and clinicians from infectious diseases by maintaining universal precautions, including hand washing, the use of barriers (i.e., gloves, masks), disinfecting equipment, and procedures for the disposal of bodily fluids (i.e., saliva, blood).

Informativeness   The degree to which a client's discourse is relevant, truthful, not redundant, and reflects plausible inferences and interpretations.

Informed consent   Providing a client with information about his or her condition, and informing the client about the relative strengths, weakness, and risks (i.e., side effects) associated with a recommended plan of action or inaction.

Inpatient rehabilitation   Therapy provided to patients who are staying in the hospital or rehabilitation center.

Input systems/device   The means by which information is entered into the computer (e.g., keyboard, mouse, joystick).

Instrumentation interface   Hooking up a device to a computer.

Integrated software   Software bundle that allows you to do many things without conflicts arising because a different program is used.

Intelligibility   The degree to which a client's speech can be understood.

Interactivity   In terms of computer applications, software that is designed to allow the user to fully interact with or control the software or hardware.

Interdisciplinary   A team approach in which professionals perform tasks within their discipline while sharing information and coordinating services.

Intermediate care facilities for persons with mental retardation (ICFs/MR)   Federally supported habilitative residential facilities for people with mental retardation and related developmental disabilities.

Internal consistency   A measure of the degree to which items on a test correlate with each other.

Interrater reliability   The extent to which two or more independent scorers are in agreement about a test score.

Intervention   A planned clinical program to change client behavior.

Interview   A process by which a clinician gathers information related to a person's communication disorder through direct verbal exchange, and through which a clinician begins to establish trust with clients while educating them about issues related to communication impairment.

Intraoperative monitoring   Continuous assessment of the integrity of the cranial nerves during surgery.

Intraoral   Within the mouth.

Joint Commission on the Accreditation of Health Care Organizations   A regulatory body that oversees the quality of care provided to patients in a variety of health care facilities.

Language difference   Expected community variations in syntax, semantics, phonology, pragmatics, and the lexicon.

Language disorders   Communication that deviates significantly from the norms of the community.

Language interference   The influence of one language on another.

Laryngectomy   A surgical procedure in which the larynx (and possibly connecting tissues) is removed, usually due to cancer. The person who has had this procedure performed on him or her is referred to as a *laryngectomee*.

Laser video disc   A type of storage device for video and audio in which the data (movies or sound) are read off of a disc by a laser beam.

Laws   Actions taken by legislative bodies and signed into law by executive officials who are responsible for their implementation and enforcement of penalties for violations.

Letters of justification   Written letters to other service providers, program administrators, insurance companies, and other agents advocating for services, supports, and equipment needed for effective client management.

Listserv   A group of individuals interested in a particular topic who exchange e-mail messages as a way of discussing topics of interest.

Local norms   The administration of standardized tests to typically developing individuals in the community in which you are working and noting the scores that they receive and the quality of their responses.

Managed care organization (MCO)   Agency that manages or controls health care expenditures by closely monitoring how service providers (e.g., hospitals, physicians) treat their patients and by evaluating the necessity, appropriateness, and payment efficiency of health services.

Maze   A type of dysfluency involving repetitions, revisions, and false starts in the flow of speech.

Mean   The arithmetic average of scores.

Measure of central tendency   Description of where the center of a distribution of scores lies. It is reported as the mean, median, and/or mode.

Medicaid   A program that combines federal and state funding to cover medical services for older individuals and for younger individuals with disabilities.

Medicare   Prepaid hospital insurance (Part A) and optional additional medical insurance (Part B) available to individuals older than 65 who are eligible for benefits or disability based on their employment before retirement and administered by the federal Health Care Financing Administration.

Medigap   Supplemental insurance designed to cover what Medicare does not.

Milieu teaching   A hybrid method of intervention that incorporates operant methods within naturalistic settings.

Misrepresentation   A type of dishonesty that occurs when truth is distorted or falsified.

MLU   Mean length of utterance; usually computed in morphemes, rather than words; used as an index of syntactic development.

Modal verbs   Auxiliary verbs used to express the subjunctive mood or future tense, including *can, will, shall, may, could, would, should, must,* and *might.*

Modifiability   Change through mediation or teaching.

Morpheme   The smallest unit of meaning in a language; can be free-standing words, inflections (bound morphemes, such as plural /s/ or past tense -ed), prefixes (re-, un-), or suffixes (-ly, -ness).

Morphology   The study of how morphemes or units of meaning are joined together to form words.

Multidisciplinary   An approach to service provision in which professionals from different disciplines work independently and report to the team.

Multimedia (and hypermedia)   Computer programs that utilize many forms to present information (e.g., video, audio, graphic, text).

Narrative   A form of connected discourse describing a temporally and causally ordered sequence of events, usually delivered in monologue form in the first (I) or third person (he or she), in which animate characters attempt to confront and resolve some problem. Narratives often convey cultural values or mores.

Nasal emission   The sound of air forcefully flowing through the nose during speech (as opposed to nasal resonance), usually due to poor differentiation between the oral and nasal cavities, as in cleft palate. *See:* Hypernasality. *Syn:* Nasal escape, snorting.

Nasogastric tube   A feeding tube inserted through the nose and ending in the stomach.

Neologism   An invented word.

Neonatal intensive care unit (NICU)   A specialized intensive care unit for newborn infants who need intensive medical treatment.

Neurologist   A specialist in the diagnosis and treatment of disorders of the neuromuscular system; the central, peripheral, and autonomic nervous systems; the neuromuscular junction; and muscle.

Neuropsychologist   A clinical psychologist with specialized training on examination of relationships between brain function and behavior.

Newsgroup   A group of individuals who are interested in a particular topic.

Newsgroup reader   A specialized software application designed for reading and responding to an Internet newsgroup.

Nodule   (specifically vocal nodules) A small group of cells causing a knot or swelling on the edge of the vocal fold.

Nondiscrimination   The nonexclusion of clients from professional practice for reasons other than whether the person needs communication services. Discrimination occurs when a clinical decision is based solely on that client's race, gender, ethnicity, religion, age, national origin, sexual orientation, or disability status.

Nonmaleficence   The deliberate avoidance of inflicting potential or actual harm or evil on others.

Norm-referenced test   Test or procedure that allows comparison of an individual's performance to the performance of a specific group.

Normal distribution   A symmetrical bell-shaped curve representing the scores of a normal population on a test. In a normal distribution, most scores fall in the middle and fewer scores are found at the high and low extremities.

Norming sample   The sample of individuals from a population to whom a test was administered to collect normative data.

Nurse   A professional who tends to the daily medical needs of the patient.

Nurse's aide   A paraprofessional who assists the nurse in management of the patient; may assist patients in performing their activities of daily living.

Obturator   A prosthesis used to close an opening of the hard palate, usually a cleft palate.

Occupational therapist (OT)   Evaluates and treats patients with upper extremity weakness, impairments in performing activities of daily living, and/or perceptual and cognitive impairments.

Odd-even reliability   A way to measure internal consistency of a test. The degree to which odd and even numbered items on a test correlate with each other.

Oncology   A division of medicine specializing in diagnosis and management of cancer.

Open-ended comment/question   A remark that encourages an elaborated reply, rather than a one-word answer (e.g., "Tell me more about that").

Openbite   Upper anterior (front) teeth are unable to meet the lower anterior teeth thus resulting in an open space between the front teeth.

Operant conditioning   A form of training that elicits desired behavior by providing a stimulus that facilitates the client's production of a response, and reinforces the appropriate response when it occurs.

Otoacoustic emissions (OAEs)   Low-level sounds produced by the cochlea that can be measured. Absence of OAEs suggests hearing loss.

Otolarnygologist   A physician who specializes in diseases of the ear, nose and throat.

Otolaryngology   Branch of medicine specializing in the diagnosis and treatment of diseases of the ear, nose, and throat.

Otoscopic   Inspection of the external auditory meatus and tympanic membrane with an otoscope.

Ototoxic   Having a poisonous action on the ear, particularly the hair cells of the cochlear and vestibular end organs.

Outpatient rehabilitation   Therapy provided to patients who live at home and are transported to a rehabilitation center.

Overall plans of service (OPS)   A formalized written plan outlining the supports and services needed to implement habilitative treatment for people with developmental disabilities living in ICF/MR residential facilities.

Overdiagnosis   Labeling someone with a communication disorder using a test standardized on a different population.

Paralinguistics   Information that accompanies a speech signal to enhance its meaning, including tone of voice, facial expressions, gestures, and so forth.

Paraphasia   Misused word.

Paresis   Partial or incomplete paralysis.

Parkinson's disease   A neurological syndrome usually resulting from deficiency of the neurotransmitter dopamine as the consequence of degenerative, vascular, or inflammatory changes in the basal ganglia: characterized by rhythmical muscular tremors, rigidity of movement, festination, droopy posture, and masklike faces.

Pediatric developmental specialist   A physician specifically trained in child development and child developmental disorders.

Percentile rank   A derived score that indicates the percentage of individuals whose score fell at or below a given raw score.

Personal ethics   One's own choices about moral behavior.

Perturbation   The variance of consecutive cycles of an acoustic wave produced by the speaker. In some cases, these measures are related to vocal disorders. Variance between waves for intensity is called *shimmer*. Variance between waves for frequency is called *jitter*.

Phonetic inventory   A list of all speech sounds (often restricted to consonant sounds) that are produced by a client in a speech sample.

Phonological processes   Systematic changes in speech sounds often used during development and seen in speech disorders. These rule-governed processes function to simplify the pronunciation of target forms.

Phonology   Study of the rules that govern the way sounds are combined in a language.

Physiatrist   A physician who specializes in rehabilitation medicine who oversees occupational therapy, physical therapy, and speech therapy rehabilitation programs.

Physical therapist (PT)   A professional who evaluates and treats patients with upper and lower extremity impairments, and who assists patients in all aspects of mobility (e.g., stair climbing, walking).

Planning and placement team (PPT)   An interdisciplinary team consisting of educators, therapists, family members, and educational support personnel charged with the development and implementation of an IEP for students ages 3–21 who receive special educational services.

Play audiometry   A technique used for testing the hearing of preschool children. The child is conditioned to perform an action, such as putting a block in a bucket, when he or she hears a sound.

Polyp   A small growth with an attached stem.

Portfolio assessment   Process of assessment in which the examiner collect a student's work over time representing a variety of tasks and assignments.

Postponement and avoidance behaviors   Behaviors that are meant to put off the onset of a difficult word or sound that the person who stutters may fear. These behaviors include circumlocutions, word substitutions, or broader behaviors such as limited verbalizations, avoidance of certain social situations, ignoring a speaker, or laughter.

Posttest   A pretest re-administered after a course of therapy to assess client progress.

Pragmatics   Study of appropriate use of language in context.

Predictive validity   A measure of the degree to which an individual's current test score can be used to estimate the person's score at a later date.

Pretest   A baseline measurement taken before the initiation of treatment on a goal.

Probe techniques   Weekly or biweekly assessment process in which the examiner determines rate and amount of learning.

Productivity software   Software designed to facilitate everyday tasks.

Productivity technology   Technology that helps a person do something better, faster, and more efficiently.

Professional ethics   Right and wrong actions in the workplace.

Professional relationships   Collegial behavior characterized by an open communication style and a climate of mutual respect and cooperation .

Prognosis   A statement that describes the likelihood that a benefit will be gained from treatment.

Progress reports   A written report summarizing a client's cumulative achievement of therapy goals and objectives across a specific period of time, and, if needed, outlining recommendations for future intervention.

Prolongation   The maintenance of a speech sound or airflow during speech when the articulators have stopped. One of the core behaviors in stuttering.

Prosody   The rhythm and melody of speech expressed by intonation, stress, pause, and juncture.

Psychiatrist   A physician who specializes in the psychiatric needs of patients.

Psychologist   A professional who evaluates and manages the psychological and/or psychosocial needs of the patient.

Public policy   Actions (e.g., laws, rules, court decisions) taken by local, state, or federal officials to address a public problem or need.

Pure tone audiometry   Audiological testing procedures used to measure hearing thresholds.

Qualitative assessment   An in-depth assessment procedure that is descriptive (rather than quantitative) in nature. This type of evaluation may include conversation analysis.

Real time   Occurring nearly instantaneously (as opposed to following a perceptible delay).

Recreational therapist   A professional who assists patients in resuming productive leisure activities.

Referral   Sending a client to another professional whose area of expertise better matches the client's needs.

Referral letters   Letters written to doctors, therapists, or other service providers referring an individual for medical or clinical evaluation and/or treatment.

Registers   Varieties of a language that depend on the context and conversational participants.

Regulations   Detailed rules for interpreting and implementing a particular law.

Rehabilitation aide   A paraprofessional who carries out specific therapeutic activities under the supervision of a licensed professional.

Reinke's edema   Swelling along the superficial layer of the lamina propria of the vocal folds. It is also called *polypoid degeneration.*

Reliability   The consistency of a test or a procedure over repeated administrations and by different examiners.

Repetitions   A sound, syllable, or word repeated more than twice. One of the core behaviors in stuttering.

Residential care facility   General term referring to health care facilities where residents receive skilled nursing care and a variety of rehabilitation services. Patients may be a permanent or temporary resident.

Resonance   The modification of laryngeal tone by altering the shape of the oral and nasal cavities.

Rugae   A fold, ridge, or crease.

Scaled score   A standard score frequently having a mean of 100 and a standard deviation of 15.

Scores of relative standing   Test scores that allow comparison among individuals of various ages and among scores on various tests taken by the same individual.

Screening   Initial assessment procedure that allows identification of individuals who require complete evaluation.

Self-contained classroom   A service provision model in which the SLP is the primary educator, providing both academic and intense speech-language remediation.

Service delivery models   The systems that are used to organize speech-language and hearing programs.

Semantics   Study of the way in which words and ideas are combined and expressed.

Signal-to-noise ratio   The ratio of intensities of foreground to background noises. It is often used as measure of vocal quality.

Skilled nursing facility (SNF)   Previously known as *nursing homes,* they include a percentage of residents who require services from such trained professionals as nurses and rehabilitation specialists.

SOAP (*Subjective, Objective, Assessment, Plan*) note   A commonly used format in medical and other service delivery settings to record and analyze data specific to a client's ongoing medical status and/or performance in therapy.

Social worker   A professional who assists patients with management of psychosocial problems and with access to various community resources.

Spasm   A sudden involuntary contraction of one or more muscle groups; includes cramps, contractures.

Specialization   The acquisition of advanced technical skills for a particular population, disorder, and/or service delivery model, through in-depth experience, advanced knowledge, and training beyond the initial CCC credential.

Spectral analysis   (or spectrographic analysis) Analysis of an acoustic signal through the study of its charted band of wavelengths.

Speech audiometry   Audiological procedures used to determine speech detection levels, speech reception thresholds, and speech discrimination.

Speech-language pathology assistant   A paraprofessional trained to assist the SLP with certain aspects of patient care.

Speech naturalness   A nine-point, equal-appearing interval scale that results in a subjective decision as to how far from normal a person speaks.

Split-half reliability   A way to measure internal consistency of a test. The degree to which scores from one half of a test correlate with scores from the other half.

Spreadsheet   A software program designed to organize and manipulate numeric information.

Standard deviation   Measure of the degree of variation in a distribution.

Standard error of measurement   The standard deviation of error around an individual's true score.

Standard score   A derived score that has been transformed into a distribution with a known mean and standard deviation.

Stimulability   The degree to which a nonmastered skill or behavior can be elicited.

Stridor   A sign of respiratory obstruction, especially in the trachea or larynx.

Stroke   A medical condition involving the interruption of blood flow within the brain.

Stuttering   A type of fluency disorder. Speech is usually marked by repetitions, prolongations, and/or pauses in speech.

Submucous   Beneath the mucous membrane.

Symmetry   Equality or correspondence in the form of parts distributed around a center or an axis at the extremities or poles, or on the opposite sides of any body.

Syntax   Study of the rules that govern the internal structure of language including grammar and word order.

Systems model of assessment   Model that emphasizes the importance of context in which an individual must function.

T-score   A standard score with a mean of 50 and a standard deviation of 10.

T-unit   Terminal units of production; used to segment utterances of school-age children and adults. A T-unit consists of an independent clause and all the dependent clauses associated with it.

Task analysis   A clinician's breakdown of an intervention goal into a series of prerequisite skills and the ordered steps that must be followed to achieve it.

Task sequence   An ordered series of steps through which a clinician plans to help a client progress toward an intervention goal.

Technology-based   Technology is the main vehicle through which material is presented.

Technology-enhanced   Technology is used to improve the presentation or form of therapy or a lecture.

Test–retest reliability   A measure of a test's consistency or stability over time.

Thread   Series of messages presented in an Internet newsgroup relating to a single topic.

Tic   Habitual, repeated contraction of certain muscles, resulting in stereotyped individualized actions that can be voluntarily suppressed for only brief periods.

Tinnitus   Sensation of ringing or other sound in the head without an external cause.

TMJ   Temporomandibular joint.

Transdisciplinary   A team approach in which members from different disciplines work collaboratively to focus on shared goals. Team members work together and may cross discipline lines.

Transdisciplinary service delivery   A service delivery format that emphasizes collaboration; role sharing; and active, ongoing communication between all team members regardless of background or specialization in order to maximize effective client intervention.

Transgendered   Exhibiting the appearance and behavioral characteristics of the opposite sex.

Transitional living center   An inpatient facility for patients needing therapy for self-management skills and community re-entry.

Treatment plan   A formal written plan outlining goals, objectives, and procedures implemented during therapy.

Tremor   Repetitive, often regular, oscillatory movements caused by alternate or synchronous, but irregular contraction of the opposing muscle groups; usually involuntary.

Tympanometry   One type of immittance testing used to measure the compliance of the eardrum relative to changes in air pressure.

Underdiagnosis   Not diagnosing a true communication disorder because all aspects of the person's communication skills are believed to be dialect/second language features.

Universal design   Built-in design that makes software accessible to the greatest number of individuals.

Universal precautions   An approach to infection control in which all human blood, tissue, and certain fluids are treated as if known to be infectious for human immunodeficiency virus (HIV), HBV, and other blood-borne pathogens.

Use   The functions of language (pragmatics).

Validity   The extent to which a test measures what it claims to measure.

Velopharyngeal   Pertaining to the soft palate (velum palatinum) and the pharyneal walls.

Velopharyngeal insufficiency   Lack of competent velopharyngeal closure.

Verbosity   Excess speech; the use of more words than is necessary to convey an idea; often exhibited in acquired aphasia.

Videostroboscopy   Instrumentation that allows visualization of vocal fold movement.

Visual reinforcement audiometry   A technique for testing the hearing of young children. The child is reinforced with lights or moving toys for looking toward a sound.

Vocal abuse   The overuse of the voice, through yelling or excessive loud talking, coughing or throat clearing, or pitching the voice too high or low; can lead to exhaustion/weakening of laryngeal muscles and, if uncorrected, to organic changes in the vocal apparatus.

Z-score   Standard score with a mean of 0 and a standard deviation of 1.

Index

Page numbers followed by *f* indicate figures; those followed by *t* indicate tables.

More informative resources for communication professionals embarking on their careers...

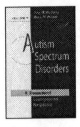

Autism Spectrum Disorders
A Transactional Developmental Perspective

Communication and Language Intervention Series

Edited by Amy M. Wetherby, Ph.D., CCC-SLP, & Barry M. Prizant, Ph.D., CCC-SLP

This cross-disciplinary reference has it all—a thorough explanation of the communication and language problems characteristic of autism as they relate to development, plus practical, research-based strategies for treatment. In Part I, experts in the field of autism consolidate recent research and analyze topics that relate to the core areas of autism spectrum disorders—communication, socialization, emotional regulation, and symbolic development. In Part II, they use this research as the framework for presenting principles and philosophies underlying treatment practices and guidelines that speech-language pathologists can use to make critical assessment and intervention decisions.

Stock Number: 4455   Price: $39.95
2000 • Vol. 9 • 448 pages • 6 x 9 • hardcover • ISBN 1-55766-445-5

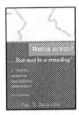

"Human services?...That must be so rewarding."
A Practical Guide for Professional Development, Second Edition

By Gail S. Bernstein, Ph.D.

The second edition of this extremely practical resource helps students and professionals be more focused and fulfilled in the work they do. Readers will learn how to approach their work more realistically and optimistically using self-analysis exercises on issues such as work-related values and conflicts, personal goals and limits, respect for consumers, and stress management. This book is an essential pre-service and in-service training text, as well as an excellent self-help resource.

Stock Number: 3327   Price: $24.95
1999 • 240 pages • 6 x 9 • paperback • ISBN 1-55766-332-7

....

Please send me   ___ copies of **Autism Spectrum Disorders** / Stock #4455 / Price $39.95
___ copies of **"Human services?..."** / Stock #3327 / Price $24.95

Name: _____

Street Address *(orders cannot be shipped to P.O. boxes):* _____ ❏ Residential ❏ Commercial

City/State/ZIP: _____

Daytime phone: _____ E-mail address: _____
❏ *Yes! I want to receive special web site offers!*
My e-mail address will not be shared with any other party.

____ Check enclosed (payable to Brookes Publishing Co.)   ____ Purchase Order attached (please bill my institution)

____ Please charge my   ____ American Express   ____ MasterCard   ____ Visa

Card No.: _____   Exp. date: _____/_____/_____

Signature *(required on all credit card orders):* _____

Within Continental U.S. Shipping Rates for UPS Ground delivery*	
If your **product** total (before tax) is:	Product Total $_____
$0.00 to $49.99 add $5.00	Maryland Orders add 5% sales tax + $_____
$50.00 to $399.99 add 10% of product total	*(to product total only)* +
$400.00 and over add 8% of product total	Shipping Rate (see chart at left) $_____
For rush orders call 1-800-638-3775 For international orders call 1-410-337-9580	Grand Total U.S. $_____

Photocopy this form and mail it to **Brookes Publishing Co.**, P.O. Box 10624, Baltimore, MD 21285-0624;
FAX **410-337-8539**; call toll-free (8 A.M. – 5 P.M. ET) **1-800-638-3775** or **1-410-337-9580** (outside the U.S.);
or order online at **www.brookespublishing.com**

Browse our entire catalog at www.brookespublishing.com

Prices subject to change without notice and may be higher outside the U.S. You may return books within 30 days for a full credit of the product price. Refunds will be issued for prepaid orders. Items must be returned in resalable condition.

Your source code is: BA 51